DEVELOPING PRACTICAL NURSING SKILLS

SECOND EDITION

EDITED BY

Lesley Baillie RGN, ONC, BA(Hons), RNT, MSc(Nurs)
Principal Lecturer (Clinical Skills Development),
London South Bank University, London, UK

Hodder Arnold
A member of the Hodder Headline Group
LONDON

First published in Great Britain in 2001 by Arnold
This second edition published in 2005 by
Hodder Education, a member of the Hodder Headline Group,
338 Euston Road, London NW1 3BH

http://www.hoddereducation.co.uk

Distributed in the United States of America by
Oxford University Press Inc.,
198 Madison Avenue, New York, NY10016
Oxford is a registered trademark of Oxford University Press

Whilst the advice and information in this book are believed to be true and
accurate at the date of going to press, neither the authors nor the publisher
can accept any legal responsibility or liability for any errors or omissions
that may be made. In particular, (but without limiting the generality of the
preceding disclaimer) every effort has been made to check drug dosages;
however, it is still possible that errors have been missed. Furthermore,
dosage schedules are constantly being revised and new side-effects
recognized. For these reasons the reader is strongly urged to consult the
drug companies' printed instructions before administering any of the drugs
recommended in this book.

British Library Cataloguing in Publication Data
A catalogue record for this book is available from the British Library

Library of Congress Cataloging-in-Publication Data
A catalog record for this book is available from the Library of Congress

ISBN   0 340 81314 8

1 2 3 4 5 6 7 8 9 10

Commissioning Editor: Clare Christian
Development Editor: Heather Smith
Project Editor: Wendy Rooke
Production Controller: Jane Lawrence
Cover Design: Amina Dudhia
Illustrator: Barking Dog Art

Hodder Headline's policy is to use papers that are natural, renewable and recyclable
products and made from wood grown in sustainable forests. The logging and manufacturing
processes are expected to conform to the environmental regulations of the country of origin.

Typeset in 10/14 Palatino Light by Charon Tec Pvt. Ltd, Chennai, India
www.charontec.com
Printed and bound in Spain

What do you think about this book? Or any other Hodder Arnold title?
Please visit our website at www.hoddereducation.co.uk

DEVELOPING PRACTICAL NURSING SKILLS

This book is dedicated to the memory of my mother, Betty Knie (formerly Chamberlain, nee Sykes), SRN, SCM, 1928–2001.

Contents

CHAPTER 1: LEARNING PRACTICAL NURSING SKILLS: AN INTRODUCTION

CHAPTER 2: THE NURSE'S APPROACH: SELF-AWARENESS AND COMMUNICATION

CHAPTER 3: PREVENTING CROSS-INFECTION

Contents

CHAPTER 7: MEETING HYGIENE NEEDS

CHAPTER 8: MEETING ELIMINATION NEEDS

CHAPTER 9: ASSESSING AND MEETING NUTRITIONAL NEEDS

Contents

Contributors

Chapter authors

Vickie Arrowsmith (Chapters 3 and 8)
RGN, BA(Hons), PGCEA
Lecturer,
The Open University

Lesley Baillie (Chapters 1, 8, 11 and 12)
RGN, ONC, BA(Hons), RNT, MSc(Nurs)
Principal lecturer,
London South Bank University

Dr Dee Burrows (Chapter 12)
RGN, RCNT, RNT, DipN(Lond), BSc(Hons), PhD
Independent nurse consultant, PainConsultants

Kay Child (Chapter 9)
RGN, RCNT, BA(Hons)
Practice placement facilitator,
Wycombe Hospital

Veronica Corben (Chapters 4 and 11)
RGN, DPNP, BSc(Hons), RNT, MSc(Nurs), Diploma Cancer Nursing
Manager, Continuing and professional education, South East London Workforce
Development Confederation

Sue Higham (Chapters 9, 10 and 11)
RSCN, RGN, DPSN, BSc(Hons), PGCEA, MA
Senior lecturer,
Thames Valley University

Janine Jones (Chapter 6)
RGN
Tissue Viability Nurse,
Buckinghamshire Hospitals NHS Trust

Sue Maddex (Chapter 10)
RGN, BSc(Hons), RNT, Post-grad. Cert. in Education and Advanced Pract
Senior lecturer,
University of Luton

Contributors

Chrissie Major (Chapter 7)
RGN, BSc(Hons)
Blood Transfusion Nurse,
Stoke Mandeville Hospital

Nicola M. Neale (Chapter 2)
RGN, RNT, MA, Post grad. Diploma Cancer Care
Senior lecturer,
Buckinghamshire Chilterns University College

Glynis Pellatt (Chapter 5)
RGN, ONC, RCNT, RNT, DipN(Lond), BA(Hons), MA
Senior lecturer,
University of Luton

Jo Sale (Chapter 2)
RMN, RGN, BSc(Hons), PGCEA, RNT, MSc(Social Psychology)
Senior lecturer,
University of Luton

Deirdre Thompson (Chapter 6)
RGN
Senior Tissue Viability Nurse Specialist,
Heatherwood and Wexham Park Hospital

Consultants

Alan Baillie (reviewed and gave guidance on mental health content: Chapters 3, 4, 5, 6, 8, 10 and 11)
RN(Mental Health), BA(Hons), MSc
Senior lecturer (Mental Health),
Buckinghamshire Chilterns University College

Rhod Broad (reviewed and gave guidance on older people with mental health needs: Chapters 7, 9 and 12)
RMN, BSc(Hons)
Community Psychiatric Nurse for Older People,
Buckinghamshire Mental Health Trust

Penny Goacher (formulated biology questions)
BSc(Hons) Human Biology, MPhil
Lecturer, School of Nursing & Midwifery,
University of East Anglia

John O'Shaughnessey (reviewed and gave learning disability input into all chapters)
RMNH, BSc(Hons), Cert.Ed.
Senior lecturer (Learning disabilities),
University of Luton

Nicky Walls (reviewed and gave learning disability input into all chapters)
RN (Learning disability), RN (Mental health), BSc(Hons)
Practice educator (Learning disabilities),
University of Luton

Preface to the second edition

The first edition of this book aimed to help students to develop a foundation in their practical nursing skills, with an emphasis on an appropriate attitude and sound underpinning knowledge. In the same year as the first edition, the Department of Health (2001) published *The Essence of Care*, which provided benchmarking statements for good practice in fundamental care. This document has, I believe, given credence and support to the view that these skills really do matter and are valued by patients/clients and their families. This is not to say that technological skills and other areas of knowledge are less important, but to recognise that fundamental skills are central to nursing practice in the very many settings where care takes place. In some environments nurses are more likely to supervise or support others than directly carry out these practical skills. However to supervise others in providing quality fundamental care requires a sound knowledge and understanding of these skills, and a commitment to their value.

This second edition retains its student-friendly approach, its interactive style, and its strong focus on applying practical nursing skills in a variety of settings. Once again, each chapter's content is applied to scenarios from all four branches, which helps students understand the necessity to apply and adapt skills across a range of settings with different client groups. The content has been fully updated throughout, with a strong evidence-based approach, and health policy documents are referred to where relevant. Further reading and useful websites and other resources are recommended where appropriate. Additional illustrations are incorporated where it was felt they would be helpful.

The first chapter provides a background to practical nursing skills, particularly in relation to theories of caring. It explains the different components of practical skills, and aims to help students think about how they can go about learning them and developing their confidence. This chapter also provides structured guidance to help students maximise their practical experience.

The skills in the following chapters strongly reflect those that students are expected to develop in their common foundation programme and those that are relevant to students in all branches of nursing. There are several additions from the first edition, in particular the inclusion of care of the body after death, more content on privacy and dignity, falls risk assessment and prevention, and colour photos in the chapter on wound care. The final chapter is new and addresses managing pain and promoting comfort across all settings. This chapter ha caring focus, linking back to the theories of caring introduced in Chapter 1. It includes both new material relating to these important skills but also draws on content from the previous chapters, demonstrating that most practical skills relate to comfort in some way.

Nurses care for people in a wide range of settings in different circumstances so no one term felt appropriate to use in every situation. A lot of the time the terms 'person' and 'people' are used, and of course 'child' and 'children'. However in some contexts the terms 'patient', 'client', 'individual' or 'service user' are referred to in relation to people nurses are caring for.

I truly hope this book will be really helpful to student nurses, and I wish all those using it in their studies a successful and rewarding nursing career. The book may also be helpful to others either learning or teaching practical nursing skills in other contexts.

Lesley Baillie
January 2005

REFERENCE

Department of Health 2001. *The Essence of Care: Patient-focused benchmarking for health care practitioners.* London: DH.

Acknowledgements

There are many people I wish to acknowledge and thank for the part they played in producing this new edition:

- The many people who read and commented on the first edition and especially all the feedback from students, which gave the encouragement to produce this second edition.
- The book's contributors for all their hard work.
- The many people who gave help, support and comments throughout the writing process. Special thanks to Maryon Pates RGN, RMN, RN(Child), for support with Chapters 8 and 12, and Rose Gallagher, Clinical Nurse Specialist, Infection Control, for reviewing Chapter 3.
- Luke Papps for help with new illustrations for Chapter 10.
- My family – Alan, Emily and Jessica – for living with a second edition and giving so much help and support in so many ways.
- Arnold publishers for supporting the production of this second edition and being so helpful and responsive.

Learning practical nursing skills: *an introduction*

Lesley Baillie

Probably no-one would dispute that caring is an essential feature of nursing, and to demonstrate caring and caring attitudes, a nurse must be a competent practitioner (Roach 2002). The focus of this book is to assist readers to develop the ability to carry out a range of practical skills with different client groups. Being able to perform a practical nursing skill involves not only the 'hands-on' (psychomotor) element, but needs evidence-based knowledge, effective interpersonal skills, awareness of the ethical dimension of care, creative and reflective thinking, and an appropriate professional attitude. These elements are considered throughout the text.

To become a registered nurse does of course require more than an ability to carry out a range of practical skills. However, developing ability to perform practical skills safely is necessary for all student nurses (Department of Health 1999; English National Board 2000; Nursing and Midwifery Council 2002), and it is this specific element of nursing which is the remit of this book. There are many other texts aimed at student nurses that comprehensively cover the other necessary subjects (see later in this chapter: 'Recommended reading').

This chapter discusses the nature of practical skills in nursing, how these skills can be learned, and how this book can help you to develop a foundation in nursing skills. There is particular emphasis on encouraging you to develop and value these practical skills as holistic, caring skills, which give you the opportunity to develop the therapeutic use of self.

This chapter includes:
- What are practical nursing skills?
- The range of practical skills used by nurses
- Practical skills included in this book, and use of practice scenarios
- Practical skills: affective, cognitive and motor dimensions
- Practical skills within the context of caring
- Therapeutic nursing and practical skills
- How can you develop your practical nursing skills?

WHAT ARE PRACTICAL NURSING SKILLS?

To be a competent nurse requires mastery of a range of skills including practical, communication and management skills. These are often integrated within the nursing role, because carrying out practical nursing skills effectively also requires skills in, for example, communication, teamwork and delegation. What, however, are practical nursing skills? Bjork (1999a) defines practical nursing skills as 'hands-on actions that promote the patients' physical comfort, hygiene and safe medical treatment (which are) … commonly referred to as procedures or psychomotor skills'. This definition appears to imply a purely physical perspective. However there is no doubt that practical skills often enhance social and psychological comfort and well-being too; oral hygiene is a good example of this. Bradshaw (1994) notes that physical, social, psychological and spiritual care is actually an integrated whole and cannot be separated. Thus while a practical nursing skill may appear to be a physical procedure, it not only results in a physical effect.

Romyn (1999) argues that deciding what constitutes a practical nursing skill is problematic as many skills that are carried out by nurses are not solely their domain, for example, injections can be given by doctors too. In this book it is assumed that practical nursing skills are skills that involve 'hands-on' care by nurses with clients, although some of these skills are also performed by other professionals. There is a vast range of practical skills that nurses use, and they must adapt these skills in different situations with differing client groups.

THE RANGE OF PRACTICAL SKILLS USED BY NURSES

Traditionally there was a hierarchy of skills within nursing, with experienced nurses undertaking more technical, medical skills such as those to do with medication, and junior staff carrying out what was sometimes referred to as 'basic nursing care', that is, assisting people with activities of daily living such as hygiene and elimination. This system has been considered biomedical and task-focused (McMahon 1998) rather than being client-focused, with a nurse delivering all the care required by that particular client. The term 'basic' has often been used in a derisory fashion, the implication being that these skills are not as important as more technical ones, and indeed student nurses have been found to view learning technical skills as more important than other aspects of care (Randle 2001).

Randle (2001) comments that engaging with the biomedical model of practice leads to deteriorating nurse–patient relationships, her research portraying ' a picture of students actively engaging with technology whilst at the same time disengaging from the emotional care of patients' (p. 162). Yet to help an older person regain the ability to wash and dress after a stroke, or to help a person with confusion to maintain continence, can be a much more complex skill than many which are apparently more technical and medically orientated, such as removal of clips from a wound. Bjork (1999b), in a longitudinal in-depth study of practical skill development, analysed the skill of mobilising a post-operative patient, and highlighted the complexity of this apparently 'simple' skill. She noted the effect of numerous individual factors, such as the patient's ability to respond to instructions and general physical and mental well-being, which affected how the skill was carried out.

The notion of delivering individualised care for clients, operationalised through the nursing process (assessing, planning, implementing and evaluating care), and based on the framework of a nursing (rather than medical) model, has become widely accepted within nursing. How nursing models are developed and chosen by practitioners is discussed by Johns (1994), and an introduction to nursing models can be found in Beretta (2003). However, with the role expansion of registered nurses (with many taking on skills previously carried out by doctors, such as intravenous cannulation), and the increasing use of health-care assistants to carry out specific skills formerly part of a nurse's repertoire of practice, it is probably unrealistic to deny that a skills hierarchy does not exist.

A respondent in a survey by Rogers *et al.* (2000) commented 'The nurses were very nice and worked very hard, but I think they have become technicians rather than providing what we used to consider "nursing care".' Nevertheless practical skills can still be client centred and delivered within the context of a caring philosophy, with value attached to fundamental as well as technical care. Poor standards of fundamental care in hospitals became the subject of a media campaign 'Dignity on the Ward', launched by the *Observer* newspaper in 1997 due to concerns about the poor quality of care delivered to older people. The campaign triggered an independent inquiry, commissioned by the UK Department of Health, into the care of older people in hospital (Health Advisory Service 2000 1998). The findings from this research led to the launching of *The Essence of Care: patient-focused benchmarking for health care practitioners* (Department of Health 2001a), which laid out benchmarking standards for fundamental care for people of all ages, as well as the National Service Framework for Older People (Department of Health 2001b), which highlights many aspects of fundamental care in relation to older people. The areas of care covered by *The Essence of Care* can be seen in Box 1.1. Where appropriate, the standards of best

---

- Principles of self-care
- Personal and oral hygiene
- Food and nutrition
- Continence and bladder and bowel care
- Pressure ulcers
- Safety of clients/patients with mental health needs in acute mental health and general hospital settings
- Record keeping
- Privacy and dignity

Box 1.1 Fundamental aspects of care included in *The Essence of Care: Patient-focused benchmarking for health care practitioners* (Department of Health 2001a)

practice are included in the relevant chapters in this book. All Department of Health publications can be downloaded from their website (www.dh.gov.uk).

PRACTICAL SKILLS INCLUDED IN THIS BOOK, AND USE OF PRACTICE SCENARIOS

This book includes the core practical skills in which students should expect to develop a foundation by the end of the Common Foundation Programme (CFP). Within the UK student nurses must achieve a range of outcomes within four domains of practice (professional and ethical practice, care delivery, care management, and personal and professional development) to enter the branch (adult, child, learning disability or mental health). They must then achieve all the 'Standards of proficiency' within each of the four domains to complete their chosen branch, and enter the nursing register. The outcomes and Standards of Proficiency are identified in the document *Standards of Proficiency for Pre-registration Nursing Programmes* (Nursing and Midwifery Council 2004). Within the care delivery domain, there is one CFP outcome explicitly connected to practical skills (see Box 1.2).

The skills included in this book are specifically related to this CFP learning outcome. Note that to meet a patient's need for comfort requires integrating a range of skills (including interventions such as wound care, pain management and respiratory care), and the book therefore ends with examining how needs for comfort can be met by combining skills which have been explored in earlier chapters. This book does not include essential first aid and emergency procedures. The skills included in these procedures are frequently updated and you need to undergo supervised practice in a classroom setting, with a qualified instructor.

For general first aid procedures you are advised to consult the most current *First Aid Manual*, at the time of writing, the eighth edition (Lee *et al.* 2002). This

---

Demonstrate a range of nursing skills, under the supervision of a registered nurse, to meet individuals' needs, which include:

- Maintaining dignity, privacy and confidentiality
- Effective communication and observational skills, including listening and taking physiological measurements
- Safety and health, including moving and handling and infection control
- Essential first aid and emergency procedures
- Administration of medicines
- Emotional, physical and personal care, including meeting the need for comfort, nutrition and personal hygiene.

Box 1.2 The Common Foundation Programme learning outcome in the care delivery domain that relates specifically to practical skills (Nursing and Midwifery Council 2004, p. 30)

manual (which can be bought at any bookseller's) is produced by the first aid organisations (St John Ambulance, St Andrew's Ambulance Association and the British Red Cross) and is very detailed and fully illustrated. The ability to perform basic life support (BLS) is an expected skill of all registered nurses. As a student nurse and a registered nurse it is mandatory for you to attend training sessions in these skills. BLS and choking procedures for adults and children are presented in detail, and regularly updated, on the Resuscitation Council website (www.resus.org.uk). This very informative website includes other interesting sections, for example 'Frequently asked questions', information about legal aspects of resuscitation and 'Do not attempt resuscitation'. Some principles underpinning moving and handling skills are covered in Chapter 5 of this book. However note that these skills are also frequently updated and you must therefore attend the training sessions provided for you, both as a student and a registered nurse, so you can update your skills under supervision.

Each chapter begins with a scenario from adult, child, learning disability and mental health care settings, and the chapter links the content back to these patients/clients, thus encouraging theory–practice links. This use of practice-based scenarios as a basis for study will be a familiar approach for many students, with the increasing use of problem/enquiry/evidence-based curricula; these have been endorsed by the English National Board (2000). The book aims to include a selection of scenarios, from a variety of settings, but it is not intended that all possible situations are represented. All scenarios have been developed from experience with similar people with health needs. Any identifying details have been changed or omitted, and pseudonyms were allocated at random.

PRACTICAL SKILLS: AFFECTIVE, COGNITIVE AND MOTOR DIMENSIONS

Activity

Almost everyone will have had an injection at some stage, and indeed you may have had recent immunizations to enter the nursing programme. You probably took it for granted that the skill would be performed competently, but try to identify the different elements that this skill entails.

You probably considered that there are technical aspects such as drawing up the correct drug accurately using sterile equipment, but may also have identified that the skill requires underlying knowledge of the drug's actions and potential side effects, and that the nurse should use a calm and friendly approach to relax you and relieve anxiety. This example illustrates that effective practical nursing skills require a skilled motor performance (the 'doing' element), a sound knowledge (based on best evidence), and an appropriate attitude towards clients. Bjork (1999a) reviews the concept of nursing practical skills and concludes that

were for many years commonly considered to comprise the art of nursing. However, she identifies that more recently these skills have been termed motor or psychomotor skills, and it has been the technical, motor element that has been emphasised.

Oermann (1990) also suggests that the motor (doing) element of a practical (psychomotor) skill is often emphasised to the exclusion of the cognitive and affective component. She highlights the importance of the cognitive base (the scientific principles underlying the performance of the skill) and the affective domain, which reflects the nurse's values and concern for the client while the skill is being performed. It can be argued that in order to provide high-quality care, nurses must be competent to apply theory and skill in each clinical situation, which includes knowledge, and mastery in each of the psychomotor, cognitive and affective domains (Fitzpatrick *et al.* 1992). These three aspects are now discussed.

THE AFFECTIVE DIMENSION

The affective domain of a practical skill includes the nurse's attitude and approach to the client as well as the ethical dimension. Bush and Barr's (1997) study of critical care nurses' experiences of caring identified the affective process as including sensitivity, empathy, concern and interest. One participant is quoted as saying: 'instead of just saying, "I'm taking your blood pressure, your temperature" you really care about what the patient is going through – how they must feel – you kind of put yourself in their position, and how you'd want to be taken care of yourself instead of just a mechanical (action)'. Bjork (1999a) argues that it is the intentional element of practical nursing skills that sets them apart from other skills. She suggests that caring intentions are necessary in practical nursing actions because 'they can transform the acts of handling and helping into tolerable or even meaningful experiences for the patient'. She goes on to suggest that within the application of a practical skill, a nurse can use the situation to convey respect for and interest in the patient, conveying the message that 'it is not just a body that is being handled'. While carrying out a practical skill, such as bathing, a nurse can take the opportunity to foster confidence and develop a trusting relationship, as being involved in such activities offers nurses opportunity to become closer to patients or clients (Wharton and Pearson 1988).

Bjork (1999a) also highlights the importance of being aware of the meaning of the practical skill for the individual, and how it fits into the person's overall experience. For example, a wound dressing may exemplify the change in body image following invasive surgery, and bathing someone may highlight their loss of independence due to physical or mental health problems. Box 1.3 details the positive experience of Dee Burrows (one of Chapter 12's authors) of being assisted with a shower post-operatively. Her story illustrates the significance of the nurse's approach while carrying out her care, and its impact on her recovery.

About 5 days after I had had major abdominal surgery, after which I had been seriously ill, a nurse got me up for the first time and took me in a wheelchair to the bathroom for a shower. I was weak, afraid of being naked in front of her, and I felt uncomfortable about my wound being on show. She helped me off with my clothes and helped me have a shower, during which she sensitively used humour to make me relaxed. She washed my body and hair, and at intervals put her hand gently on my shoulder in a comforting way. At one point she knelt down and gently put her hands either side of my large wound and said 'It looks beautiful – it's going to heal up really well. You'll be back in a bikini within a month'. (I was!) I got this tremendous sense of relief that even though I had this massive scar I would still be me again. She had encouraged me to accept my scar. By the end of the whole episode of care I felt wonderfully clean from top to toe, relaxed, and had begun to recover a sense of self. The fear had just disappeared.

Box 1.3 Illustrative example of the significance of the nurse's approach to a patient while assisting with showering

Each time you carry out a practical skill with a patient/client, you convey a message about your state of being (Paterson and Zderad 1988); for example are you anxious, in a hurry, distracted or uninterested? Chapter 2 considers the nurse's approach to clients during practical nursing skills application.

Valuing people

An important document that all nurses should be familiar with is *Valuing People: A new strategy for learning disability for the 21st century* (Department of Health 2001c). This document identifies that people with learning disabilities have often encountered prejudice and discrimination and their access to health services has been poor, with health needs often unmet. *Valuing People* stresses that people with learning disabilities are people first and there should be a focus on what they can do rather than what they cannot. All people with learning disabilities should have a health facilitator (who may often be a nurse) appointed from the local community learning disability team to ensure they get the health care they need, and a Health Action Plan. An individual's Health Action Plan includes details of health interventions, oral health and dental care, fitness and mobility, continence, vision, hearing, nutrition, emotional needs, medication, and records of screening (p. 64). The UK Department of Health website (www.dh.gov.uk) gives more details. Any nurses carrying out practical skills with people with learning disabilities, or supporting their carers in doing so, should do so with an appropriate attitude and with reference to their Health Action Plan.

THE COGNITIVE DIMENSION

This reflects the 'thinking' element behind the skill, including the application of research to practice and problem solving, and is what makes the nurse a 'knowledgeable doer'. Being able to adapt a skill in the practice setting requires a sound underlying knowledge of why it is being performed and the rationale for each stage. For example, understanding the principles behind the administration of oxygen therapy enables nurses to choose a method of administration that is acceptable to clients in specific clinical situations. There is increasing emphasis on 'evidence-based care' throughout health care with the aim that all health care professionals should be applying best evidence to their practice. Nurses need to choose best options when implementing care, and be reflective decision makers (Watkins 1997). In many cases this knowledge will be derived from empirical evidence – research, but it may also be based on experience, and knowledge gained through reflection on practice. In Benner's (1984) work she identifies that practice is always more complex and presents many more realities than theory ever can, and she highlights the value of theory derived from practice (see later section: 'Learning from experience and reflection').

Various theorists have tried to explain the nature of knowledge within nursing. One of the first of these theorists was Carper (1978), who identified four 'ways of knowing': empirics (scientific knowledge); aesthetics (the art of nursing); personal (knowledge of self); and ethical. As an example a nurse carrying out a wound dressing would use all four ways of knowing in the following way:

- **Empirical knowledge** is that based on tested theory, such as research conducted to trial the effect of a specific wound dressing on wound healing. The nurse might use clinical guidelines (based on best evidence) to select a particular dressing. Clinical guidelines may be informed by systematic reviews, which are where research studies about a particular topic have been evaluated by experts according to criteria, and recommendations for practice made. These are a sounder source on which to base practice than individual research studies, which though informative, will inevitably have limitations.
- **Aesthetic knowledge** is based on the nurse's intuitive grasp of the whole unique situation, for example, the meaning of the patient's wound to that individual. The nurse would use this knowledge to skilfully individualise care.
- **Personal knowledge** involves the nurse knowing her/his self and the effect they are having on the interaction with the patient who is having their wound dressing.
- **Ethical knowledge** focuses on moral decision making and values. The nurse would use this knowledge if the patient refused to have the dressing done, for example.

Bearing in mind the position of a registered nurse as an accountable practitioner, it is important to be able to explain the knowledge base for practical skills. The difference between practical and theoretical knowledge is discussed by Benner (1984). She cites philosophers such as Kuhn (1970) and Polanyi (1958) who have observed that 'knowing-how' (for example, how to take a temperature) is different from 'knowing-that' (for example, what a normal temperature recording is and what might cause a low or high reading). Benner (1984) goes on to explore how expert nurses develop knowledge from their practice, learning to recognise, for example, subtle changes in clients' conditions. Not all nursing skills have a firm evidence base on which to implement practice, but in many areas such research-based knowledge is obtainable. Within this book, authors have searched for up-to-date evidence on which to base practical skills and systematic reviews have been used wherever available. Health service users should be able to assume that practical skills carried out by nurses are based on sound evidence if it is available, rather than on ritual or unsubstantiated knowledge.

Increasingly NHS Trusts and other health care organisations are developing their own clinical guidelines, based on best evidence, to assist nurses and other health care professionals to implement evidence-based practice. If you yourself are searching for evidence, an excellent source of information is the National Electronic Library for Health (www.nelh.nhs.uk). This includes access to centres which are examining evidence from which to produce recommendations for practice. Examples of these are the Cochrane Library, the University of York: NHS Centre for Reviews and Dissemination (www.york.ac.uk/inst/crd), and the National Institute for Clinical Excellence (NICE) (www.nice.org.uk). The standards in the National Service Frameworks, mentioned earlier, are also based on best evidence, and these are all accessible on the UK Department of Health website (www.dh.gov.uk).

THE MOTOR DIMENSION

Mastering the motor dimension of a skill is important for achieving a good outcome as lack of a skilled motor performance can jeopardise both safety and comfort. Knowing how to do a practical skill can be termed 'know-how' type of knowledge – practical expertise and skill that is really acquired through practice and experience (Manley 1997). The characteristics of a skilled motor performance were identified by Quinn (2000) and are shown in Table 1.1, applied to the administration of an injection. Nursing skills are performed in a changing clinical environment, with people who respond and react in different ways, so nurses need to adapt skills accordingly. This need for adaptability in practical nursing skills means that they can never be wholly automatic in nature.

Three types of motor skills have been identified (Oermann 1990): (1) fine motor skills are precision orientated tasks, for example drawing up and giving an injection; (2) manual skills are repetitive and often include eye–arm act

Table 1.1 Characteristics of a skilled motor performance, from Quinn (2000) applied to injection administration

Criteria	Explanation	Illustration
Accuracy	Performed with precision	The injection is drawn up accurately, maintaining asepsis and the needle is inserted into the correct body area
Speed	Movements swift and confident	The injection is performed confidently and without hesitation
Efficiency	Movements economical, leaving spare capacity available	The nurse gathers all equipment at the start and positions her/himself and equipment to avoid awkward movement
Timing	Accurate timing and correct sequential order	The steps in preparing the injection and administration are in the correct order, and the time given to each stage is appropriate
Consistency	Results are consistent	The injection is performed in this manner on each occasion
Anticipation	Can anticipate events quickly and respond accordingly	The nurse anticipates that the client may become tense or move suddenly, and is able to respond effectively by steadying the injection and using appropriate communication
Adaptability	Can adapt the skill to current circumstances	The nurse adapts injection administration, taking into account factors such as age, level of anxiety and physical build of the client
Perception	Can obtain maximum information from a minimum of cues	The nurse quickly takes in factors that could affect the injection. For example he/she perceives the client's anxiety about having an injection from minimal observation and questioning

such as washing someone, and (3) gross manual skills involve the whole body such as when assisting a person to walk. Quinn (2000) also explains that a motor skill may involve continuous adjustment and corrections to stimuli (e.g. removing sutures), while a discrete skill is a one-off movement (e.g. switching off an alarm on an electronic pump).

PRACTICAL SKILLS WITHIN THE CONTEXT OF CARING

You were probably asked to state reasons for wanting to study nursing in your application, and might well have cited a desire to care, amongst them. That caring is inherent within nursing is a theme to be found in many nurse theorists' work. Watson (1979) stated that 'the practice of caring is central to nursing' (p. 9). Benner and Wrubel (1989) consider that the 'nature of the caring relationship is central to most nursing interventions' (p. 5). They identify that the same act done in a non-caring way, as opposed to a caring way, has very different consequences, thus 'nursing can never be reduced to mere technique' (p. 4). Roach (2002) identified caring both as a natural concomitant of being a human and as the core of nursing. McMahon (1998) considers that in Britain it is widely accepted that the concept of care is the nurse's domain. Bjork (1999b) presents a model of practical skill performance, which includes aspects such as sequence and fluency, but also includes caring comportment. She views this as being how the nurse creates a respectful, accepting and encouraging atmosphere, which includes concern for the whole person.

THE EXPERIENCE OF NON-CARING VERSUS CARING

The detrimental effects of skills being implemented without a caring context are identified in a study by Halldorsdottir (1991). The in-depth interviews she conducted with former patients highlighted the vulnerability of patients who found uncaring encounters with nurses to be discouraging and distressing. Patients described being initially puzzled and disbelieving, followed by experiencing feelings of anger and resentment, and then despair and helplessness. She found that dependent people being uncared for developed feelings of a sense of loss, and of being betrayed by those counted on for caring. Non-caring nurses were described as being 'cold human beings, like computers'. Box 1.4 illustrates the effect on an individual of feeling uncared for. Halldorsdottir describes this feeling as dehumanisation, with the person feeling that they have no value as a person and are 'an object': 'I was … a piece of dust on the floor'. The uncaring nurse, Halldorsdottir found, did carry out the routine tasks (as the nurse in Box 1.4 did leave a vomit bowl for Jane), but was perceived as not 'caring about the patient as a person'. In a study by Thorsteinsson (2002) participants reported that poor-quality nursing care made them feel angry and stressed. One person said: 'It made me mad – I did not feel that I deserved it. When you are in my position you are unable to defend yourself – it was an unpleasant feeling.'

With application of this research to practical skills, to carry out observation of blood pressure in a technically competent manner would not, in itself, be perceived

---

Jane, aged 14, was in hospital following orthopaedic surgery. During the night she felt very sick and then started to vomit. She was unable to reach her call bell. Eventually a nearby patient called a nurse. The nurse told her off for not pressing her call bell, left a bowl on her table and walked away. Jane described feeling 'upset, unwanted and a waste of space'.

Box 1.4 Illustrative example of feeling uncared for

as caring. In Thorsteinsson's (2002) study nurses perceived as giving high-quality care were described as 'joyful, warm, tender, smiling, positive, polite and understanding'. It is notable that all these attributes are to do with the nurse's approach; clinical competence was also expected but did not lead to an experience of high-quality care unless accompanied by these other aspects. Kralik *et al.*'s (1997) research identified that patients saw nurses as being either engaged or detached in their care. Care by detached nurses was viewed negatively by patients. They felt that they were treated as if they were a number or an object, the nurses were sharp/cold in their approach to their care, and were rough with their physical care. Nurses who were engaged with their care however, were friendly and warm, behaved as if nothing was too much trouble and had a gentle touch.

Woodward's (1997) analysis of the literature on professional caring identifies these two elements as instrumental caring (the technique comprising skills and knowledge) and expressive caring (the emotional element which includes respect for the individual). It is expressive caring which, she suggests, transforms nursing actions into caring. Halldorsdottir (1991) identifies a 'life-sustaining mode of being with a patient' which includes 'compassionate competence, genuine concern for the patient as a person, undivided attention when the nurse is with the patient, and cheerfulness'. This approach is described as 'professional caring'. Participants in the research felt relief when they felt cared for, and believed that this diminished anxiety gave them time to concentrate on getting better.

Roach (1992) has made a study of caring in relation to nursing and developed a framework: the 5Cs. These are compassion, competence, confidence, conscience and commitment. In her more recent work (Roach 2002) she includes a sixth aspect: comportment. She explains that her theory developed over time in response to the question: What is a nurse doing when she or he is caring? The 6Cs are a broad framework 'suggesting categories of human behaviour within which professional caring is to be understood' (Roach 2002, p. 66).

ROACH'S 6CS: A FRAMEWORK FOR CARING

Compassion

Compassion is defined by Roach (2002) as 'a way of living born out of an awareness of one's relationship to all living creatures. It engenders a response of participation in the experience of another; a sensitivity to the pain and brokenness of the other and a quality of presence that allows one to share with and make room for the other' (p. 50). Compassion is 'a simple unpretentious presence to each other, a gift that we seem to have lost even as we have developed sophisticated techniques in our efforts to acquire it' (Roach 2002, p. 51). Roach (2002) argues that compassion is needed more than ever to humanise the ever-increasing cold and impersonal technology used within health care. Box 1.5 illustrates this with a nurse's act of compassion that occurred in the highly technical environment of the intensive therapy unit.

James was in the final stages of heart and lung failure and his nurse, about to go home after a 12-hour shift and knowing that she would not see him again, asked him if there was anything she could get him before she left. He replied 'Oh a port and brandy please!' Phone calls around the hospital were unsuccessful in locating any and the nurse went off shift. She returned half an hour later with a small glass of port and brandy brought from home. As James was unable to swallow she dipped sponge mouth sticks into the drink and put them in his mouth for him to suck. James grinned and said it was 'wonderful'. This act of compassion brought tenderness to this patient's final hours and made an immeasurable difference to his relatives' feelings about his death.

Box 1.5 Compassion: an illustrative example from an intensive therapy unit

Competence

To ensure safe and effective care, practical skills must be carried out competently. Roach (2002) defines competence as having the 'knowledge, judgement, skills, energy, experience and motivation required to respond adequately to the demands of one's professional responsibilities' (p. 54). Roach goes on to state that 'while competence without compassion can be brutal and inhumane, compassion without competence may be no more than a meaningless, if not harmful, intrusion into the life of a person or persons needing help' (p. 54). Wallis's (1998) in-depth study of patients' experiences of being cared for in a coronary care unit, found that patients viewed competence as essential in a caring nurse: 'You have got to have a competent nurse to start with'. It seemed that technical competence was reassuring to patients, and that this competence then allowed the nurse to 'transcend' the technology and become close to patients. Competence also requires that health and safety factors are maintained – for nurses as well as for clients.

Confidence

Confidence is defined by Roach (2002) as 'the quality that fosters trusting relationships' (p. 56). Roach (2002) discusses the importance of not deceiving clients and states that 'Caring confidence fosters trust without dependency, communicates truth without violence and creates a relationship of respect without paternalism or without engendering a response borne out of fear or powerlessness' (p. 58). Consider a situation whereby a person who has had a hip fracture due to a fall is regaining mobility and independence. The client may lack confidence and be afraid of falling again, but the nurse's approach enables a trusting relationship to be built. The nurse can help the client to set and reach realistic goals in mobilisation, giving them praise for achievements, and helping them to believe in their abilities.

Conscience

Conscience is, according to Roach (2002), a 'state of moral awareness' (p. 60) and this is exuded throughout the nurse's approach when undertaking practical skills. She considers that conscience grows out of experience, 'out of a process of valuing self and others' (p. 61). Nurses can demonstrate whether they value people and respect their rights to dignified and humane care. Nurses will also speak out if they feel that the care is compromised in any way.

Commitment

Commitment is defined by Roach (2002) as 'a complex affective response characterised by a convergence between one's desires and one's obligations, and by a deliberate choice to act in accordance with them' (p. 62). This very much conjures up a picture of duty; nurses may sometimes not want to carry out certain practical skills but commitment means that if it is necessary then they will do so. The situation in Box 1.5 that exemplified compassion also demonstrates commitment from the nurse to James, in her decision to bring in the drink from home despite just finishing a 12-hour shift.

Comportment

In considering this attribute of caring, Roach (2002) asks the question: 'Are dress and language of caregivers consistent with the belief that the patient – client is of incalculable worth, and that the caregiver him/herself is a person of intrinsic worth and dignity?' (p. 65) She proposes that how nurses present themselves represents their beliefs about the worth of those they are caring for. She argues that 'Caring is reflected in bearing, demeanour, dress and language' (p. 65), and that 'we usually dress and use language consistent with our attitude towards the person or the occasion' (p. 64). Thus we would not usually wear jeans to a funeral, and it might be considered offensive for a health visitor visiting families in an area of extreme poverty to wear a great deal of expensive jewellery.

Roach's 6Cs act as a useful framework when considering how practical skills can be carried out in a caring manner.

Activity

Think about the skill of assisting someone with eating a meal in a caring manner. Can you think of relevant points in relation to compassion, competence, confidence, conscience, commitment and comportment?

A few points in relation to each of the 6Cs are discussed below, but you may well have thought of other issues. A **compassionate** approach entails being understanding and empathetic in manner, showing insight into the individual's experience of being assisted with eating, and using effective communication to convey this. This would include sitting at the person's level and not appearing rushed. **Competence** means that the nurse has knowledge about what nutrients the person needs, and can help the person to make informed menu choices. The competent nurse is aware of any potential problems such as swallowing difficulties, and ensures that the person is positioned so as to minimise problems. The nurse has the knowledge and skill to deal with choking if it occurs and if the person's nutritional input is being monitored, ensures that the meal is recorded accurately. The nurse also has knowledge about any special utensils deemed necessary. **Confidence** means that the nurse is honest about their ability to regain independence in eating. Realistic goals are set and the nurse encourages the client to work towards them. The nurse's **conscience** promotes awareness of moral dimensions, such as the approach to take if the person refuses food. **Commitment** on the nurse's part is shown by being there to assist the client on time so that the food does not become cold, and, if the meal is unsuitable for the client, making the effort to contact the kitchens and ensure that a more acceptable meal is provided. **Comportment** means that the nurse is dressed according to the ward or unit dress code and has a good standard of personal hygiene. Assisting someone with eating involves quite close contact (as do many other nursing skills). If the nurse has an unpleasant body odour (smelling of stale cigarettes for example), bad breath or dirty nails it will not enhance the person's appetite, as well as being unhygienic. Self-awareness is an important attribute that you will explore in Chapter 2.

TRANSCULTURAL CARING

Like many countries, Britain is a multicultural society, and practical nursing skills must be carried out with sensitivity and in a culturally appropriate manner for each individual and family. The American nurse and anthropologist, Madeleine Leininger, has studied transcultural caring over many years, and identified how acts of caring such as comforting and physical care, and the meaning attached to them, can vary between cultures (Leininger 1981). Leininger suggests that culture and caring cannot be separated within nursing actions and decision making. An overview of her theory can be found in Reynolds and Leininger (1993). Papadopoulos *et al.* (1998) developed a model for the development of transcultural skills, consisting of four linked elements: cultural awareness, knowledge, sensitivity and competence.

- Cultural awareness includes examining and questioning one's personal value system (see Chapter 2), thus leading, the authors suggest, to the exploration of different views.
- Cultural knowledge may be drawn from sources such as sociology and research, and from experience of people. Where appropriate to specific practical skills, cultural variations (particularly related to religious beliefs) are considered in this book. However there are often individual and regional variations, and it is important to avoid stereotyping and making ethnocentric judgements; these are barriers to cultural sensitivity.
- Cultural sensitivity, the third dimension of Papadopoulos *et al.*'s model, can be achieved by nurses working with clients as partners, offering choices i

> Ellen had terminal cancer, was severely visually impaired and was being nursed in a side room. A plate of food was left in front of her wordlessly. When the nurse returned to collect the plate some while later, she remarked 'Oh you weren't hungry today then?' Ellen had not even known that the food was there. She could not see it, and would have been unable to reach it or feed herself anyway. She told the nurse that she had not known the food was there as she could not see. The nurse said 'Oh', picked up the tray and walked out.

Box 1.6 Non-therapeutic nursing: an illustrative example

care. Very important here are communication skills, respect and empathy (see Chapter 2).

■ Cultural competence is achieved when practice is both antidiscriminatory and anti-oppressive. Papadopoulos *et al.* (1998) include a number of useful exercises aimed at promoting the development of transcultural caring skills.

THERAPEUTIC NURSING AND PRACTICAL SKILLS

The term therapeutic nursing can be defined as nursing that 'deliberately leads to beneficial outcomes for the patient' (McMahon 1998, p. 7). At first glance it might seem obvious that this is what nursing seeks to attain, and if you look back to the discussion of feeding above, the care described should certainly have a positive effect on the client. However, read through Box 1.6, which illustrates how care relating to nutrition can be non-therapeutic. Under the headline 'Nurses "failed to feed us", patients say', an article in the *Nursing Times* ('This Week' 2000) stated that a Community Health Council had reported that nurses 'placed food out of patients' reach and failed to help them eat'. Unfortunate examples such as these illustrate that nursing does not always have a therapeutic effect on an individual. Indeed it might be said that some patients get better despite their nursing care, not because of it (McMahon 1998).

McMahon (1998) identifies a number of activities in nursing (see Box 1.7) which can be considered therapeutic. Note that complementary health practices include such activities as massage, aromatherapy and reflexology. These require qualifications which are not usually included as part of pre-registration education, as the courses are quite extensive. NHS Trusts usually have protocols for implementing complementary health practices. It is likely that they will only be performed by registered nurses holding the appropriate qualifications.

McMahon's (1998) framework will now be discussed in relation to bathing. Bathing a client is an ideal time to develop the nurse–patient relationship as it involves being physically close to the person, and giving one-to-one care. The nurse can use effective communication skills throughout the process to value the person. A bath can be comforting and make the person feel cared for as long

- Developing
  - partnership
  - intimacy
  - reciprocity in the nurse–patient relationship
- Caring and comforting
- Using evidence-based physical interventions
- Teaching
- Manipulating the environment
- Adopting complementary health practices.

Box 1.7 Therapeutic activities in nursing (McMahon 1998)

as it is done considerately, without being rushed, and with the nurse aiming to meet individual preferences. An evidence-based physical intervention could be the use of particular moving and handling techniques to transfer the person safely into and out of the bath. Bathing can provide a good opportunity for education, for example if the person is at risk of pressure ulcers, the nurse could explain about how to check for signs of redness. The nurse can promote a conducive environment for bathing, by ensuring that the bathroom is warm enough, and that privacy is maintained throughout.

Work by Ersser (1998) identified three core categories which he found reflected views about nurses' therapeutic actions. These were presentation of the nurse, such as non-verbal communication and greeting the patient, relating to patients as when developing rapport, and specific actions of the nurse, which are largely instrumental or procedural such as doing a wound dressing. When carrying out any practical nursing skill you need to consider how your actions can be therapeutic. For example, what will turn taking someone to the toilet into a therapeutic action, as opposed to simply assisting with elimination?

Reflecting on your practice can help you to identify how you could provide a more positive outcome for patients and clients (see later section: 'Learning from experience and reflection').

HOW CAN YOU DEVELOP YOUR PRACTICAL NURSING SKILLS?

In order to make the most of opportunities to learn practical skills it is helpful to think about how skills are learned.

Activity

To understand how nurses acquire practical skills, reflect back on a practical skill which you have learned, for example learning to drive. How did you learn this skill?

You may recall that you had to build up the skill in step by step stages, learning each sub-skill one at a time. You could probably focus only on the skill, and found that it was difficult to do anything else (e.g. have a conversation) at the same time. Benner (1984) identified that when learning any new skill, the performance is initially 'halting and rigid' (p. 37) and that one must pay careful attention to the explicit rules relating to the skill.

It is important to realise that as a student you are not expected to be an expert in your practical skills! Benner's (1984) research adapted a skill acquisition model by Dreyfus and Dreyfus (1980) to describe different levels of performance in nurses. She conducted paired interviews with beginners and experienced nurses as well as using participant observation to study nurses with various levels of experience. The five stages of performance identified are outlined below.

STAGES OF SKILL PERFORMANCE

Stage 1: Novice

Novice nurses have no experience on which to draw (this applies not only to new students but also to experienced nurses moving to an unfamiliar area of practice). Benner describes the novice as being 'rule governed' in behaviour. By this she means that the novice needs explicit guidelines about what to do and in which sequence. However, these guidelines need to be adapted to the actual situation, and novice nurses need help and guidance to do this.

Stage 2: Advanced beginner

At this stage nurses can use previous experience and apply it in practice but continue to need adequate support, particularly with aspects that are situational, such as prioritising. They have difficulty seeing a situation as a whole and focus on the specific skill to be carried out, regardless of additional situational factors.

Stage 3: Competent

Competent nurses are able to carry out conscious and deliberate planning, and prioritise and manage their work. However they lack the flexibility and speed of proficient nurses.

Stage 4: Proficient

Proficient nurses perceive situations holistically, recognise important and less important elements, and make decisions quickly. Benner found proficiency in nurses who have worked in an area for some time.

Stage 5: Expert

Expert nurses have a deep understanding and an intuitive grasp of situations, gained from substantial experience in the practice setting. You may observe this level in some practitioners with whom you work. In her book Benner gives many examples of expert nurses' care for clients. Such nurses may be excellent and inspirational role models but it is important not to feel inadequate or overawed by such expertise.

DEVELOPING THE AFFECTIVE, COGNITIVE AND MOTOR ELEMENTS OF A SKILL

A detailed review of theories about learning psychomotor skills can be found in Knight (1998).

Woodward's (1997) analysis indicates that developing the affective domain of a skill requires practice and perseverance, just as will the motor element. Roach (1992) suggested that while nursing students may start their course with rudimentary expressive caring skills, these sometimes go unrecognised and unvalued and may be eroded rather than developed further. This book includes activities throughout which focus on the affective dimension, asking you to think about, for example, how a patient might be feeling in a particular situation. Chapter 2 concentrates on the affective dimension of practical skills, and will help you to understand the concept of self-awareness and how your values might affect how you carry out your care.

Developing the cognitive domain of a skill involves you in undertaking activities to acquire and understand the underpinning knowledge and rationale. Throughout this book research findings relating to nursing practice are discussed, but there are also activities encouraging you to access other sources of knowledge, such as reflection on experience. It is hoped to encourage you to develop an enquiring and problem solving approach to your nursing practice.

To learn the motor dimension of a psychomotor skill requires practice – the opportunity to try out and repeat performance (Oermann 1990). It is only with practice that movement becomes refined and a smooth co-ordinated performance can be developed. The amount of practice needed varies according to motivation to learn the skill, previous related skills learning, familiarity with equipment, level of anxiety, and the physical resources and co-ordination of the learner (Oermann 1990). More complex skills need more practice. Motivation affects mastery as many skills are initially difficult but highly motivated students will persevere. If you have had previous experience of a related skill, some component parts of the skill will be familiar, so then your practice can focus on parts of the skill not already learned. Familiarity with equipment also eases the learning of a new skill. The stages that learners move through when acquiring a new skill are identified in Box 1.8. Quinn (2000) suggests that levels 3 or 4 are an appropriate aim for students learning nursing skills. Achieving the higher levels in many skills is only possible for qualified nurses who have practised for some time.

If you understand the different stages that you are likely to go through when learning new skills, you can be systematic and realistic in your approach. For example, you will understand that you will initially need guidance and that being adaptable and creative is unlikely to be possible until you have mastered the routine stages of the skill. You may find that people who have reached stage 7, origination, carry out skills in such a fluent manner that they find it difficult to break skills down into sub-skills at all. It may also mean that you see the same

1. **Perception**: at this stage the learner has watched the skill and can perceive what it is going to entail
2. **Set**: physically and psychologically, the learner is ready to attempt the skill
3. **Guided response**: the skill is performed under guidance
4. **Mechanism**: becomes habitual
5. **Complex overt response**: a typical skilled performance
6. **Adaptation**: the skill can be adapted to each individual situation
7. **Origination**: creation of original movement patterns. The skill can be carried out creatively

Box 1.8 The stages which a learner moves through when learning a new skill (Simpson 1972, cited by Quinn 2000)

- Provide an atmosphere conducive to learning
- Carry out a skills analysis
- Determine sequence
- Assess student's prior knowledge
- Demonstrate the skill at normal speed
- Teach sequence
- Teach skill by either whole learning or part learning
- Allocate sufficient time to practise
- Provide feedback
- Prompt student to self-evaluate
- Encourage transfer of skills.

Box 1.9 How a facilitator can help a student learn a practical skill (adapted from Quinn 2000)

skills carried out in different ways by different nurses with different clients, due to the adaptations which they have made. An understanding of the cognitive and affective dimensions enables adaptations to be made which enhance rather than compromise practice. There are key points a facilitator can do to help when you are learning a new skill (see Box 1.9).

You yourself can be active about promoting these conditions. For example, the time to ask a nurse to supervise you drawing up an injection is probably not in the middle of an emergency situation, as the stress and anxiety in the environment are unlikely to be conducive to learning. Thus when asking to be supervised carrying out a skill for the first time, pick the right moment! You can be open about your prior knowledge, saying explicitly that you have, for example, observed a number of injections, and now feel ready to be supervised administering one.

De Tornyay and Thompson (1987) highlight some other issues too. They identify that learners need to handle equipment as this diffuses anxiety;

therefore always take opportunities to become familiar with equipment that you are likely to use. This book will help by explaining what type of equipment is used for the skills discussed and includes illustrations of equipment. There is also advice about where you might be able to access equipment with which to become familiar. De Tornyay and Thompson (1987) suggest that adult learners can be self-conscious when trying out new skills. You need to be supervised when practising a new skill, but you may wish to ensure that there won't be too big an audience if you feel that you will be self-conscious! A warm and accepting learning environment helps to reduce excess anxiety that might adversely affect your performance. Although supervisors should avoid the temptation to 'take over', they will need to do so if client safety is compromised. De Tornyay and Thompson (1987) also suggest that when learning a new skill feedback is crucial – to reinforce correct behaviour and eliminate error.

THE IMPORTANCE OF OBTAINING FEEDBACK

Gaining feedback when you are developing skills is important for your learning. From whom can you gain feedback? Obviously nurses supervising you can give you feedback. It is best if the comments are as specific as possible rather than a general comment such as 'very good', or 'you need to be quicker'. It will help your supervisor if you identify any aspects in particular that you want feedback about. For example, you might state that when performing the skill last time, the supervisor had said that you needed to give a clearer explanation to the client, and ask that they give you feedback on this aspect in particular. Clients may also give you feedback. They may make spontaneous comments, such as that they feel 'much more comfortable now', but you can also seek feedback specifically, by asking how they feel at different stages. If you are approachable in the way you seek feedback, clients are more likely to give honest responses. Your observation of clients while you are carrying out practical skills will also give you feedback; for example, you can observe for facial expressions that might indicate fear or discomfort.

The sources of feedback outlined so far will provide 'extrinsic feedback'. Combined with intrinsic feedback, this should give you a balanced view of your performance. Intrinsic feedback involves you reflecting on your performance, and asking yourself what were the strengths and weaknesses and how you could improve your performance next time.

LEARNING FROM EXPERIENCE AND REFLECTION

Becoming skilled at learning from experience is essential for you to benefit fully from your practice experience. We have already established that to develop competency, practice is necessary. But is it inevitable that experience leads to learning, and improved performance? Bjork's (1999b) study followed the progress of four newly qualified nurses' practical skill development. Her focus was on the skill of mobilising a post-operative patient. In fact their skills performance did not necessarily improve over time. Some aspects in some nurses improved while other aspects deteriorated. Bjork's findings led her to question how it could be that nurses with 8–14 months' experience 'do not give the patient sufficient physical support during ambulation, or that basic attention to the patient's clothing and comfort is missing?' She also found that nurses became quicker and seemingly more efficient, but learned to cut corners in a way that was culturally acceptable, such as not washing hands. Andrews *et al.* (1998) suggest that continued repetition of skills may lead to merely habitual behaviour, rather than conscious analysis of actions.

Bjork (1999b) theorises a number of possible reasons why these nurses' performance did not necessarily improve with experience. She questions whether their knowledge base was adequate, believing that some skills are inadequately described in nursing text books. She identifies therefore that nurses cannot use in practice knowledge that they do not have, but equally, they may not use in practice the knowledge that they do have. However, she also identifies lack of reflection on experience as a possible cause. She suggests that nurses are often intent on long-term outcomes and that opportunity to reflect and learn from practice is delayed or embedded in a broader context. The results of our actions in everyday life are often clear and direct, therefore making an obvious connection between our action and its result. For example, if you leave a cake in the oven too long it will burn, so you might take more care next time. The result of nurses' failure to wash their hands after dealing with patients is unlikely to be immediately obvious.

Dewey, an educational theorist, has argued that we do not 'learn by doing' but by 'doing and realizing what came of what we did' (Dewey 1929, p. 367). Dewey's theories were developed further by Kolb and Fry (1975), and then more fully by Kolb (1984). The theory of how we learn from experience is often referred to as experiential learning, and is portrayed as a cycle. The process starts at the point of a concrete experience or event, after which observations and reflections occur, followed by abstract conceptualisation, where new ideas are developed, linked to other knowledge and experience, and then the new knowledge arising from the experience is tested out in a new situation. This new experience then starts the experiential learning cycle once again.

Honey (1982) proposes that students tend to have a preferred learning style, and may be stronger in one component of the learning cycle than the others. The four learning styles identified are: **activists**, who are open to new experiences; **reflectors**, who are cautious and like to observe; **theorists**, who are logical and rational; and **pragmatists**, who like to experiment and try out new ideas. Identifying your preferred learning style can give you useful insights. It can also help you to focus on developing your skills in the other learning styles, thus enabling you to learn from experience more effectively.

Reflection enables you to consider what you did and why, and provides opportunities to develop knowledge from experience and link theory and practice.

Johns (1994) defines reflective practice as involving 'the practitioner paying attention to "significant" aspects of experience in order to make sense of it within the context of their intention' (p. 7). Andrews *et al.* (1998) emphasise that reflection is not just recalling events but is a purposeful activity, which requires the nurse to want to change behaviour. Knowledge gained as a result of reflection on practice has been termed 'practical knowledge' (Schon 1987). It has been asserted that reflection can enable the uncovering of knowledge embedded in practice (Lawler 1991). Furthermore, Johns (1994) considers that reflection can enable practitioners to become aware of conflicts between aims of care and the reality of practice, and these insights can enable nurses to become more effective.

How guided reflection can help nurses to learn from their experience and 'assert and realise caring as an everyday reality' is explored in Johns (1996). Schon (1983) suggested that there is also such a thing as reflection-in-action. In relation to practical skills this means that rather than dealing with a client's incontinence and reflecting on your care afterwards, gaining new insights for application on the next occasion, you would reflect and acquire knowledge while you are carrying out the care. Reflection-on-action is usually a conscious act but reflection-in-action may not be, making it difficult to articulate knowledge gained in this way. An analysis of both experiential learning and reflection is discussed in some detail by Powell (1998), who suggests that it is unrealistic for nurses to use reflection on every occasion; rather reflective techniques can be applied to specific situations.

To think over or mull over an event is commonplace, but without an analytical and purposeful approach it may not lead to new ways of thinking or behaving (Andrews *et al.* 1998). To help you to develop your reflective skills you will probably be encouraged to keep a reflective journal, recording and reflecting on significant events which you experience in your nursing practice. This activity can assist you in developing evaluative and decision-making skills, and help you to link theory and practice (Howard 1999). It is essential, however, that you do not identify patients or clients (either by name or by using other identifying material) in your reflective writing, to maintain confidentiality. You are also likely to take part in reflective activities within the classroom setting where you will be encouraged to reflect on specific incidents from practice. You may be recommended to use a reflective model, which can help you to be more structured and systematic about your reflection.

THE SKILLS LABORATORY

As it is recognised that students need opportunities to rehearse skills in a safe environment and to handle equipment, most universities have skills laboratories or centres (formerly called practical rooms). These vary in complexity, but usually contain equipment for practising technical procedures. Some skills, such as blood pressure recording, can be practised safely on your peers and there may be models for simulation of other skills. Some skills laboratories organise volunteer 'patients' for students' practice (Smith 1995). Universities have different systems for learning in skills laboratories, which you need to become familiar with. There may be compulsory sessions, optional workshops, and formal or informal sessions. Activities within the chapters of this book often suggest that you access equipment to practise with. You will need to find out about your local policies/procedures for use of equipment in the skills laboratory.

At one stage in nurse education, learning skills in the classroom setting went out of favour (Knight and Mowforth 1998). Some educationalists felt that skills could only be learned in the practice setting with actual patients/clients, and that skills learned in the classroom could not in any case be readily transferred to the practice setting (Neary 1997). However, without any classroom-based practical skills learning, students often reported feeling unprepared and lacking in confidence (Neary 1997). Practice staff do not always have the time to teach skills 'from scratch', and can be reluctant to involve students in practical skills that they have not been 'taught'. When skills are taught in the practice setting, the focus is usually on the physical procedure and manual dexterity, while the cognitive and affective dimensions are omitted. This is probably due to time constraints on practitioners. Students have also reported anxiety about practising skills in the clinical setting without previous experience (Neary 1997). McAdams *et al.* (1989) in a survey of fifty-nine students, found that students believed classroom-based skills learning reduced anxiety, increased feelings of mastery, enhanced patient safety and provided hands-on, pre-clinical experience. Some would consider that it is only fair to patients/clients that students should have had some prior preparation before practising on such vulnerable people. Clinical practice on patients must certainly be carried out safely (McAdams *et al.* 1989).

Some researchers have attempted evaluation of whether practice in skills laboratories does actually enhance performance in the clinical setting (Erickson Megel *et al.* 1987; Gomez and Gomez 1987; Hallal and Welch 1984; Love *et al.* 1989; McAdams *et al.* 1989) with varied results. Knight's (1998) critical review of some of these studies casts doubt on some of their conclusions. Gomez and Gomez (1987) explain the difference between 'open' and 'closed' psychomotor skills. An example of a closed psychomotor skill within nursing is making an unoccupied bed. This skill is not greatly affected by situational variables and is therefore easier to transfer from the classroom to the clinical setting. Skills performed in dynamic environments such as taking a patient's blood pressure are called 'open' psychomotor skills as there are many different factors affecting how this skill has to be performed. Noise within a ward setting, relatives looking on and a patient who has difficulty in fully straightening their arm, for example, are all unpredictable variables that are not present when the student practises this skill in the classroom setting. Thus practising the skill of taking a blood pressure in the classroom, while beneficial in leading to familiarity with equipment and the sequence of steps in the procedure, has recognised limitations. To actually become competent and confident in this skill requires repeated practice in the clinical setting.

Knight's (1998) extensive review of the literature on learning psychomotor skills in nursing supports the use of a controlled and safe environment to facilitate initial skills practice. She identifies that learning a skill requires a structured and systematic approach, which enables practice in a safe environment. Overall, most educationalists support the view that students should have classroom preparation for practical skills, and these facilities are now generally available. The use of skills laboratories is endorsed by the English National Board (2000), as a means to enable students to become safe and effective in practice. Their use in no way replaces the need for practice of skills within clinical placements. However, the classroom provides a more controlled environment for familiarisation with practical skills than the clinical setting, and if students are familiar with some skills and equipment they can focus on learning aspects which cannot be simulated in the classroom (Hallal and Welch 1984). Some skills laboratories include video equipment so that students can analyse their performance afterwards (Knight and Mowforth 1998; Smith 1995). Watching the video objectively and identifying your strengths and areas for improvement will help you to enhance your skills performance. Increasingly students are also being tested in the classroom, often through a system termed 'objective structured clinical examination' (OSCE). OSCEs require students to carry out practical skills with simulated patients, in response to a given scenario, and their performance is assessed against pre-set criteria (Nicol and Freeth 1998).

LEARNING IN THE PRACTICE SETTING

Clinical experience is 'central to the development of nursing practice skills' (Nolan 1998). Indeed, actual practice with clients in the clinical environment is essential to enable competence to be developed. It is important, however, not to see clients as just people to be practised on, therefore objectifying them (Roach 1992). Roach (1992) suggests that instead, students should see themselves as being 'in a helping therapeutic relationship with clients who freely collaborate in the educational enterprise' (p. 120). Practical skills development and practice should therefore take place within the context of the relationship between you and the client, as part of their holistic care. I was once told of a student who refused to help a patient to wash because she said she already knew how to do that! Obviously you should take every opportunity to develop new skills, but not within a task-orientated framework that is dehumanising and objectifies clients. Learning practical skills should thus occur within the total care required for each individual.

In Nolan's (1998) qualitative study about learning in clinical practice, she cites a student starting a new placement as saying: 'You are so scared and wondering, Oh God, I want to do this right'. When starting a new clinical placement you may well feel anxious or even fearful and it is important to be aware that you are not alone in these feelings. Starting a new clinical placement has been likened to starting a new job! Each practice setting has its own culture and you need to familiarise yourself with the environment, staff and routines

(Nolan 1998). Until you 'settle in' and start to feel part of the team, effective learning can be difficult. Some practice settings send you information prior to your placement to help you feel welcome and reduce anxiety, and often a pre-placement visit is encouraged. Alternatively this information may be available to you on the intranet; do make sure you access it and make good use of this facility. The English National Board (2001) details standards for all aspects of student nurses' practice experience, including the learning environment, student support and assessment of practice.

When students enter a new practice setting they can sometimes feel overwhelmed by the range of learning opportunities. To help you to focus on the specific opportunities available in your placement, the English National Board (2001) suggests that each placement area identifies what opportunities are available, and these will of course include practical skills.

In any practice setting you will have an assigned mentor, whose remit includes supporting you in:

1. Identifying your learning needs.
2. Addressing these learning needs through enabling you to practise, and giving feedback.
3. Assessing your performance at the end of the placement.

Your role should be an active one throughout this process.

Identifying your learning needs

When, with support from your mentor, you identify your learning needs you should take into account:

- The learning outcomes for your stage of the course.
- Your prior learning, from previous practice placements, and any relevant experience prior to entering nurse education.
- Any learning needs which were identified during your previous practice placements.
- The specific learning opportunities identified by this placement.

Your mentor will discuss these learning needs with you, and can advise you of the learning opportunities in the practice area that can help to meet these learning needs, but it will be up to you to be honest about your strengths and areas needing improvement. Your learning needs are likely to include practical skills but will include a range of other needs too.

Addressing learning needs

Unfortunately some studies found that students do not always learn while in practice settings as effectively as they could do (Ashworth and Morrison 1989; Melia 1987). The earlier section 'Learning from experience and reflection' gives you insight into how you can most benefit from your clinical experience. Further suggestions are given below.

You need to be active in seeking out your learning opportunities. Being aware of how practical skills are learned will help you to make the best use of opportunities available, ensuring that you observe a skill first, and ask for supervised practice until you feel confident to practise the skill independently. While some skills need minimal practice, others are much more complex and need repeated practice. It is very important not to attempt a skill unsupervised unless you are confident of your ability. You will be given formative feedback during practice placements to guide your learning. As discussed before, the practical skills you develop should be considered within the holistic care of patients, and not as isolated tasks which you have learned to perform.

You can be more proactive about learning in the practice setting if you are aware of different learning methods. There is much you can learn from observing others in the practice setting but you need to distinguish between 'good' professional role models and 'poor' ones. In some practice settings there may be formal teaching sessions organised. This might be particularly appropriate when there are several students in a placement area, and where workload is predictable so a specific time can be set aside for teaching sessions. Formal teaching sessions enable you to prepare, by pre-reading for example. Informal teaching occurs more spontaneously 'on the spot'. Such sessions can be particularly meaningful as they are likely to be directly linked with the clinical practice occurring at that time. This type of learning is called 'action learning' (Howard 1999). Sometimes a critical incident can be used as a basis for reflection in the practice setting. This might be a situation that has occurred which was difficult or challenging, such as where a relative has complained about lack of care by staff. Critical incident analysis can aid reflection and learning from such a situation.

An example of how you might employ different learning methods in the practice setting is now given. When taking part in drug administration, you can actively observe a qualified nurse, either asking questions at the time (if appropriate) or making a note of questions for later or of specific drugs you want to find out about. The nurse you are with might ask you questions in order to check your understanding and encourage you to think about what is happening. You may be able to take part in practical elements such as dispensing of tablets or preparing a nebuliser. If a difficult situation occurs, for example a patient refuses his tablets, you could use this incident to reflect afterwards and develop knowledge from this experience. You could consider, for example, whether a different approach to the patient would have made any difference, or whether an adequate explanation about the tablets was given. You could also follow up later by looking up information about drugs that you encountered and were not familiar with.

RECOMMENDED READING

As stated earlier, the remit of this book is to help you to develop a foundation in practical nursing skills. For guidance about reading material for other aspects you should refer to the recommended reading list for your course. Hinchliff *et al.*'s (2003) book addresses the four domains of practice and their identified competencies.

Many practical nursing skills require an underlying biological knowledge base. For example, when taking and recording blood pressure it is necessary to understand what blood pressure is and how it is maintained. A foundation in biology is not, however, within the scope of this book and it is assumed that students will gain their biological knowledge from one or more of the texts available, many of which are aimed specifically at student nurses. When working through each chapter of this book it is sensible to have an understanding of the related biology, so each chapter includes biology questions. You are advised to use your recommended text to check your biological knowledge by finding out the answers to the questions posed. Studying the relevant biology and then working through the chapter can help to make the biology more comprehensible and memorable, as you can see its immediate relevance and applicability to nursing practice.

CHAPTER SUMMARY

All registered nurses are required to be competent in a range of practical nursing skills and the Nursing and Midwifery Council (2004) has identified skills that student nurses should acquire as a foundation prior to entering their chosen branch of nursing. There is a vast range of practical skills; this book addresses skills that are applicable to all branches of nursing and are expected to be achieved by students prior to entering their chosen branch. Practical nursing skills should be carried out therapeutically and within the context of caring. They include motor, affective and cognitive dimensions, and to become competent requires all three aspects to be developed. To develop competence requires practice and experience, which should include gaining feedback and reflection, thus maximising learning from experience. Through classroom preparation in a skills laboratory or equivalent setting students can develop familiarity with equipment and the sequential steps of a skill, and the cognitive and affective domains can also be introduced. Carrying out practical skills in the dynamic and variable environment of the clinical setting is affected by many factors. Repeated practice in the clinical setting is needed in order to become competent and confident in practical skills, and students need to be proactive in seeking out opportunities for learning.

REFERENCES

Andrews, M., Gidman, J. and Humphreys, A. 1998. Reflection: does it enhance professional nursing practice? *British Journal of Nursing* **7**, 413–17.

Ashworth, P. and Morrison, P. 1989. Some ambiguities of the student's role in undergraduate nurse training. *Journal of Advanced Nursing* **14**, 1009–15.

Benner, P. 1984. *From Novice to Expert*. Massachusetts: Addison-Wesley.

Benner, P. and Wrubel, J. 1989. *The Primacy of Caring*. Massachusetts: Addison-Wesley.

Beretta, R. 2003. Assessment: the foundations of good practice. In Hinchliff, S., Norman, S. and Schober, J. (eds) *Nursing Practice and Health Care*, fourth edition. London: Arnold, 122–46.

Bjork, I.T. 1999a. What constitutes a nursing practical skill? *Western Journal of Nursing Research* **21**, 51–70.

Bjork, I.T. 1999b. Practical skill development in new nurses. *Nursing Inquiry* **6**, 34–47.

Bradshaw, A. 1994. *Lighting the Lamp: The spiritual dimension of nursing care*. Harrow: Scutari Press.

Bush, H.A. and Barr, W.J. 1997. Critical Care Nurses' lived experiences of caring. *Heart and Lung* **26**, 387–98.

Carper, B.A. 1978. Fundamental patterns of knowing in nursing. *Advances in Nursing Science* **1**, 13–23.

Department of Health 1999. *Making a Difference: Strengthening the nursing, midwifery and health visiting contribution to health and health care*. London: DH.

Department of Health 2001a. *The Essence of Care: Patient-focused benchmarking for health care practitioners*. London: DH.

Department of Health 2001b. *National Service Framework for Older People*. London: DH.

Department of Health 2001c. *Valuing People: A new strategy for learning disability for the 21st century*. London: DH.

de Tornyay, R. and Thompson, M.A. 1987. *Strategies for Teaching Nursing*, third edition. New York: Delmar Publishing.

Dewey, J. 1929. *Experience and Nature*. New York: Grove Press.

English National Board for Nursing, Midwifery and Health Visiting 2000. *Education in Focus: Strengthening pre-registration nursing and midwifery education*. London: ENB.

English National Board for Nursing, Midwifery and Health Visiting 2001. *Placements in Focus: Guidance for education in practice for health care professions*. London: ENB.

Erickson Megel, M., Wilken, M.K. and Volcek, M.K. 1987. Nursing students' performance: administering injections in laboratory and clinical area. *Journal of Nursing Education* **26**, 288–93.

Ersser, S. 1998. The presentation of the nurse: a neglected dimension of therapeutic nurse–patient interaction? In McMahon, R. and Pearson, A. (eds) *Nursing as Therapy*, second edition. Cheltenham: Stanley Thornes, 36–63.

Fitzpatrick, J.M., While, A.E. and Roberts, J.D. 1992. The role of the nurse in high-quality patient care: a review of the literature. *Journal of Advanced Nursing* **17**, 1210–19.

Gomez, G.E. and Gomez, E.A. 1987. Learning of psychomotor skills: laboratory versus patient care setting. *Journal of Nursing Education* **26**, 20–4.

Hallal, J.C. and Welch, M.D. 1984. Using the competency laboratory to learn psychomotor skills. *Nurse Educator* **9**, 34–8.

Halldorsdottir, S. 1991. Five basic modes of being with another. In Gaut, D.A. and Leininger, M.M. (eds) *Caring: The compassionate healer*. New York: National League for Nursing Press, 37–49.

Health Advisory Service 2000, 1998. *'Not because they are old': An independent inquiry into the care of older people on acute wards in general hospitals*. London: Health Advisory Service 2000.

Hinchliff, S., Norman, S. and Schober, J. (eds) 2003. *Nursing Practice and Health Care: A foundation text*, fourth edition. London: Arnold.

Howard, A. 1999. Strategies for meeting learning needs. In Hinchliff, S. (ed.) *The Practitioner as Teacher*, second edition. Edinburgh: Baillière Tindall, 107–21.

Honey, P. 1982. *The Manual of Learning Styles*. Maidenhead: Honey and Munford.

Johns, C. 1994. A philosophical basis for nursing practice. In Johns, C. (ed.) *The Burford NDU Model: Caring in practice*. Oxford: Blackwell Science, 3–19.

Johns, C. 1996. Visualising and realising caring in practice through guided reflection. *Journal of Advanced Nursing* **24**, 1135–43.

Knight, C. 1998. Evaluating a skills centre: the acquisition of psychomotor skills in nursing – a review of the literature. *Nurse Education Today* **18**, 441–7.

Knight, C.M. and Mowforth, G.M. 1998. Skills centre: why we did it, how we did it. *Nurse Education Today* **18**, 389–93.

Kolb, D.A. 1984. *Experiential Learning: Experience as the source of learning and development*. London: Prentice Hall International.

Kolb, D.A. and Fry, R. 1975. Towards an applied theory of experiential learning. In Cooper, C.L. (ed.) *Theories of Group Processes*. London: John Wiley, 33–57.

Kralik, D., Koch, T. and Wotton, K. 1997. Engagement and detachment: understanding patients' experiences with nursing. *Journal of Advanced Nursing* **26**, 399–407.

Lawler, J. 1991. *Behind the Screens: Nursing somology and the problem of the body*. London: Churchill Livingstone.

Lee, T., Newman, L., Crawford, R. *et al.* 2002. *First Aid Manual*, eighth edition. London: Dorling Kindersley.

Leininger, M. 1981. Transcultural nursing: its progress and its future. *Nursing and Health Care* **2**, 365–71.

Love, B., McAdams, C., Patton, D.M. *et al.* 1989. Teaching psychomotor skills in nursing: a randomised control trial. *Journal of Advanced Nursing* **14**, 970–5.

Manley, K. 1997. Knowledge for nursing practice. In Perry, A. and Jolley, M. (eds) *Nursing: A knowledge base for practice*, second edition. London: Arnold, 301–33.

McAdams, C., Rankin, E., Love, B. and Patton, D. 1989. Psychomotor skills laboratories as self-directed learning: a study of nursing students' perceptions. *Journal of Advanced Nursing* **14**, 788–96.

McMahon, R. 1998. Therapeutic nursing: theory, issues and practice. In McMahon, R. and Pearson, A. (eds) *Nursing as Therapy*, second edition. Cheltenham: Stanley Thornes, 1–20.

Melia, K. 1987. *Learning and Working: The occupational socialisation of nursing*. London: Tavistock Publications.

Neary, M. 1997. Project 2000 students' survival kit: a return to the practical room (nursing skills laboratory). *Nurse Education Today* **17**, 46–52.

Nicol, M. and Freeth, D. (1998) Assessment of clinical skills: a new approach to an old problem. *Nurse Education Today* **18**, 601–9.

Nolan, C.A. 1998. Learning on clinical placement: the experience of six Australian student nurses. *Nurse Education Today* **18**, 622–9.

Nursing and Midwifery Council 2002. *Requirements for Pre-registration Nursing Programmes*. London: NMC.

Nursing and Midwifery Council 2004. *Standards of Proficiency for Pre-registration Nursing Education*. London: NMC.

Oermann, M.H. 1990. Psychomotor skill development. *The Journal of Continuing Education in Nursing* **21**, 202–4.

Papadopoulos, I., Tilki, M. and Taylor, G. 1998. Developing trans-cultural skills. In Papadopoulos, I., Tilki, M. and Taylor, G. (eds) *Trans-Cultural Care: A guide for health care professionals*. Dinton, Salisbury: Quay Books, Mark Allen Publishing, 175–211.

Paterson, J. and Zderad, L. 1988. *Humanistic Nursing*. New York: League for Nursing.

Powell, J. 1998. Reflection and the evaluation of experience: prerequisites for therapeutic practice. In McMahon, R. and Pearson, A. (eds) *Nursing as Therapy*, second edition. Cheltenham: Stanley Thornes, 21–36.

Quinn, F. 2000. *The Principles and Practice of Nurse Education*, fourth edition. Cheltenham: Stanley Thornes.

Randle, J. 2001. Past caring? The influence of technology. *Nurse Education Today* **1**, 157–65.

Reynolds, C.L. and Leininger, M. 1993. *Madeleine Leininger: Cultural Care Diversity and Universality Theory*. Newbury Park: Sage Publications.

Roach, M.S. 1992. *The Human Act of Caring: A blueprint for the health professions*, revised edition. Ottawa: Canadian Hospital Association Press.

Roach, M.S. 2002. *Caring, the Human Mode of Being: A blueprint for the health professions*, second revised edition. Ottawa: Canadian Hospital Association Press.

Rogers, A., Karlsen, S. and Addington-Hall, J. 2000. 'All the services were excellent. It is when the human element comes in that things go wrong': dissatisfaction with hospital care in the last year of life. *Journal of Advanced Nursing* **31**, 768–74.

Romyn, D.M. 1999. Commentary. *Western Journal of Nursing Research* **21**, 64–70.

Schon, D. 1983. *The Reflective Practitioner*. London: Temple Smith.

Schon, D. 1987. *Educating the Reflective Practitioner*. San Fransisco: Jossey-Bass.

Smith, K. 1995. All taped. *Nursing Times* **91** (1), 16.

This Week 2000. Nurses 'failed to feed us', patients say. *Nursing Times* **96** (1), 9.

Thorsteinsson, L. 2002. The quality of nursing care as perceived by individuals with chronic illnesses: the magic touch of nursing. *Journal of Advanced Nursing* **11**, 32–40.

Wallis, M.C. 1998. Responding to suffering: the experience of professional nurse caring in the coronary care unit. *International Journal for Human Caring* **2**, 35–44.

Watkins, M. 1997. Nursing knowledge in nursing practice. In Perry, A. and Jolley, M. (eds) *Nursing: A knowledge base for practice*, second edition. London: Arnold, 1–31.

Watson, J. 1979. *Nursing: The philosophy and science of caring.* Boston: Little Brown.

Wharton, A. and Pearson, A. 1988. Nursing and intimate physical care – the key to therapeutic nursing. In Pearson, A. (ed.) *Primary Nursing: Nursing in the Burford and Oxford Nursing Development Units*. London: Chapman and Hall, 117–24.

Woodward, V.M. 1997. Professional caring: a contradiction in terms? *Journal of Advanced Nursing* **26**, 999–1004.

USEFUL WEBSITES

- Department of Health (www.dh.gov.uk)
- National Electronic Library for Health (www.nelh.nhs.uk)
- National Institute for Clinical Excellence (www.nice.org.uk)
- Nursing and Midwifery Council (www.nmc-uk.org)
- Resuscitation Council (UK) (www.resus.org.uk)
- The University of York: NHS Centre for Reviews and Dissemination (www.york.ac.uk/inst/crd)

The nurse's approach:
self-awareness and communication

Joanne Sale and Nicola M. Neale

> Other people's behaviour doesn't happen in a vacuum. When they relate to us, they are relating to *us*, to the people we are. Their behaviour towards us is a response, in no small measure, to our behaviour towards them.
>
> *(Fontana 1990, p. 24)*

As Fontana suggests, any interaction is a two-way process and therefore it is important for nurses to be aware that their approach to clients/patients in any setting will affect the outcome. This book addresses practical skills required by nurses and in this chapter we focus on the nurse–patient interactions while carrying out these skills.

This chapter includes:
- ■ Developing self-awareness
- ■ Communication skills in a range of care settings with a variety of clients.

The above sections will incorporate ethical considerations when caring for individuals and their families.

PRACTICE SCENARIOS

The following scenarios, taken from later chapters in this book, will be referred to during the text.

Cerebrovascular accident (CVA)
Cerebral damage caused either by decreased blood flow or haemorrhage. Effects vary but often causes paralysis down one side of the body (hemiplegia), and speech and swallowing difficulty. Commonly termed a 'stroke'.

Adult

Mr Jack Jones is a 78-year-old man who has been admitted to a medical ward from the Accident and Emergency (A&E) department with a right-sided hemiplegia following a **cerebrovascular accident** (CVA). He is well nourished and his general condition is good. He is conscious but his speech has been affected.

Child

Tracey Livingstone is 12 years old. She has fallen off her horse and fractured her sixth cervical vertebra. She has no sensation below the level of the injury, has

Neurogenic bladder and bowel
Damage to the neurological pathways that regulate bladder and bowel function.

Health Action Plan
A personal action plan developed for each individual with a learning disability, containing details of their health interventions, medication taken, screening tests etc. See *Valuing People* (Department of Health 2001a).

Alzheimer's disease
Also referred to as dementia of Alzheimer's type (DAT), this is the most common form of dementia. It is commoner in older people and is thought to result from neurological changes in the brain (Cheston and Bender 1999). Dementia is chronic and progressive in nature, has many causes and commonly presents with memory and language impairment, decline in self-care ability, and behavioural and personality changes (Jacques and Jackson 2000).

Osteoarthritis
A degenerative joint disorder where there is progressive loss of articular cartilage, new bone formation and capsular fibrosis. Main symptoms are pain, stiffness and restricted movement.

some arm and hand function but no movement in her legs. She has a **neurogenic bladder** which is managed by a supra-pubic catheter and a **neurogenic bowel** which is emptied daily, so she is usually continent. She is up in a wheelchair undergoing her rehabilitation programme.

Learning disability

Ian is 25 years old and has a severe learning disability. He lives in a staffed group home where he is usually continent. However in unfamiliar surroundings he can become incontinent. He has been admitted to a surgical ward via A&E with abdominal pain, for monitoring and further investigations. A carer has accompanied him to hospital and the home is intending to supply a staff member as much as possible. However there may not be anyone able to stay overnight. Ian's **Health Action Plan** has been brought with him and the care staff have informed the community nurse for learning disability of his admission to hospital.

Mental health

Violet Davies, aged 76, with advanced **Alzheimer's disease**, has been admitted to a nursing home as her husband is physically and emotionally exhausted and unable to cope. He has refused help in the past as he has been determined to look after his wife himself but he has now agreed to her admission. Violet is physically well but she is also known to have **osteoarthritis** in her right hip. She looks permanently worried and agitated and keeps repeating the same phrase over and over again. Mr Davies looks shaky and tearful.

DEVELOPING SELF-AWARENESS

According to Burnard (1999, p. 68), 'Self awareness is the evolving and expanding sense of noticing and taking account of a wide range of aspects of self'.

LEARNING OUTCOMES

By the end of this section you will be able to:

1. Reflect upon the importance of self and self-awareness in a caring context.
2. Understand the terms self-concept and body image and recognise their relevance to nursing practice.
3. Show insight into the relevance of understanding aspects of personality.
4. Discuss attitudes, values and beliefs and their impact in the care environment.

Learning outcome 1: Reflect upon the importance of self and self-awareness in a caring context

 Activity
- Describe yourself. Spend 5 minutes writing down the aspects of yourself that you would like a stranger to know.
- Highlight what you see as your strengths and weaknesses.

Check out what you have written with a friend:

- Does their view match yours?
- Were there things that you did not know about yourself?
- What do any differences tell you about yourself? (the authors accept no responsibility for the break up of friendships!).

Figure 2.1 shows a model called the Johari window, which was developed by Luft and Ingram (1955) to help individuals to identify aspects of self. This model suggests that through self-disclosure, i.e. telling others about yourself and seeking feedback from others, like the exercise that you have just completed, there will be an effect on your awareness of self. This occurs because there is an increase in the size of the public area in relation to the other three – so you will acquire a greater understanding of your own strengths and weaknesses.

	You know	You don't know
Others know	Public area	Blind area
Others don't know	Hidden area	Unknown area

Figure 2.1 Johari window (Luft and Ingram 1955).

 Activity
How might this understanding of these aspects of self affect you as a caregiver when carrying out practical skills?

You may have considered several different aspects. For example, if you have had an argument at home you may well understand why you feel impatient with a client who appears to lack motivation to assist with hygiene needs. Both Mrs Davies and Ian may be unable to express their needs. This may cause frustration in you, as the carer, and could potentially increase your feelings of anger. However as a result of acknowledging your emotional state this will help you to understand why you are angry and the effect it has on the care you are giving. This increased awareness may highlight the need for you to adapt your behaviour accordingly.

It is important that health care professionals develop an appreciation of how and why they behave in particular ways in certain circumstances and as suggested by Irving and Hazlett (1999, p. 270), 'self awareness is an important precursor of effective communication'. The crucial point about self-awareness is that it affects our communication with others, and therefore can help us to recognise how our behaviour affects others.

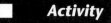**Activity** | Think of a recent situation where you think that your behaviour had an impact on the outcome of a particular incident.

Were you able to recall your thoughts, feelings and emotions related to this incident? Do you think that these may have affected your actions, your choice of words or your relationship with others? In what way do you think your behaviour may have influenced the situation?

■ If you were angry at the time, did you shout? Did you say things you regret? Did you 'storm off'?

■ If you were sad, did you cry? Were you too emotional to speak? Were you able to listen?

It is helpful for nurses to reflect and analyse their own behaviour and the factors that influence it. In Chapter 1, reflection was discussed in some detail, suggesting that it is a conscious activity that usually involves a change in behaviour. Reflection, therefore, should help to increase awareness of how psychological, sociological, physical and contextual factors impact upon our relationship with others.

Learning outcome 2: Understand the terms self-concept and body image and recognise their relevance to nursing practice

■ **Self-concept** can be defined as the information and beliefs that individuals have about their own nature, qualities, and behaviour (Rogers 1961).

■ **Body image** is the individual's interpretation of their 'bodily self' and includes aspects such as their physical characteristics – tall, short, fat, thin, brown eyed, blond haired (Gross 2001).

It is generally accepted that there are three components to the self-concept: self-image, self-esteem and ideal self (Gross 2001).

Self-image

Self-image is the way in which we would describe ourselves. Kuhn and McPartland (1954) (cited by Gross 2001) suggest that this can be found by asking a person to answer the question 'who am I' twenty times. The answer might include **social roles**, **personality traits** and **physical characteristics** (as in body image).

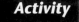**Activity** | Look back to your strengths and weaknesses, as identified earlier. Do any of these match up with the above three categories? Adams and Bromley (1998) suggest three additional categories: **sexuality**, **spirituality** and **lifestyle**. You may find that some of your responses fit into these more readily.

However, how many of your strengths and weaknesses relate to physical characteristics? Price (1990) identifies three aspects of body image:

■ **Body ideal** is how we would like to look. Sometimes this is guided by society's views and is a dynamic process. A recent survey found that Kylie

Minogue was considered to have the most attractive body shape for a woman and David Beckham for a man (*Observer* 2003). The ideal woman emerged as being short, slim, with long hair and tanned skin. Neither author accurately reflects this body ideal!

- **Body presentation** is how we present ourselves – so, we need to go out and spend some time on tanning beds and buy long-haired wigs if we want to live up to perceptions of body ideal.

- **Body reality** is the way we are, which may be far from our body ideal! The *Observer* survey found that we judge our own bodies more harshly than we do others, and nearly half of us feel uncomfortable undressing in a communal changing room.

Another aspect of body presentation is how we behave. It is likely that you would not only choose different clothes to wear to a party than for a job interview, but that you would also probably act differently. In relation to the above discussion about body presentation, nurses are expected to have a certain standard of dress when on duty and to conform to a certain standard of behaviour. Chapter 1 explains that this aspect of caring is referred to by Roach (2002) as 'comportment'. The NMC (2002a) suggests that nurses should behave in a way that upholds the reputation of the profession and also highlights the individual's responsibility for their behaviour. Consider what effect you think that having dirty nails when carrying out the monitoring of vital signs would have. It is unlikely to demonstrate a 'professional' manner, and might well affect the client's confidence in the nurse and the interaction that follows.

Activity

For each of the scenarios, how might the person's perceptions of their self-image be influenced by what they are experiencing?

Mr Jones might have been very independent prior to admission but now, because of his CVA, he will be reliant upon health care professionals for his essential needs. Thinking about his sudden loss of speech, he will also find it difficult to ask for help. This may cause frustration and therefore possibly anger; this is often related to a loss of control and will impact on self-concept.

Thinking about Tracey's situation, how do you think her self-image may be affected? Body image is a dynamic process and Tracey is particularly vulnerable because adolescence is already a period of major changes. You might have identified that Tracey is now coping with devastating unexpected changes to her physical functioning, leading to a loss of independence, a loss of control and a loss of privacy. At the same time, as an adolescent, she is already in a period of transition and is having to cope with new social and emotional roles. Russell (1999) suggests that adolescence is a significant life stage that may affect the stability of 'self'.

Ian, who has a learning disability, has had to cope with being seen as different from his peers. The Department of Health (2001a), in the white paper *Valuing People*, acknowledges that people with learning disabilities have often felt excluded and marginalised. New approaches aim to improve this situation but

Ian's experiences to date may not have been positive. In addition he has been used to the familiar environment of the group home but now, being in hospital, he may feel increasingly disorientated and vulnerable, especially if he does not understand what is happening. He could experience a range of emotions, such as fear or anger, and could be disempowered and deskilled in the hospital setting.

Mrs Davies's increasing dementia might have affected her sense of self from the physical, psychological and social perspectives. For example, physical changes in her brain might have changed her perception. At some point in her illness she might have had insight and been aware of her loss of intellectual functioning. She might also have noted changes in other people's reactions to her and interactions with her.

Self-esteem

Self-esteem is the extent to which we value and approve of ourselves, relating to how much we like the person we are. These judgements can be global or specific (Gross 2001). For example, we might like ourselves on the whole but might not like a particular aspect, say the size of our nose, or our tendency to be short tempered. Self-esteem and self-image are connected; if your self-image is positive then it is likely that you will also have good self-esteem and vice versa.

The ideal self

The ideal self is the person we would like to be. Although this is similar to Price's concepts discussed earlier, it is not just about physical characteristics, but also considers wider issues such as personality and relationships. We might want to change some aspects of ourselves or we might wish we were a different person altogether, perhaps kinder, less judgemental or more intelligent. Rogers (1961) suggests that the greater the gap between our self-image and our ideal self, the lower our self-esteem.

Activity — Think about how illness might affect someone's ideal self and/or self-esteem.

Some of the things that you might have thought of are:

- Disfigurement
- Loss of dignity (consider Ian's possible incontinence in an unfamiliar environment)
- Loss of hair due to treatment
- Loss or gain of weight (as a result of treatment or the illness process)
- Loss of self-worth (e.g. Tracey will be affected by her new disability and people's reactions to her; it is likely that she is further away from her ideal self than ever before)
- Loss of function (e.g. Mr Jones, due to his CVA).

It is likely that all of the individuals in the scenarios will have changes to their self-concept and body image to a greater or lesser extent as a result of their illness experiences. Thus the approach of nurses while carrying out care can do much to either reinforce these views or to improve self-esteem or self-worth.

Learning outcome 3: Show insight into the relevance of understanding aspects of personality

■ **Personality** can be defined as 'those relatively stable and enduring aspects of individuals which distinguish them from other people, making them unique, but which at the same time allow people to be compared with each other' (Gross 2001, p. 610). This is just one of many attempts to define personality.

Activity

Go back to your list of strengths and weaknesses. Which of these would you describe as being relatively stable and secure aspects of your personality?

Eysenck (1965, cited in Gross 2001), proposed that there were two principal dimensions of personality: introversion/extroversion and neuroticism/stability, and that each individual lies within one of the four quadrants as shown in Fig. 2.2. Where do you think you would lie in this diagram?

An introverted nurse may find communicating with clients or colleagues in a group setting more stressful than an extrovert one. However on a one-to-one basis there may be little difference. The personality of the client is important too, as this will affect any interaction. The behaviour that you observe may give only a small indication as to the person's personality, but it would be an important glimpse. For example in the practice scenario above, Tracey may be quiet and uncommunicative. What conclusions would you draw from this? You might decide that Tracey is an introverted, shy girl, or that she is thoughtful and polite.

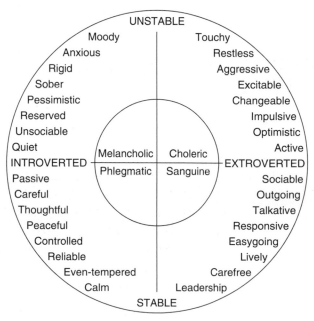

Figure 2.2 Dimensions of personality (Eysenck 1965, cited in Gross 2001).

Conversely you might think that Tracey is unusual for a girl of her age and therefore you might put her behaviour down to her physical condition. All of these views would say something about her personality, as you see it.

Shaw (1999) proposes that an understanding of personality is important because personality appears to have an impact on individuals' coping styles and psychological wellbeing. This suggests that whether Mr Jones was extrovert or an introvert, stable or unstable (see Fig. 2.2) would affect how he adapted to his new situation. As you saw from the definition of dementia earlier in this chapter personality changes can be one effect of Alzheimer's disease. Mr Davies may find such changes hard to cope with in his wife.

Learning outcome 4: Discuss attitudes, values and beliefs and their impact in the care environment

■ A **value** can be defined as the judgement that a person places on the desirability, worth or utility of obtaining some outcome (Adams and Bromley 1998).

■ A **belief** is an opinion held about something – the information, knowledge or thoughts about a particular thing (Stahlberg and Frey 1994, cited in Adams and Bromley 1998).

Our values and beliefs feed into our attitudes and these are of interest because they can, and do, affect how we behave with others.

■ **Attitudes**: These are 'constant feelings that give order and shape to our lives' (Tschudin 1998, p. 16). For example, what is your opinion about smokers receiving health care? You may value life but believe in the right to freedom of choice, therefore your attitude towards smokers receiving care may be ambivalent.

Hoveland and Rosenberg (1960, cited in Gross 2001) suggest that there are three components to attitudes. The **affective** component is how the individual feels about a person, object, etc. The **cognitive** component concerns those thoughts and perceptions that the individual holds toward the person, object, etc. Finally the **behavioural** component reflects how we act toward the person, object, etc.

Activity

Consider the following scenarios (be as honest with yourself as possible). Would you feel any differently about Mrs Davies if you found out that her dementia was related to alcohol abuse in the past? How would you feel if you were told in handover that Tracey's father had been verbally aggressive towards staff?

The sort of responses you may have thought of might include:

■ With Mrs Davies, you may feel less keen to care for her because you believe her condition is her own fault, or you may even openly criticise her behaviour.

■ With Tracey's father you may be wary of him and also avoid anything but basic contact with Tracey when her father is present. You may believe that he presents a danger to you.

Morrison and Burnard (1997) propose that those in caring roles are constantly making decisions about whether or not individuals are deserving of care and cite Rajecki (1982) who suggests that attitudes play a crucial part in influencing caring behaviours. However 'The Essence of Care' (Department of Health 2001b) within the section on Privacy and Dignity, suggests that in order to meet 'best practice' all patients/clients should 'feel that they matter all of the time' (p. 182). Therefore, nurses should use their professional judgement to ensure that the care given is focused upon respect for the individual at all times.

■ **Activity** | Are there other illnesses or disorders where health professionals may decide that the individual or their lifestyle is responsible for the health problem?

Some examples we have thought of are:

■ A person who is HIV positive as a result of unsafe sex (in contrast with someone infected as a result of an infected blood transfusion).
■ A chest infection in a child from a travelling family (as opposed to one from the local boarding school).
■ A person who has deliberately taken an overdose (in comparison to someone who has mistakenly taken an overdose).
■ A prisoner who has drug-related psychosis (as opposed to a non-prisoner with non-drug related psychosis).

The examples above are linked to social position and diagnosis, however in reality there are many subtle, social factors that influence our judgements in client-centred relationships (Johnson and Webb 1995). You may have thought of other examples, but the main consideration is to be aware of how our values, beliefs and attitudes are central to how we behave.

We will come back to some of these issues in the section about stereotyping and labelling.

■ **Activity** | In the practice setting listen to how nurses and other health care professionals talk to each other about clients and their families. Are value judgements being made and are these affecting caring relationships? If so, how?

Summary

■ Developing self-awareness will improve how nurses approach patients/clients.
■ Aspects of self-awareness include self-concept and body image.
■ Personality and attitudes are influential in affecting the nurse–patient relationship.

COMMUNICATION SKILLS IN A RANGE OF CARE SETTINGS WITH A VARIETY OF CLIENTS

LEARNING OUTCOMES

By the end of this section you will be able to:

1. Discuss interpersonal perception and its relevance to communication.
2. Understand the terms stereotyping and labelling.
3. Discuss relevant aspects of communicating with people who are anxious, angry or confused.

Learning outcome 1: Discuss interpersonal perception and its relevance to communication

- **Interpersonal perception** can be defined as 'how we try to explain and predict other people's behaviour. It seems impossible to interact with other people without trying to make sense of their actions, and to anticipate how they are likely to act' (Gross 2001, p. 325).
- A general definition of **communication** is 'social interaction through messages' (Fiske 1990, p. 2). It involves 'transmitting not only information from one person to another, but also in communicating a relationship' (Thompson 2003, p. 10).
- **Social skills** are 'a set of goal directed, interrelated, situationally appropriate social behaviours (that can be learned and are under the control of the individual)' (Hargie 1997, p. 12).
- **Interpersonal skills** include 'communication and listening, observation of verbal and non-verbal behaviour and planning and problem-solving' (Russell 1999, p. 7).

All of the above are linked and contribute to effective nursing practice. How nurses perceive others is fundamental to skilful interactions but often our perceptions are influenced by our own thoughts, feelings and attitudes. Misinterpretations in perceptions can lead to errors in communication, for example we might assume that Tracey's father's anger is directed at health care professionals due to his dissatisfaction with Tracey's care. Yet there may be many other reasons for his behaviour. Hargie *et al.* (1994) suggest that where negative emotions are directed towards the carer they can interfere with effective listening and act as a barrier in the interaction.

Activity

Make a list of the factors that might affect your perceptions of behaviour in a social setting. You might like to observe people in a variety of different social settings and try to analyse what you saw and heard and how the setting influenced the behaviours.

You may have found it difficult to differentiate between what you actually observed and how you interpreted these observations. Kagan *et al.* (1986) suggest that as we grow up we develop schemata that help us to organise, interpret and remember social information. Schemata are cognitive or mental frameworks and these are formed from knowledge of ourselves, others and our past experiences. For example, our past experiences may lead us to accept verbally abusive behaviour at a football match but not in the A&E Department. The demands of these situations are different as interpreted by our memory.

As we have seen, communication is a two-way process whereby one individual sends a message and another person receives it.

Activity | Write down as many different ways that you can think of to send a message.

You may have thought of talking to someone either face to face or on the telephone, by writing a note, a text message or sending an e-mail. Did you think of sign language too? Petrie (1997) suggests that there are two forms of interpersonal communication: verbal and non-verbal. Sign language can be viewed as a form of verbal communication (Williams 1996).

Activity | List under the headings 'Verbal' and 'Non-verbal' as many aspects of communication as you can think of.

For the verbal aspects you may have thought of tone of voice, pitch (or loudness), use of silence and pauses. These verbal components express our emotions and communicate information about our interpersonal attitudes. Sometimes clients' speed of speech may indicate their emotional state – someone who is depressed may speak in a slow, flat, monotone voice. Mrs Davies, who is increasingly agitated, keeps repeating the same phrase over and over again and her speech may become faster and increase in volume. Sometimes the way we use these aspects can alter the meaning of the words we use. For example, consider the different ways the question 'What do you want?' can be said.

Non-verbal aspects that you may have thought of include proximity, posture, body movements, touch, eye contact, facial expression and gesture.

Many verbal and non-verbal behaviours are culturally determined (Arnold and Bloggs 1999). For example, in some religions and cultures chanting and outpouring of emotions at funerals is the norm. In relation to non-verbal behaviour, some religions consider that eye contact is inappropriate and that individuals should lower their eyes to avoid contact. Whilst we must never make assumptions about culturally determined behaviours they are still important factors to consider when delivering care.

Several authors have developed models or frameworks of the communication process, for example the linear model of Shannon and Weaver (1949) (cited in Adams and Bromley 1998). This tends to suggest that communication is something that people do to one another, rather than a process where there is

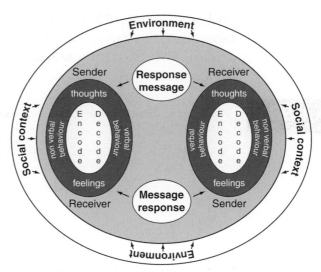

Figure 2.3 A framework for communication.

continual receiving, responding and interacting. Many frameworks now incorporate wider aspects in relation to communication. Figure 2.3 shows one such framework for communication, developed by this chapter's authors.

This illustrates that the social context and environment encompass and influence all areas of the interaction process. It also shows that at any given moment, the sender of a message is also the receiver. Aspects such as our thoughts, feelings and behaviour (verbal and non-verbal) will influence our interpretation and therefore our response to the message and its perceived meaning. Encoding entails turning our thoughts and feelings into a recognisable message (in many cases this is reflected in our responses). Decoding is about how we interpret a message we have received, to make sense of it. Therefore we are continually receiving and sending messages in this dynamic process of interaction. We discuss some of these issues further in this chapter.

Activity   List some of the relevant factors that affect the communication process.

You should have included aspects like attitudes and intra-personal issues as we have discussed these earlier. However, did you consider the environment or context? Thompson (2002) suggests that the emotional climate is as important as the physical in relation to effective communication. Did you also think about age or gender? For example, when helping Tracey with hygiene needs, we may want to consider the effects of her age on the interpersonal relationship and how comfortable she may feel if talking to an older or a male nurse.

The effects of differences in culture are a factor often overlooked in the nurse–client interaction. A study by Vydelingum (2000), which included Hindu, Sikh and Muslim clients, highlighted how communication difficulties led to patients feeling isolated due to language barriers. Significantly, nurses did not provide sufficient information, for example in relation to diagnosis or medication

(Vydelingum 2000). This was supported by a study by Gerrish (2001), who found that 'patients who spoke little English were disadvantaged' (p. 571).

Long (1999) suggests that interpersonal skills form the tools necessary for effective communication.

■ **Activity**	Think about a recent experience in practice when you were performing a practical skill, for example when helping an agitated client to use the toilet (perhaps like Mrs Davies), or when recording blood pressure (for example Mr Jones). Try to identify at least five interpersonal skills that you used.

There are many skills that you may have identified. Hargie *et al.* (1994) propose the following:

- Being able to initiate an interaction successfully
- Listening
- Non-verbal communication
- Giving clear explanations
- Questioning appropriately
- Praising others and accepting praise
- The ability to reflect others' thoughts and feelings
- Being assertive
- Effective group-work
- Being able to finish interactions appropriately.

We will explore the first five areas in more detail in the following section.

Initiating a successful interaction

■ **Activity**	Imagine you are meeting the people from the scenarios at the beginning of the chapter. Write down how you think you would introduce yourself to each of them.

You may introduce yourself giving your first name, for example 'Hello, I'm Jane' or 'I'm Jane Smith' or perhaps you may say 'Hello I'm student nurse Smith'. You need to be aware that if you offer your first name you may make it difficult for clients not to give you their's. Some clients may prefer to be called by their formal titles, for example Mr Jones. Usually if the person wants you to call them by their first name, they will give you permission sometime in the relationship. The use of a formal title is a sign of respect while the use of first names implies intimacy or familiarity. Think back to the first time you met the practitioner in charge of a recent placement – how did you address him/her? It is likely that you adopted a formal approach until told otherwise.

With children or younger people it is usually more appropriate to use their first names as a way of putting them at ease. However it is still important to find out their preferred manner of address. For example with Tracey she may like to be called 'Trace' or perhaps a nickname. It is an essential aspect of beginning a relationship with any patient/client that you respect their wishes regarding their chosen names.

Here again, cultural aspects need to be considered. It is important that what may seem to be a trivial aspect of the relationship is given due attention. For example it would be very disrespectful for a nurse to call a Sikh man by his first name or to ask him for his 'Christian' name. As highlighted earlier, cultural norms determine all aspects of the communication process, including the verbal and non-verbal.

Activity — Imagine that you have been asked to measure Mr Jones's blood pressure. You are meeting him for the first time – how would you establish rapport?

Knapp and Vangelisti (1992, cited in Hargie and Tourish 1997) suggest that relationships develop in a number of stages, the first of which is **initiating**. In this stage, they propose that opening introductions and reactions often involve a degree of small talk. You might, for example, note that Mr Jones comes from a local village with which you are familiar and comment: 'I see you come from Whitchurch. That's a lovely village – have you lived there long?' This conversation should put Mr Jones at ease, thus enabling your assessment of him to be more accurate, and also helping you to assess his level of consciousness (see Chapter 10, Monitoring vital signs).

Listening and non-verbal communication

There are many different definitions of listening emphasising the aural (hearing), oral (spoken) and environmental aspects. However Stein-Parbury (2000) underlines the importance of recognising listening as an active process that requires concentration and effort to enable the development of the appropriate skills.

Activity — Reflect on the last occasion you were speaking to a friend in a social setting, speaking to a colleague at work or speaking to a client.
What can you recall about:
- Verbal ways that you showed that you were listening
- Body positions: your's and their's
- Eye contact and facial expression
- Other non-verbal skills?

What can you remember about the content?

Weaver (1972, cited in Bostrom 1997) suggests that our attitudes and culture determine the selection, perception and retention of any received message – do you consider these aspects are relevant to your examples? Was it easier to remember what you discussed with your friend rather than a colleague? This exercise may demonstrate to you how important attention and memory are within the listening process.

Egan (1990) uses the acronym 'SOLER' to help us to remember how to use our body position to help us to focus on the skill of listening:

- **S**it squarely in relation to the client
- Maintain an **O**pen position
- **L**ean slightly towards the client

- Maintain reasonable **E**ye contact
- **R**elax.

Were these aspects of body language apparent in your examples? You may also have reflected on your or others' use of space, silence, touch and gestures, such as nodding the head in agreement or the use of facial expression to show interest or understanding. You may also be aware of how you or others used verbal signals to indicate that you were listening, for example the use of 'umm', 'aah', 'uh-huh', 'oh' or 'I see'. There is always a danger that when we are supposed to be actively listening, we can slip into automatic pilot and are not really fully responsive to the message. Stein-Parbury (2000) suggests that there are many barriers to effective listening, both external and internal, for example our own thoughts, value judgements and feelings.

When we are with clients it may be particularly useful to develop the skill of 'reflecting'. Stein-Parbury (2000) proposes that this is the ability to demonstrate to the speaker that we have heard and understood both the emotional and factual content of the message. This, she suggests, is not always correct and often requires validation and further clarification from the client. This means that we must also be alert to any non-verbal messages, for example, Tracey, when asked, may say that she is 'OK'. However you may determine from her non-verbal cues that she is very anxious.

In order to recognise this incongruence between the verbal and non-verbal message, the development of sensitive observational skills and an empathetic approach is required. Empathy entails thoughts and emotions related to understanding the client's position, and may be portrayed non-verbally and through the nurse's words and actions (Baillie 1996). The skills of empathy thus include appropriate use of skills mentioned earlier – touch, eye contact and use of voice. Vocal features may encompass not only the words we use but, just as importantly, the tone and manner – perhaps through the use of a calm and soothing voice.

Another skill of listening that relates to verbal aspects is called 'paraphrasing'. This is the ability to put what an individual has said into different words without losing the original meaning. For example, when you suggest to Tracey that she might like to have a wash and clean her teeth, she may say: 'No thank you. I'm not bothered about having a wash today. I'm not dirty anyway'. You could respond to Tracey using paraphrasing.

Another issue that this scenario highlights is that of Tracey's right to refuse care. Consider why Tracey might be refusing care. There may be many reasons – for example:

- She may be shy.
- She may prefer another nurse or her parents to help her but feel that she cannot tell you.
- She may be afraid that washing will cause her discomfort.
- She may simply just not want a wash today.

The Code of Professional Conduct (Nursing and Midwifery Council 2002a, p. 3) states that the nurse has 'a duty of care to your patients and clients, who are entitled to receive safe and competent care'. In relation to the above example, Tracey would not suffer undue physical harm if she went without a wash. However due to the high risk of pressure ulcers, her skin must be checked for signs of pressure regularly, and she will need repositioning. For Mr Jones skin care will also be a necessary part of his management. So if either Tracey or Mr Jones were to refuse this care their nurses would need to have an understanding of why, as there may be an underlying psychological need that requires addressing.

Giving clear explanations

Perhaps what Tracey or Mr Jones would need in this situation is clear explanations, for example as to why their skin needs to be observed and cared for. One of the key elements of the NHS Charter (Department of Health 1998) is the aspect of effective communication, and it suggests that individuals should receive comprehensive information about all aspects of their care. In providing explanations, nurses should take into account language (e.g. if the person does not speak English), age, child development and, particularly with clients with learning disability, their usual methods of communication. Methods of communication for people with learning disabilities might include non-verbal, pictures and use of signing. Sometimes the person concerned might have developed their own unique language. The nurses on Ian's ward must work closely with Ian and his carers to explain things to him in an understandable manner. *Valuing People* (Department of Health 2001a) emphasises that people with learning disabilities should be able to access health care as easily as any other member of the public, and this includes matters of communication. The onus is on staff to adapt and use different approaches to meet people's needs. Regarding children, Colson (2000) emphasises providing sufficient and understandable information so that informed consent can be obtained from children and parents, and recommends that play activities can help with children's understanding.

An important part of giving information is paying attention to the words that we use and as nurses we need to develop an understanding of the power of language. Crawford (1999) argues that language shapes relationships and Thompson (2002) suggests that it is a powerful tool for reinforcing social and cultural divisions. He also emphasises that it is not just the words we use that exert an effect, but the way we use them.

One response to Tracey could have been: 'Come on, don't be a baby – you're old enough to be sensible – what would your mother say?' It would be easy to take a dominant stance and make it difficult for Tracey to assert herself. The way that nurses talk to clients can be beneficial and supportive or it can be detrimental by being patronising or debilitating. Imagine that Mr Jones needed to wear an incontinence pad, and the nurse said 'Come on Grandad – let's put your nappy on'. How do you think he would feel? How would you feel if someone spoke to your father or grandfather in this way? Crawford (1999, p. 49) emphasises the unacceptability of 'secondary baby talk' and the harmful effects it may have on the nurse–client relationship. The way that we use language is also an important aspect of labelling and this is discussed later.

Questioning appropriately

There are many different types of questions that have been identified.

Activity   Make a list of some different types of questions and give an example for each.

Niven and Robinson (1994) suggest the following types of questions:

- **Closed questions** (e.g. 'Do you want a cup of tea?' 'Have you got pain?'): These are useful for gaining factual information but they do not allow further exploration or elaboration. Often this type of question may be used in the initial assessment of a patient and can lead on to the second major type of question.
- **Open questions** (e.g. 'How is your diet?' 'How would you describe your pain?'): These allow a fuller response and enable people to reply in their own manner. Sometimes open questions can precipitate a long and not necessarily relevant response and it may be appropriate to use a closed question to refocus the conversation. Thus both closed and open questions are extremely valuable when interviewing clients.
- **Probing questions** (e.g. 'You say that the pain is worse in the mornings. Tell me when else it is particularly bad?'): The use of probes or prompts can assist clients in talking about their thoughts and feelings and enable them to address their concerns.
- **Leading questions** (e.g. 'You don't look as if you are in pain – are you?'): These are better avoided as they can pressure the client to respond in a particular way. However, nurses are often unaware of using them.
- **Affective questions**: These are specifically used to address the emotions of clients and indicate our concern. For example, if Tracey is quiet and uncommunicative she may need to be asked how she feels about being in hospital. In order to ask this kind of question we need to have established a good rapport and should ensure that we can give time for her response. We should also know our own limitations in terms of helping responses.

Privacy and dignity

The above section has looked at some of the interpersonal skills that are an essential part of client care. Respect for people's dignity and privacy are principles emphasised in 'The Essence of Care' (Department of Health 2001b), and should be central to any client–nurse interaction. Privacy is defined as 'freedom from intrusion' and dignity is defined as 'being worthy of respect' (Department of Health 2001b, p. 182).

Maintaining client dignity is recognised as an essential component of professional nursing practice (Nursing and Midwifery Council 2002a) and has been specifically highlighted in 'The National Service Framework for Older People' (Department of Health 2001c). Calnan *et al.*'s (2003) study of 72 hospital patients (mean age, 72 years) suggested that concerns for lack of dignity were related to:

■ Lack of privacy
■ Mixed sex wards
■ Loss of independence
■ Forms of address.

Walsh and Kowanko (2002) outline several elements that nurses attributed to the concept of dignity. These were respect, privacy, control and time and were very similar to the patients' views, however the themes of humour and matter-of-factness were also evident in the interviews with patients.

■ Activity — Can you think of any specific issues that may be important to consider in relation to maintaining dignity and privacy for the clients outlined in the scenarios?

Recognising the individual needs of Tracey, Mr Jones, Ian and Mrs Davies is important at all times. For all four of them admission to a hospital or nursing home environment could lead to loss of privacy, particularly where accommodation is shared with others, as in wards. Specific examples relating to each of these clients are:

■ Tracey's age, stage of development and the sudden and traumatic nature of her hospitalisation could all lead to loss of dignity. In addition, because of the nature of her injuries she will require help with intimate body functions. A sensitive approach will be essential while ensuring that she retains control over as much of her life as possible.
■ Mr Jones will also experience a loss of control and independence and is unable to communicate his needs clearly.
■ Ian is particularly vulnerable due to possible disorientation in unfamiliar surroundings and may need perceptive assistance to maintain his usual independence and control. This would be achieved by working closely with Ian and his carers, identifying how the environment can be adapted to meet Ian's needs.
■ Mrs Davies may have had a level of independence in her own familiar environment which could be lost in the strangeness of the nursing home. She will require time and patience in order to overcome her agitation and anxiety. Mr Davies's needs should also be considered.

Thus when carrying out practical skills it is important to be aware of, and to maintain, clients' privacy and dignity and this is often promoted through verbal and non-verbal communication.

Written communication

Written communication is an important but often neglected area in nursing. It is increasingly emphasised in relation to documentation and record-keeping. The Nursing and Midwifery Council (NMC) (2002b, p. 7) states that 'record-keeping is an integral part of nursing and midwifery practice. It is a tool of professional practice and one that should help the care process'. The NMC (2002b, p. 8) outlines seven crucial principles in relation to documentation that should be adhered to. Below we have listed some of these, with discussion related to the scenarios as examples of application of these principles.

Patient and client records should:

- **Be factual, consistent and accurate**: For Mrs Davies it would be important to document her behaviour in an unbiased and non-judgemental way.
- **Be written as soon as possible after the event has occurred, providing current information on the care and condition of the patient or client**: For Tracey, who is undergoing a rehabilitation programme, it would be vital for her progress to be documented immediately after each session. Equally, with Mr Jones, any change to his level of consciousness would need to be recorded and acted upon appropriately.
- **Be written clearly, in such a manner that the text cannot be erased**: Pencil and correcting solutions should not be used and any errors should have a single line drawn through them and should be dated, timed and signed.
- **Not include abbreviations, jargon, meaningless phrases, irrelevant speculation and offensive subjective statements**.

Activity

What do the following abbreviations mean: CF, CPA, PID, TPR, BP, OE, RXT, ABC, ETA, DTA, DNA, ABS, DOA, GCS, HAP? All these can be found in health care settings. Discuss them with a friend or colleague.

How many of these did you know without further investigation? Were there any that could have more than one meaning – if so which one would you use, and why? One example is that PID can mean either 'prolapsed intervertebral disc' or 'pelvic inflammatory disease'. Other examples are that BP could mean 'blood pressure' or 'bedpan', and DOA might mean 'dead on arrival' or 'date of admission'. You might think DNA is to do with genetics but it is often used to abbreviate the phrase 'did not attend'. The context of the clinical environment may influence your interpretation of an abbreviation. Generally, although abbreviations are part of everyday life (particularly with the popularity of text messages) there are few that are acceptable in health care practice, especially in written records.

When completing nursing records nurses need to have a comprehensive awareness of all the pertinent issues contained in the NMC guidelines (2002b) as these are professional standards for practice.

Learning outcome 2: Understand the terms stereotyping and labelling

■ **Stereotyping** is the assigning of individuals to categories as a result of assumptions that have been made (Tourish 1999).

■ **Labelling** is a form of stereotyping where we categorise people by, for example, aspects such as their behaviour, their dress or their age.

As previously discussed, when we were considering attitudes, the judgements we make of others may affect the care we give. Sometimes we make these judgements as a result of our personal bias, and as a result we fail to see the individual as a unique human being. This can lead to the nurse being prejudiced in the care that is given. Prejudice means 'to pre judge'.

Activity

You are to admit a new patient. The only information you have is the patient's name 'Albert Higginbottom' and limited background information, i.e. that he is aged 67 years, lives in a hostel, has fallen while under the influence of alcohol, is reluctant to be admitted, and has a fractured right femur. Describe how you might imagine Albert to be, e.g. his personality and his physical characteristics.

You may have decided that Albert is elderly, scruffy, has an alcohol problem, has no supporting relatives, and is possibly uncooperative. You would thus already be starting to form judgements about the patient and this might affect how you approach him when he arrives on the ward. On the other hand, you might have decided to keep a completely open mind!

There are two manifestations of prejudice – direct and indirect (Pettigrew and Meertens 1995). Direct or open prejudice is just that: it is blatant and obvious. An example of this might be a patient refusing to be looked after by a nurse who is black. Indirect or closed prejudice, on the other hand, is subtle; a nurse who does not approve of a patient who acquired HIV through their lifestyle, for example, might give them the minimum acceptable level of care and not talk to them or make eye contact with them.

Activity

Consider the practice scenarios. How might both direct and indirect prejudice manifest itself?

You may have felt that Tracey would be seen as a young girl and therefore she may not be involved in decisions about her care. Mr Jones, on the other hand, may be seen as an older man who would not understand the implications of possible treatment choices, and could therefore be excluded from the process. Ian may be judged as a result of his learning disability, and as a result, care staff may not tell him what they are doing when performing practical skills as they may assume he won't understand. Mrs Davies may be avoided by staff if she is agitated and confused, as they may consider her 'difficult' and as a result her physical needs may not be fully met.

We make attempts at ordering the world around us in an effort to understand what is happening but, as we have already seen, at times this leads us to erroneous perceptions. This can then affect the care that is delivered, usually negatively though sometimes in a positive way. Included in this is how we communicate with our patients/clients as this can reflect our underlying prejudices.

At one time labelling of patients was thought to be fairly fixed in nature, so that once labelled, this would remain with the patient/client (Stockwell 1972). However Johnson and Webb (1995) found that labels were more flexible and transient, and could change with time and experience. Therefore when approaching people to undertake a practical skill you need to aware of whether your behaviour is affected by any labels or stereotypical views held about the person.

Hannigan (1999) suggests that negative representations and attitudes about mental illness are prevalent in the media and community. This is associated with violence and is sensationalised, and leads to a reduction in the quality of life of individuals living within the community. Social inclusion is currently high on the UK Government agenda as a way of improving integration and acceptance of those with a learning disability or a mental illness (Department of Health 1999, 2001a). Nurses in any sector may find themselves caring for people with learning disabilities or a history of mental health problems, and if they hold stereotypical or prejudiced views this could affect their approach to care and their interactions.

Learning outcome 3: Discuss relevant aspects of communicating with people who are anxious, angry or confused

Anxiety

Many people are anxious when admitted to hospital or faced with a new situation or uncertainty about the future. Anxiety is defined as 'a palpable but transitory emotional state or condition characterised by feelings of tension and apprehension and heightened autonomic nervous system arousal' (Speilberger *et al.* 1968, cited in Adams and Bromley 1998, p. 15).

Anxiety is one of our basic emotions and can range from mild to very severe. It can serve as a warning and a certain amount can help us to cope with threatening situations, but if it becomes excessive this may become detrimental and can interfere with normal functioning. Sometimes anxiety is referred to as either 'state' or 'trait'. State anxiety means that it is the state the person is in that causes the state of anxiety. Trait anxiety refers to the fact that some people are naturally more anxious than others. For example, Mrs Davies may be anxious because of her admission to the nursing home or she may be a naturally anxious person.

Activity

(a) What are the cues that may lead you to think a person is anxious?
(b) What aspects of their situations may give rise to anxiety for Ian, Mr Jones or Tracey?

For activity (a) you might have considered facial expression, restlessness, wringing hands and profuse sweating, which are some indicators that an individual is anxious. You will find out more about the effects of anxiety upon the vital signs when reading Chapter 10 (Monitoring vital signs).

For activity (b), anxiety about illness and the implications for the future are often linked to fearfulness and/or uncertainty, and these could be relevant to Ian, Mr Jones or Tracey. Recipients of health care may have:

■ Fear of needles and pain – depending on previous experience, Ian might associate hospitals with needles and pain
■ Fear of finding out something is wrong, with blood pressure for example
■ Fear of being harmed, for example, use of the hoist or falling when being helped – Mr Jones might be anxious about mobilising
■ Fear of the unknown environment – Ian may feel particularly vulnerable outside his usual surroundings
■ Fear of the future – the uncertainty of both Mr Jones's and Tracey's situation may cause them anxiety.

It is important that we make no assumptions about what may be causing an individual's anxiety. Careful assessment and development of a trusting relationship enables nurses to more accurately identify the cause for people's anxiety.

Once a nurse has recognised that a person is experiencing anxiety, there are some steps that can be taken to help to reduce the symptoms. Anxiety management techniques include the following:

■ Explanation of the process of anxiety and the symptoms experienced
■ Breathing control
■ Relaxation therapy
■ Challenging of cognition (thoughts)
■ Assertiveness training.

In many instances to implement these techniques successfully the nurse would first need to establish a trusting relationship with the person concerned. For someone with a learning disability, the nurse would also need to know how the person communicates and ensure that communication entails using methods appropriate to that individual. A transitional object, which is something familiar and important like a photo, can be helpful in preventing and relieving anxiety.

If anxiety is not addressed then it can impact on physical and emotional well-being. Adams and Bromley (1998) suggested the following examples of outcomes of unmanaged anxiety: angina, migraine, aggravation of skin disorders, disturbance in bowel movement, unstable diabetes, vulnerability to infections and cognitive impairment including poor concentration, memory and motivation. The factors relating to impairment of thinking may be particularly important to be aware of if you need to teach a patient a practical skill. Anxiety can also act as a barrier to communication.

Activity Identify other factors that may act as barriers to your communication and relationship with clients.

It is sometimes helpful to think about barriers in terms of whether they are physical, psychological or social.

- **Physical barriers** could include visual impairment, auditory impairment, pain or how the surrounding environment is organised (a desk between two participants, one person sitting while the other is standing or a loud television in the background).
- **Psychological barriers** may relate to aspects that we have discussed earlier, such as personality (e.g. if someone is very shy), attitudes, beliefs and labelling (either the caregiver's or the client's), the emotional state of either party (e.g. anxiety) and cognition, which may affect language and/or understanding. For example Ian, who has a learning disability, might understand what is said to him but be unable to express his comprehension, or may not understand but use language or gestures that imply that he does.
- **Social barriers** may include aspects such as culture (including the culture of the ward, for example whether it is considered acceptable to sit and talk to a patient), religious beliefs and social status.

This list is not exhaustive and the distinction between the physical, psychological and social aspects are not always clear cut. However, we need to be aware of these barriers and the effect that they may exert.

Anger

Anger is a natural human emotion associated with displeasure; it is often passionately felt and can be expressed in a number of ways, if expressed at all (Adams and Bromley 1998). Nurses are sometimes confronted with people who are displaying strong emotions such as anger and aggression. It is very important for nurses to employ good interpersonal skills at these times. This can help to minimise the psychological impact of the emotions.

Activity How would you recognise that a client was becoming angry?

You may be able to divide your answers into the following categories: verbal and non-verbal. Examples of verbal indications may be a raised voice, fast speech or the use of obscenities. Non-verbal indications include changes in body language – the person may display exaggerated movements, clenched fists, pace back and forth, throw or kick objects. There may be changes in facial expression, for example, frowning, and eye contact may be negligible or it might be extended – glaring.

These are just some of the indications that an individual is becoming angry. It is important that a nurse who has recognised these signs acts to disperse the anger. This can be done by:

- Listening actively to what the person has to say, thus showing a non-judgemental stance. However it is also important that eye contact is not held for too long as this may be seen as threatening (Williams 1996).
- Acknowledging the anger. This demonstrates empathy with what the client is feeling (Williams 1996).
- Encouraging the client to identify the cause of the anger – this is done through skilful questioning.
- Where possible, empowering the person to resolve any causes.

Thus the aim is the peaceful resolution of the situation. However, if a nurse confronts anger with anger through direct confrontation, defensiveness or questioning of the client's feelings, then this will probably lead to an escalation in anger, maybe to aggression. You may find it useful to reflect upon situations where you have encountered anger and try to identify possible causes.

Confusion

Confusion is defined as 'any condition in which there is a loss of orientation or difficulty … with memory, attention span or other cognitive function' (Adams and Bromley 1998, p. 179).

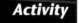 **Activity**   On arrival at the nursing home Mrs Davies appears confused. Identify what could be the possible causes of this.

Confusion may be a relatively permanent feature of her condition, related to dementia. However, again we must avoid making assumptions as her confusion may be due to physical factors such as malnutrition, dehydration, constipation or an acute infection. She may also be disorientated by having been taken away from the familiar environment of her home. This would be compounded if she had a visual or hearing impairment.

 Activity   You think that Mrs Davies needs to use the toilet as she is becoming more agitated. Suggest some strategies you could use in helping her in this confused state.

Strategies to consider include:

- Orientation to time and place, for example 'Mrs Davies, I'm student nurse Smith and I'm here to help you'.
- Use of appropriate and understandable language.
- A calm and clear voice.

- A calm manner, for example avoiding sudden or exaggerated movements.
- The use of active listening skills.

Sometimes, despite all attempts to help a patient, their confusion may make it difficult for them to make their needs known and for the nurse to identify the appropriate interventions. In these situations the safety of the patient will be paramount and continued observation and assessment will be crucial. Aspects of dignity and privacy should be observed in line with the benchmark for best practice in *The Essence of Care* (Department of Health 2001b) and attention should be paid to protecting modesty.

In the above section, we have included some key aspects when caring for people who are anxious, angry or confused. However this discussion is not exhaustive and there are other ethical and clinical considerations to be taken into account too.

Summary

- Communication takes many forms and has verbal and non-verbal components.
- Nurses need to be able to use a range of interpersonal skills effectively. In relation to practical nursing skills, initiating interaction, listening, non-verbal communication, questioning and giving explanations are all of particular importance.
- Stereotyping of people can detract from an individual approach to care and impact on the nature of nurse/client interactions.
- There are many situations where communication is challenging, for example when people are anxious, angry or confused, and this requires nurses to be skilled and empathetic.

CHAPTER SUMMARY

In conclusion, this chapter aimed to provide some insights into the importance of the nurse/client relationship. It has included a discussion about the impact of self within this relationship, and how this will inevitably affect communication and thus the care of people. It has also highlighted some principles of communication and their applications in a variety of care settings with a range of different clients, linked to the scenarios. As suggested by Niven and Robinson (1994) one of the most crucial features of communicating with others is that we understand ourselves as well as those with whom we are communicating.

In the following chapters, specific practical nursing skills will be focused on and the importance of the approach of the nurse while carrying out these skills cannot be over-emphasised.

REFERENCES

Adams, B. and Bromley, B. 1998. *Psychology for Health Care: Key terms and concepts*. London: Macmillan Press.

Arnold, E. and Bloggs, K. 1999. *Interpersonal Relationships: Professional communication skills for nurses*, third edition. London: Saunders.

Baillie, L. 1996. A phenomenological study of the nature of empathy. *Journal of Advanced Nursing* **24**, 1300–8.

Bostrom, R.N. 1997. The process of listening. In Hargie, O. (ed.) *Handbook of Communication Skills*, second edition. New York: Routledge, 236–58.

Burnard, P. 1999. *Counselling Skills for Health Professionals*, third edition. London: Chapman and Hall.

Calnan, M., Woolhead, G. and Dieppe, P. 2003. Older people. Courtesy entitles. *Health Service Journal* **113**(5843), 30–1.

Cheston, R. and Bender, M. 1999. *Understanding Dementia: The man with the worried eyes*. London: Jessica Kingsley.

Colson, J. 2000. Concepts. In Huband, S. and Trigg, E. (eds) *Practices in Children's Nursing: Guidelines for hospital and community*. Edinburgh: Churchill Livingstone, 1–12.

Crawford, P. 1999. Nursing language: uses and abuses. *Nursing Times* **95**(6), 48–9.

Department of Health 1998. *The NHS Charter*. London: DH.

Department of Health 1999. *The National Service Framework for Mental Health*. London: DH.

Department of Health 2001a. *Valuing People: A new strategy for learning disability for the 21st century*. London: DH.

Department of Health 2001b. *The Essence of Care: Patient-focused benchmarking for health care practitioners*. London: DH.

Department of Health 2001c. *The National Service Framework for Older People*. London: DH.

Egan, G. 1990. *The Skilled Helper: A systematic approach to effective helping*, fourth edition. California: Brooks/Cole.

Fiske, J. 1990. *Introduction to Communication Studies*, second edition. London: Routledge.

Fontana, D. 1990. *Social Skills at Work*. Leicester: The British Psychological Society and Routledge Ltd.

Gerrish, K. 2001. The nature and effect of communication difficulties arising from interactions between district nurses and South Asian patients and their carers. *Journal of Advanced Nursing* **33**, 566–74.

Gross, R. 2001. *Psychology: The science of mind and behaviour*, fourth edition. London: Hodder and Stoughton.

Hannigan, B. 1999. Mental health care in the community: an analysis of contemporary public attitudes towards, and public representations of, mental illness. *Journal of Mental Health* **8**, 431–40.

Hargie, O. 1997. Communication as a skilled performance. In Hargie, O. (ed.) *A Handbook of Communication Skills*, second edition. London: Routledge, 7–21.

Hargie, C.T. and Tourish, D. 1997. Relational communication. In Hargie, O. (ed.) *A Handbook of Communication Skills*, second edition. London: Routledge, 358–82.

Hargie, O., Saunders, C. and Dickson, D. 1994. *Social Skills in Interpersonal Communication*, third edition. London: Routledge.

Irving, P. and Hazlett, D. 1999. Communicating with challenging clients. In Long, A. (ed.) *Interaction for Practice in Community Nursing*. Basingstoke: Macmillan Press, 260–85.

Jacques, A. and Jackson, G.A. 2000. *Understanding Dementia*, third edition. Edinburgh: Churchill Livingstone.

Johnson, M. and Webb, C. 1995. Rediscovering unpopular patients: concept of social judgement. *Journal of Advanced Nursing* **21**, 466–75.

Kagan, C., Evans, J. and Kay, B. 1986. *A Manual of Interpersonal Skills for Nurses, an Experiential Approach*. London: Harper and Row.

Long, A. 1999. Introduction. In Long, A. (ed.) *Interaction for Practice in Community Nursing*. London: Macmillan Press, 1–23.

Luft, J. and Ingram H. 1955. *The Johari Window: A graphic model of interpersonal relations*. Los Angeles, CA: University of Los Angeles Press.

Morrison, P. and Burnard, P. 1997. *Caring and Communicating: The interpersonal relationship in nursing*, second edition. Basingstoke: Macmillan Press.

Niven, N. and Robinson, J. 1994. *The Psychology of Nursing Care*. London: Macmillan Press.

Nursing and Midwifery Council 2002a. *Code of Professional Conduct*. London: Nursing and Midwifery Council.

Nursing and Midwifery Council 2002b. *Guidelines for Records and Record-Keeping*. London: Nursing and Midwifery Council.

Observer 2003. The poll: body uncovered. 26th October, 14–23.

Petrie, P. 1997. *Communicating with Children and Adults: Interpersonal skills for early years and playwork*, second edition. London: Arnold.

Pettigrew, T. and Meertens, R. 1995. Subtle and blatant prejudice in Western Europe. *European Journal of Social Psychology* **25**, 55–75.

Price, B. 1990. *Body Image: Nursing concepts and care*. London: Prentice Hall.

Roach, M.S. 2002. *Caring, the Human Mode of Being: A blueprint for the health professions*, second edition. Ottawa: Canadian Hospital Association Press.

Rogers, C.R.1961. *On Becoming a Person*. Boston: Houghton Mifflin.

Russell G. 1999. *Essential Psychology for Nurses and Other Health Professionals*. London: Routledge.

Shaw, C. 1999. A framework for study of coping, illness behaviour and outcomes. *Journal of Advanced Nursing* **29**, 1246–55.

Stein-Parbury, J. 2000. *Patient and Person – Developing interpersonal skills in nursing*, second edition. London: Churchill Livingstone.

Stockwell, F. 1972. *The Unpopular Patient*. London: Royal College of Nursing.

Thompson, N. 2002. *People Skills*, second edition. Hampshire: Palgrave Macmillan.

Thompson, N. 2003. *Communication and Language: A handbook of theory and practice*. Hampshire: Palgrave Macmillan.

Tourish, D. 1999. Communicating beyond individual bias. In Long, A. (ed.) *Interaction for Practice in Community Nursing*. London: Macmillan Press, 190–216.

Tschudin, V. 1998. *Managing Yourself*. London: Macmillan.

Vydelingum, V. 2000. South Asian patients' lived experience of acute care in an English hospital. *Journal of Advanced Nursing* **32**, 100–7.

Walsh, K. and Kowanko, I. 2002. Nurses' and patients' perceptions of dignity. *International Journal of Nursing Practice* **8**, 143–51.

Williams, D. 1996. *Communication Skills in Practice: A practical guide for health professionals*. London: Jessica Kingsley.

Preventing cross-infection

Vickie Arrowsmith

Preventing cross-infection is an essential activity for all nurses in their everyday practice. For nurses there is an ethical and legal duty to protect patients against infection (Cochrane 2000; Fletcher and Buka 1999) but within hospital and residential situations, where many nurses work, the risk of cross-infection is high. In any health care setting, unless adequate care is taken, nurses can unwittingly transmit microorganisms from one person to another. The media regularly report on standards of hospital hygiene and such coverage is often uncomplimentary, reflecting both public and governmental concerns about lack of cleanliness and associated infection rates in hospitals and health care.

Hospital-acquired infection, sometimes referred to as nosocomial infection, is a serious problem, with as many as 5000 patients dying each year as a result of hospital-acquired infection in the UK (Pratt *et al.* 2001). Rapid improvements in medical technology and the consequent changes in the way care is delivered have increased the risk of infection and the subsequent personal and financial costs. As hospitals take in people from ever-wider catchment areas, mixing them and frequently moving them around within the hospital, the risk of infection increases. Unfortunately the antibiotic therapy that revolutionised the treatment of infections can destroy helpful as well as harmful bacteria in people's bodies (Wilson 2000) and some antibiotics that were once considered life saving are now ineffective because of the increasing problem of antibiotic resistant microorganisms.

With an emphasis on community care, including GPs' surgeries and care homes carrying out invasive procedures, and the trend for early discharge of patients from hospital settings, hospital-acquired infection often first becomes evident in the community, thus the term 'health care-associated' infection needs to replace the more traditional term 'hospital-acquired infection' (Pratt *et al.* 2001).

This introduction gives some of the reasons why skills in preventing cross-infection are both important and necessary in all health care settings.

Preventing cross-infection

This chapter includes:

- Principles for preventing hospital-acquired infection and health care-associated infection
- Hand hygiene
- Use of personal protective equipment including gloves, aprons and gowns
- Non-touch technique
- Specimen collection
- Source isolation
- Sharps disposal
- Clinical waste disposal.

Recommended biology reading:

These questions will help you to focus on the biology underpinning the skills required to prevent cross-infection. Use your recommended textbook to find out:

- What are microorganisms? Where are they found? Are all microorganisms harmful?
- Identify some of the beneficial roles of microorganisms.
- How do microorganisms enter the body?
- How are microorganisms classified?
- What are the structure and properties of bacteria, viruses, prions, fungi, yeasts and protozoa?
- How do bacteria grow and multiply?
- What factors influence the proliferation of microorganisms?
- What is meant by the terms: commensal, pathogen, normal flora?
- Distinguish between endogenous and exogenous sources of infection.
- What mechanisms does the body employ to defend itself from infection? (Think about non-specific defences, e.g. secretions, reflexes, barriers, etc. as well as specific mechanisms). Review the structure of the skin.
- How does the body fight infections?
- What are the clinical signs of infection? What role does histamine play?
- Which cells are involved in the specific immune response? Where are they found?
- What is the difference between humoral and cell-mediated immunity?
- What are antibodies? How do they help protect us from infection?
- How do we achieve an immunological memory?
- What factors can affect an individual's immune system?

PRACTICE SCENARIOS

As discussed above, prevention of cross-infection is part of the nurse's role in all practice settings. The following scenarios will be referred to throughout the text, when discussing the practical skills covered in this chapter.

Adult

Rheumatoid arthritis
This is an inflammatory disease often affecting a number of joints (initially smaller ones), causing pain, swelling, stiffness and deformity. It is often accompanied by systemic ill health.

Mrs Winifred Lewis, aged 87, was widowed many years ago and lives in war-dened accommodation. She has a history of **rheumatoid arthritis** and type 2 diabetes, and recently fell and fractured her hip. This was operated on in hospital but the wound developed an **infection**, which grew **MRSA**. She was discharged home, under the care of the district nursing team and intermediate care, but her wound deteriorated and the surrounding skin showed signs of infection. Mrs Lewis appeared unwell and dehydrated, so her GP requested readmission. She is now being isolated in the side room of a surgical ward, and an intravenous infusion and intravenous antibiotics have been commenced. She has a commode in the room and can transfer with help.

Infection
The successful invasion, establishment and growth of microorganisms within the tissues of the host.

MRSA
Methicillin-resistant *Staphylococcus aureus* is a highly resistant microorganism and is discussed in the section on source isolation.

Child

Chickenpox
An infectious disease caused by a virus (varicella-zoster virus, a member of the herpesvirus family). It results in skin lesions that are intensely itchy and that can result in permanent scarring if scratched, with resulting bacterial infection.

Laura Cox is 4 years old and is in hospital with a chest infection but has developed **chickenpox**. She is being nursed in the isolation area of the children's ward and has to remain in the cubicle at all times. Laura has many skin lesions all over her body, some of which are beginning to crust over. Lesions on her vulval area sting when she passes urine, making her reluctant to go to the toilet. Consequently, she sometimes wets the bed when she is asleep. She is pyrexial, lethargic and reluctant to eat or drink anything. The family decided that Laura's father would remain with her in hospital while her mother would care for Molly, Laura's 8-month-old sister, at home. Both Laura's parents have had chickenpox but her sister has not.

Learning disability

Health Action Plan
A personal plan developed for each individual who has a learning disability, detailing their health interventions, medication, oral health, nutrition etc. (DH 2001).

James Smith is a 59-year-old man with a learning disability who lives alone in a farm cottage and works on the adjacent farm. Following an accident James has an open wound on his lower left leg that shows signs of infection. There is a large amount of exudate, which has an offensive odour. The district nurse has been visiting the farm to carry out dressings and a wound swab has been taken. James is keen to carry on with his usual work on the farm. The district nurse is liaising with the community nurse for learning disabilities to help to teach James how to care for his leg in between dressings. This information is now included in James's **Health Action Plan**. As the district nurse runs a clinic at the local GP's surgery James is being encouraged to attend this for dressings instead of receiving visits at his home.

Mental health

Stacey is 28 years old and has been addicted to opiates for 6 years. She is living with her parents who are very supportive. Recently Stacey began a community-based detoxification programme with support from her local drug and alcohol team. During detoxification Stacey experienced severe withdrawal symptoms including very high blood pressure and vomiting. As a result she was admitted as an emergency to the acute mental health admission unit. She arrived feeling very unwell, and soon after arrival vomited over her bed. She was prescribed intramuscular metoclopramide (an antiemetic) to stop her vomiting. Stacey is known to have hepatitis B.

PRINCIPLES FOR PREVENTING HOSPITAL-ACQUIRED INFECTION AND HEALTH CARE-ASSOCIATED INFECTION

In 2001 guidelines were published, commissioned by the Department of Health (England), which laid out standard principles for preventing infections in hospitals (Pratt *et al.* 2001). These were the first phase of national evidence-based guidelines, systematically developed to provide broad statements or principles of good practice that can be used by practitioners and incorporated into local protocols. The standard principles are:

1. Hospital environmental hygiene
2. Hand hygiene
3. The use of personal protective equipment
4. The use and disposal of sharps.

In this chapter you encounter each of these principles and the focus is on the skills that are associated with them. These principles are consistent with and build on the 'universal precautions' that were established in the 1980s in response to the growing problems of blood-borne infections. Universal precautions recognised a few simple practices that could be used to care for all patients to minimise the risk of cross-infection to patients and staff alike. The National Institute for Clinical Excellence (NICE) (2003) has now produced guidelines for preventing health care-associated infection in primary and community care. These apply the Department of Health standard principles of hand hygiene, use of personal protective equipment and sharps disposal to various aspects of community-based care.

The first principle – 'Hospital environmental hygiene' – states that hospitals must be visibly clean, free from dust and soilage and acceptable to patients, their visitors and staff (Pratt *et al.* 2001). It should be remembered that many microorganisms exist but not all cause infection in individuals. Those that cause disease are called **pathogens**. When pathogens are acquired from another person, or from the environment, they are described as **exogenous**. The transmission of pathogens, between people and across environments, is termed **cross-infection**. When microorganisms **colonise** one site on the host and enter another site on the same person causing further infection, this is called self-infection or **endogenous** infection.

Colonisation

The establishment of pathogenic microorganisms at a specific body site with little or no host response. Can lead to a large number of microorganisms, forming a reservoir for infection and cross infection.

| **Activity** | Now read Table 3.1 that lays out the routes by which pathogenic microorganisms can be transmitted or spread between people. Then quickly reread the practice scenarios. Although you do not know the details of the pathogenic organisms involved in each of the case studies, by examining Table 3.1 can you work out which route of transmission would feature mostly strongly throughout the scenarios? |

Table 3.1 Routes of transmission (adapted from Parker 1999)

Route	Explanation	Example
Direct or indirect contact	Transfer from body surface to body surface **directly** between an infected or colonised person and a susceptible host, or **indirectly** via an intermediate object	**Direct**: Patient to patient, e.g. through touch, or staff to patient when carrying out patient care activities such as moving and handling. **Indirect**: Patient touched by a nurse's unwashed hands or gloves that have not been changed, after contact with an infected/ colonised patient
Inanimate objects and equipment (fomites)	Susceptible host is infected by an object which is contaminated with microorganisms	Beds, curtains, toys, bedpans, tables can all be contaminated and spread infection, (e.g. via hands of staff) acting as transmitters
Droplet	Microorganisms transmitted through the air within droplets, mainly saliva	Coughing, sneezing, talking and singing can transmit, as can procedures e.g. bronchoscopy or suctioning
Air-borne	Microorganisms carried in droplet nuclei (small particle residue), or by dust particles (made of e.g. dead skin scales, clothing fibres)	Carried by air currents in the environment and breathed in by a susceptible host, or they settle on horizontal surfaces. Some bacteria form spores and survive for months in such conditions
Ingestion	Ingested into the body with food or water causing gastrointestinal infections and excreted in faeces. Known as the faecal–oral route	Food may be contaminated when hands that have been in contact with faeces transfer the organisms onto food that someone then eats
Vector	Transmission via insects or rodents	Cockroaches, rats, mice and ants can contaminate food. Mosquitoes spread malaria and yellow fever; ticks spread Lyme disease and typhus

It is likely that direct or indirect contact via hands of carers is the principal cause of spread. For Mrs Lewis, infection can be spread via the air-borne route but direct and indirect contact transmission is likely. Laura has chickenpox (varicella-zoster virus) and this is secreted in the vesicles on the skin but it is primarily an infection of the respiratory tract and large amounts of the virus are found in respiratory secretions. So, droplet transmission is important, but direct and indirect contact by hands with secretions is also possible. Stacey has hepatitis B and this is transmitted via blood and serum-derived fluids such as vaginal secretions, so direct and indirect contact with these fluids is a major source of transmission. Hands would also be likely to spread infection from James's leg wound, especially since there is a large amount of exudate.

Whilst all routes of transmission are important, this short activity points out that the most common route of spread is via hands. The Department of Health (2003) identifies that health care workers are a major route through which patients become infected and that high levels of compliance with hand hygiene protocols are essential.

The next section examines how the risk of transmission by this route can be greatly reduced.

HAND HYGIENE

A number of standard principles relating to hand hygiene were identified by Pratt *et al.* (2001) and these are referred to throughout this chapter, with application to practice and this chapter's scenarios. The term 'hand decontamination' is used throughout these principles and this is defined by the National Institute for Clinical Excellence (2003) as 'the process for the physical removal of blood, body fluids, and transient microorganisms from the hands – that is, handwashing and/or the destruction of microorganisms – hand asepsis' (p. 46). Thus handwashing is the key skill used in achieving hand hygiene and this is looked at in detail in this section. Hand decontamination can also be achieved, in some circumstances, by using an alcohol handrub, containing 70 per cent isopropyl alcohol. This preparation, which is rubbed over the hands and dries quickly, does not remove microorganisms but rapidly destroys them. Alcohol based handrubs are not effective in removing physical dirt or soiling but they can be used as an alternative to handwashing on visibly clean hands free of dirt and organic material.

LEARNING OUTCOMES

By the end of this section you will be able to:

1. State the purpose and importance of hand decontamination for the care and safety of both patients and nurses.
2. Assess when hand decontamination is needed.
3. Carry out handwashing effectively.
4. Understand the factors that influence effective handwashing practice.

Learning outcome 1: State the purpose and importance of hand decontamination for the care and safety of both patients and nurses

Hungarian obstetrician Ignaz Semmelweis (1815–1865), succeeded in reducing the death rate of his patients from around 1 in 8 to 1 in 79 by the simple action of persuading his colleagues and medical students to wash their hands in a solution of chlorinated lime. However, he failed as a communicator, alienated his colleagues and had to leave his post (Meers *et al.* 1995). Since that time, however, it has become widely recognised that the hands of those employed in health care settings are an important route for the transmission of infection (Naikoba and Hayward 2001, Pratt *et al.* 2001). People requiring health care are often more vulnerable to infection for a variety of reasons, meaning that infection control measures, like hand hygiene, are central to their care.

Activity

Discuss with a colleague the people in the scenarios and the factors that make them susceptible to cross-infection.

Individuals vary widely in their ability to resist infection. However patients are especially vulnerable to infection if they have underlying disease. Mrs Lewis's chronic diseases of rheumatoid arthritis and diabetes and Stacey's hepatitis B will render them more susceptible. Mrs Lewis's impaired defence mechanisms could have led to her infection being more severe than in healthy people, and hospital strains of bacteria can be difficult to treat (Meers *et al.* 1995). Additionally, serious diseases, such as cancer, and associated treatments such as powerful drugs including steroids and chemotherapy, affect the immune system. Local factors, such as a poor blood supply to a wound, increase the likelihood of infection developing, and people who have diabetes, like Mrs Lewis, can have impaired circulation.

Age, especially the very young and the very old, and previous exposure to infection and vaccinations, all affect levels of risk (Wilson 2000). Mrs Lewis, as an older adult, and Laura, as a young child, are both therefore more vulnerable to infection. Infants and small children are susceptible as their immune systems are not yet fully developed (Simpson 1998/9).

The presence of a wound, as in the cases of Mrs Lewis and James, increases susceptibility to infection as the skin, which is an important normal defence, is breached. Mrs Lewis has an intravenous infusion in progress and this can provide a route for bacteria and other microorganisms to enter the body directly. Additionally you may have thought of other reasons for susceptibility to infection such as poor nutrition, which could apply to any of the people in the scenarios, and you should look out for underlying susceptibilities when you are in clinical practice.

Microorganisms are important in an ecological balance on earth; some live in humans and other animals and are needed to maintain health. However as some microorganisms cause disease, how individuals interact with the environment is important. The environment James is working in may not have been conducive to keeping his wound free from infection, especially if not kept adequately covered, although as you will read in Chapter 6 'Principles of wound care', traumatic wounds are nearly always contaminated so infection poses a high risk in these situations. Like everyone in the general population, James requires a basic knowledge of hygiene and infection control, including handwashing to reduce his susceptibility to infection. Now that he has an infected wound the community nurse for learning disabilities would need to check that he has the cognitive and physical dexterity to care for his wound in between dressing changes, and this includes ensuring that he is able to carry out handwashing. These steps can help to reduce the risk of infection being transferred to other sites in his body or to prevent reinfection. His Health Action Plan should include this information and the other care associated with his leg, documenting the role of the different professionals involved in his care.

A structured behavioural programme may be necessary in order to teach James effective handwashing techniques. With some people, depending on their developmental level, this may require the use of backward chaining techniques. This involves teaching the final stage of the skill first, and then working consecutively backwards. Encouragement and reinforcement by nurses are very important. These techniques for teaching self-help skills such as handwashing are covered in detail by Carr and Wilson (1987).

Bacteria on hands

In a series of classic studies, Price (1938) discovered two populations of bacteria present on hands: resident organisms and transient organisms. **Resident microorganisms**, sometimes called normal flora, lie deep in the stratum corneum of the skin and are difficult to remove, and are therefore less likely to be implicated in cross-infection. **Transient microorganisms** are acquired from the environment and are carried temporarily on the hands. These organisms may be transferred between nurse and client, resulting in cross-infection as the nurse moves from one person to another, or handles different sites on the same person. The aim of hand hygiene is to remove transient bacteria to below the level likely to cause infection.

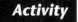 **Activity**   Try to think of some of the ways in which you might pick up transient microorganisms on your hands during everyday nursing practice.

You might have thought of:

1. Following the care of a person who has been incontinent.
2. When emptying urine bags and bedpans.
3. When handling the bedlinen of a person who has an infection or has been incontinent.
4. When bed bathing and handling wash bowls.

5. When touching furniture, such as lockers or beds.
6. During bed making.
7. When taking a patient's pulse or temperature.

Ayliffe *et al.* (2001) state that studies in their laboratories, using finger impressions, indicate that significant contamination can follow activities 1, 2, 3 and 4 and less so 5, 6 and 7. However it is important to note that you can pick up microorganisms in any of these ways that involve direct or indirect contact with patients/clients.

Transferring bacteria from your hands to a patient can lead to them acquiring infection. In the second national prevalence survey of infections in hospital, the prevalence of hospital-acquired infection (HAI) was found to range from 2–29 per cent, with an average of 9 per cent (Emmerson *et al.* 1996). The most common infection sites identified were the urinary tract (23.2 per cent), lower respiratory tract (22.9 per cent), surgical wounds (10.7 per cent) and the skin (9.6 per cent). In special care baby units the HAI rate is estimated as 14.2 per cent (5.2 per cent septicaemia), but in children's wards, the rate is 5.6 per cent (Simpson 1998/9). Effective hand hygiene can reduce the incidence of HAI in all settings.

Learning outcome 2: Assess when hand decontamination is needed

Activity

With a colleague, make a list of the times when you think it is important to decontaminate your hands in the practice setting.

Your answers could include:
Generally:

■ Before and after direct contact with patients/clients (especially those who are immunosuppressed) and after any activity or contact that potentially results in hands becoming contaminated.

More specifically:

■ Before aseptic procedures.
■ Before and after handling invasive devices.
■ Before and after handling food.
■ After removing gloves.
■ When hands become visibly soiled.
■ After using the toilet.
■ When leaving the clinical area.

Pathogens are likely to be acquired on the hands in greatest numbers when handling moist, heavily contaminated substances, such as body fluids. Hand decontamination must be carried out at this time. However there is a key message. The standard principle you should adhere to is that you should decontaminate your hands immediately 'before each and every episode of direct patient contact/care and after any activity or contact that potentially results in hands becoming contaminated' (Pratt *et al.* 2001, p. 23).

Learning outcome 3: Carry out handwashing effectively

Most people learn about washing their hands at an early stage in their lives as part of personal health and hygiene. However, because of the susceptibility of people in health care settings, particular care must be taken to decontaminate hands carefully and thoroughly. Lowbury (1991) describes three levels of handwashing:

1. Social handwashing uses soap and water to render hands socially clean, and is effective under most circumstances with 99 per cent of transient microorganisms removed or killed in this way (Ayliffe *et al.* 2001, Pratt *et al.* 2001).
2. Hygienic hand disinfection aims to decontaminate hands and remove transient microorganisms. This is the level that nurses and other clinically based health care workers use throughout everyday practice. The physical process and the time spent are factors in achieving this. Although soap is sufficient in most circumstances, antimicrobial solutions are sometimes used (see later discussion).
3. Surgical scrubbing removes or destroys transient organisms, reduces resident microorganisms and confers a prolonged effect. The nails are scraped or brushed and the hands and forearms are washed with an antimicrobial agent for a minimum of 2 minutes. This technique is used before invasive procedures, especially surgery.

As you have read, hygienic hand disinfection to decontaminate hands is fundamental to everyday nursing practice. Next you consider when hands should be decontaminated.

Activity

For each of the practice scenarios, identify when nurses would decontaminate their hands.

Now check your answers:

■ **Mrs Lewis**: You could have thought of many situations, for example before and after any direct contact such as assisting with personal hygiene, before and after using gloves (this is discussed further in the next section), when dealing with a used commode and when carrying out her wound dressing.
■ **Laura**: Again hand decontamination would be needed before and after any direct contact, before and after using gloves and when dealing with body fluids.
■ **James**: Nurses should decontaminate their hands when carrying out his wound dressings.
■ **Stacey**: Hand decontamination would be necessary before and after dealing with her vomit and soiled bedlinen and before and after giving her intramuscular injection.

The nurses caring for Stacey may be aware that she has hepatitis B but in many other situations this information is not known. Therefore, following the principles of hand decontamination and the other principles discussed in this chapter (personal protective clothing, use and disposal of sharps) for each and every patient will protect you and other patients from the unwitting transmission of dangerous pathogens such as hepatitis B. In addition the Department of Health (2003) recommends that all appropriate health care staff should be up-to-date with immunisations for hepatitis B, tuberculosis (TB), influenza and chickenpox.

A standard principle, illustrated in the above activity and discussion, is that you should apply an alcohol-based handrub or wash your hands with liquid soap and water to decontaminate your hands between caring for different patients, or between different caring activities for the same patient (Pratt *et al.* 2001). Next we look at the merits of the various hand cleaning preparations.

Hand cleaning preparations

Pratt *et al.* (2001) reviewed hand cleaning preparations, considering the evidence related to plain soap and water, antimicrobial handwashes (e.g. chlorhexidine) and alcohol-based handrubs. They found no clear evidence to favour the general use of antimicrobial handwashing agents over soap and water, finding that soap and water is equally effective for removing transient microorganisms and decontaminating hands. However antimicrobial handwashing agents remove resident microorganisms more effectively than preparations not containing an antimicrobial agent. They also found that although alcohol-based handrubs are not effective in removing physical dirt and soiling they are more effective in destroying transient microorganisms, and give a greater initial reduction in hand flora, than handwashing with either soap or antimicrobial handwashing agents. Thus Pratt *et al.* (2001) advise that when deciding which hand decontamination preparation to use, the need to remove transient and/or resident hand flora should be considered, but that for everyday clinical practice, preparations with a residual effect are not usually needed. They go on to recommend that for general clinical contact and most clinical care activities effective handwashing with a liquid soap is sufficient. Alcohol handrubs are advantageous in situations where handwashing facilities are absent or poor, such as in some community settings, or to reduce the need to leave patients during procedures, like wound dressings, to carry out handwashing.

Effective handwashing technique involves three processes: preparation, washing and rinsing, and drying. The Department of Health recommendations for these are summarised in Box 3.1. These processes are now discussed.

Preparation for handwashing

Activity | What do you think you would need to do to prepare for handwashing?

Remove all wrist and (ideally) hand jewellery and cover all cuts/abrasions with waterproof dressings at the start of each shift.

Preparation
- Wet hands under running water before applying liquid soap or an antimicrobial preparation.

Washing
- The handwash solution must come into contact with **all** the surfaces of the hand.
- The hands must be rubbed together vigorously for a minimum of 10–15 seconds.
- Particular attention must be paid to the tips of the fingers, the thumbs and the areas between the fingers.

Drying
- Hands should be rinsed thoroughly prior to drying with good-quality paper towels.

Box 3.1 Steps for an effective handwashing technique (Pratt *et al.* 2001)

You should remove all wrist and ideally hand jewellery at the beginning of each shift and before you begin to handwash (Pratt *et al.* 2001). You are probably aware that in most health care settings the only hand jewellery allowed is a wedding ring and staff are encouraged to keep nails short. Preparation also includes covering cuts and abrasions with a waterproof dressing to prevent the risk of acquiring infections such as hepatitis B and C and human immunodeficiency virus (HIV), and this may also prevent infection from bacteria and fungi. Preparation before handwashing also requires that you wet your hands under tepid running water **before** applying liquid soap or an antimicrobial cleaning agent.

Next think about the handwashing process itself.

Washing and rinsing

Activity

Find out if you can access pink dye handwashing solution. This may be available in the skills laboratory or via the infection control nurse. Wash your hands with this solution in your usual fashion and then take note of those areas that you have not covered with the dye.

Figure 3.1 shows a diagram of the areas most commonly missed (Ayliffe *et al.* 2001). How does this compare with your handwashing result?

Ayliffe *et al.* (2001) emphasise the need to wash thoroughly covering **all** surfaces of the hands, which may be more important than the time spent on the

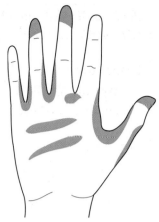

Figure 3.1 Areas commonly missed with poor handwashing (Ayliffe *et al.* 2001).

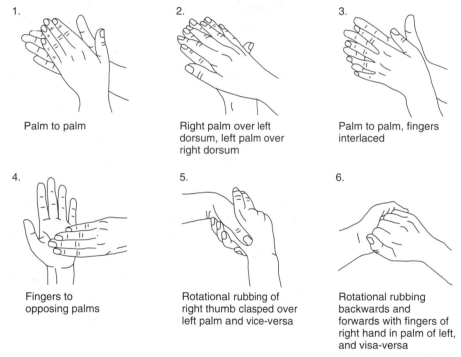

1. Palm to palm

2. Right palm over left dorsum, left palm over right dorsum

3. Palm to palm, fingers interlaced

4. Fingers to opposing palms

5. Rotational rubbing of right thumb clasped over left palm and vice-versa

6. Rotational rubbing backwards and forwards with fingers of right hand in palm of left, and visa-versa

Figure 3.2 An example of handwashing technique to cover all skin surfaces.

handwashing or the agent used. Figure 3.2 is an example of a technique that can help you to cover all surfaces of your hands during hand decontamination.

Activity

Re-wash your hands using the principles in Box 3.1 and the technique in Fig. 3.2 as a guide. If available, use pink dye for this activity so you can note any improvement: did you manage to cover all areas of your hands this time? Ensure you time your handwashing with a watch and adhere to the recommendation of a minimum of 10–15 seconds.

The amount of time you wash your hands for is important, as the mechanical action helps to remove bacteria. As you can see, the Department of Health guidelines (Pratt *et al.* 2001) for hand hygiene suggest you spend a minimum of 10–15 seconds; when timing this in the last activity did this feel longer than usual? Hands should be rinsed thoroughly prior to drying, and how diligently you do this influences the effectiveness of the whole handwashing procedure.

Drying

The Department of Health guidelines (Pratt *et al.* 2001) state that hands should be dried with good-quality paper towels.

■ Activity | Why do you think using paper towels to dry your hands is recommended rather than other methods like linen towels or hand dryers?

In a study by Gould (1994) paper towels were found to be most effective for the following reasons: not only are these inexpensive and effective in drying hands, but they also continue the mechanical action which promotes further removal of transient bacteria and loose dead skin cells. Linen towels can spread infection and are expensive to launder. Hot-air hand dryers become heavily contaminated with bacteria and recontaminate hands and the air. They are also expensive to run. In the community, as when the district nurse was carrying out James's dressing at home, it may be necessary to carry paper towels for hand drying. Note that when disposing of paper towels, foot-operated pedal bins are preferred as they reduce the risk of recontaminating hands after washing.

Alcohol-based handrubs

■ Activity | Do you think the principles for performing handwashing and drying that you have read about above are any different when using an alcohol-based handrub? If so how?

The principles are similar but as you have read, to be effective handrubs can only be used on hands that are free of dirt and organic material. Organic materials contain carbon and carbon chains form the basis of most living cells (Tortora *et al.* 1998). The preparatory measures for handwashing discussed apply equally to prior to decontamination of hands with alcohol-based handrubs. The standard guideline principles (Pratt *et al.* 2001) state that just in the same way as using soap or an antimicrobial agent and water, when using handrubs all surfaces of the hands must be covered. You should remember that the alcohol contained in most handrubs lacks viscosity and this can result in insufficient contact (Gould and Brooker 2000). In exactly the same way as when using soap or an antimicrobial agent and water, hands must be rubbed together vigorously, paying particular attention to the tips of the fingers, the thumbs and the areas between the fingers (Pratt *et al.* 2001). The technique in Fig. 3.2 is therefore applicable. Hand drying is not needed as handrub solutions are used until they have evaporated and hands are dry.

Learning outcome 4: Understand the factors that influence effective handwashing practice

According to the Department of Health (2003) it is widely believed that failure to wash hands is due to laziness or carelessness; however, there are a number of other barriers to proper hand hygiene.

Activity

What factors can you think of that might influence effective handwashing? In particular think about when you would need to wash your hands either in the community or in a hospital setting. Referring to the scenarios will help you.

By referring to the scenarios you will probably have noted how frequently nurses need to wash their hands. Frequent handwashing can cause damage to skin, especially if antiseptic solutions are used, or if hands are not dried properly. Cracked skin may harbour more bacteria and increase the risk of cross-infection. Department of Health guidelines (Pratt *et al.* 2001) state that you should apply an emollient hand cream regularly to protect skin from the drying effects of regular hand decontamination. They also state that if a particular soap or antimicrobial handwash or alcohol-based product causes skin irritation, then occupational health advice must be sought.

Other reasons you may have thought of that could deter nurses from washing their hands include:

- Inadequate and inconveniently placed handwashing facilities. Lack of time may deter handwashing when facilities are some distance away. Water may be too hot and no mixer taps present (Dancer 2002). Taps and dispensers should be elbow operated and good facilities should exist for dispensing and disposing of paper towels.
- Lack of education concerning the importance of handwashing.
- Lack of emphasis on handwashing by peers and managers.
- The use of gloves, incorrectly seen as obviating the need for handwashing.

Summary

- Effective hand hygiene is an essential tool in the prevention of cross-infection.
- There are different decontamination agents and techniques and nurses need to be aware of which are appropriate in different situations, e.g. alcohol-based handrubs are an acceptable alternative to handwashing when hands are not visibly soiled.
- Handwashing must be performed thoroughly, paying attention to preparation, washing and rinsing, and drying, and for an adequate length of time.
- Hands must be dried carefully with paper towels.
- There are a number of barriers to effective handwashing but these must be overcome to prevent cross-infection.

USE OF PERSONAL PROTECTIVE EQUIPMENT, INCLUDING GLOVES, APRONS AND GOWNS

Protective equipment, including aprons, gowns, gloves, eye protection and face masks, should be used on the basis of: 'an assessment of the risk of transmission of microorganisms to the patient, and the risk of contamination of health care practitioners' clothing and skin by patients' blood, body fluid, secretions and excretions' (Pratt *et al.* 2001, p. 29). In this section gloves, aprons and gowns are discussed.

LEARNING OUTCOMES

On completion of this section you will be able to:

1. Identify the procedures for which gloves, sterile or non-sterile, are recommended and key factors in their usage.
2. Show awareness of the materials commonly used in the manufacture of disposable gloves, their relative values and costs.
3. Discuss when plastic aprons and gowns should be worn, stating the rationale.

Learning outcome 1: Identify the procedures for which gloves, sterile or non-sterile, are recommended and key factors in their usage

Pratt *et al.* (2001, p. 29) identify that gloves are worn for two main reasons:

■ To protect hands from contamination with organic matter and microorganisms.
■ To reduce the risks of transmission of microorganisms to both patients and staff.

They go on to advise that gloves should not be worn unnecessarily as prolonged and indiscriminate use can lead to adverse reactions and skin sensitivity. Therefore risk assessment should be carried out considering who is at risk and whether sterile or non-sterile gloves are needed, the potential for exposure to blood, body fluids, secretions and excretions, and the likelihood of contact with non-intact skin or mucous membranes. In the next activities you consider situations where sterile gloves are needed, situations where non-sterile gloves are sufficient, and situations where no gloves are needed.

Sterile gloves

■ Activity

Referring to each scenario at the beginning of the chapter, write down those clinical procedures and situations for which you think sterile gloves should be worn.

You may have identified the following:

- **Mrs Lewis and James Smith**: A non-touch technique (see later section) using sterile gloves will be necessary to clean and dress their wounds to reduce the risk of cross-infection. Although sterile forceps can be used for wound dressings (see discussion in later section), gloves are more likely to be used in these scenarios as their high quality gives nurses the necessary protection from the infected wound exudate.
- **Stacey and Laura**: None, from the information given in the scenarios.

From the above activity you can conclude that sterile gloves are used most frequently for invasive procedures and for direct contact with non-intact skin (O'Toole 1997). Examples of other procedures where sterile gloves are necessary are urinary catheterisation, and for insertion of a chest drain.

Non-sterile gloves

Activity | Look again at the practice scenarios and list those clinical procedures and situations when nurses and other ward-based staff should use non-sterile gloves.

Your list might include:

- **Mrs Lewis**: As she has MRSA present in her wound, gloves should be used for all contact by nurses, doctors and other health professionals, such as the physiotherapist. Additionally, gloves must always be worn when there is potential contact with faeces, urine or any other body fluid (Pratt *et al.* 2001). Non-sterile gloves must therefore be worn when dealing with her commode. Additionally the domestic cleaner should be instructed to wear gloves (and apron) when cleaning the room and to discard them before leaving.
- **Laura**: As Laura is a potential source of infection to others, non-sterile gloves should be worn for any contact with body fluids, especially respiratory secretions and contact with skin lesions.
- **James**: Probably none. However when the district nurse removes James's soiled dressing, any outer layers (such as a cotton bandage keeping the dressing in place) might be removed using non-sterile gloves, with sterile gloves preserved for the aseptic dressing procedure itself.
- **Stacey**: Contact with vomit, as a body fluid, necessitates the use of non-sterile gloves. Whether gloves would be worn for other procedures with Stacey depends on individual risk assessment and local policy but non-sterile gloves may be worn for carrying out her injection (due to the small risk of bleeding occurring) and for when she has blood taken.

In addition to the points above, it is worth noting that local policy concerning the handling and preparation of specific drugs, such as antibiotics and cytotoxic materials, may necessitate the use of gloves in order to protect the nurse.

Key factors in using gloves

All gloves can perforate and should therefore be checked for defects, and finger-nails should be kept short to avoid perforations. Pratt *et al.*'s (2001) standard principles include the following points:

- Gloves should never be reused and washing them rather than changing them is not safe.
- Gloves are single-use items and must be put on immediately before an episode of care and discarded after each care activity for which they were worn. This is to prevent the transmission of microorganisms to other sites in that individual or other patients.
- Hands should be decontaminated before putting on gloves and after removing them.
- Removal of used gloves should be carried out in such a way as to avoid skin contamination and all gloves should be disposed of as clinical waste.

Situations where gloves are not necessary

Activity

With reference to the scenarios, make a list of the procedures and situations for which gloves are usually unnecessary. Think particularly of all the individuals who may come into contact with the patient/client and try to decide if they need to wear gloves.

You may have identified the following:

- **Mrs Lewis**: As noted in the activity above there are many occasions when gloves should be worn when attending to Mrs Lewis. However, the risk to visitors is minimal as most do not have contact with body fluids and do not therefore need to wear gloves. Nevertheless, they should be instructed to wash their hands before leaving the room. If Mrs Lewis visits another department (e.g. X-ray), whether their staff require gloves depends on their level of contact with her. As porters transferring Mrs Lewis are unlikely to be in contact with her directly, gloves are not needed.
- **Laura**: Again, Laura's visitors do not need to wear gloves but both her parents need a clear explanation of the importance of hand hygiene while caring for Laura and they should be encouraged to be proactive in ensuring that any other social visitors wash their hands on entering and leaving the cubicle. The infection control nurse and local policy can also give specific guidance in situations like these.
- **James**: Gloves are only needed when changing wound dressings so for any other aspects of his care they are not required.
- **Stacey**: Gloves are unnecessary except where contact with blood, faeces, vomit or other body fluids is possible. Thus for most of Stacey's care, for example checking her blood pressure, administering oral medication and giving psychological support, gloves are not required.

Learning outcome 2: Show awareness of the materials commonly used in the manufacture of disposable gloves, their relative values and costs

■ Activity | When next in the clinical area take note of the different types of gloves available to practitioners.

There are two main types of disposable gloves:

1. Latex, which is derived from the sap of the Brazilian rubber tree
2. Vinyl – PVC (polyvinylchloride).

Polythene gloves should not be used due to their permeability and tendency to damage. From reviewing the literature, Pratt *et al.* (2001) concludes that latex gloves generally offer more protection than vinyl, but latex contains a large number of different proteins, some of which can be allergenic. Hypersensitivity is increased due to residual accelerators (chemicals added to latex in order to assist the manufacturing process). Patients, staff and visitors should be educated about the potential problem of allergic reactions and alternative gloves must be made available (Pratt *et al.* 2001). The guidelines for standard principles (Pratt *et al.* 2001) state that gloves conforming to European Community standards and of an acceptable quality must be available in all clinical areas. They recommend that alternatives to natural rubber latex (NRL) gloves must be available for use by practitioners and patients with NRL sensitivity.

The starch powder used in certain gloves can also cause allergens to leak from the rubber and bind to the starch. There is considerable evidence that cornstarch powder used to assist in the putting on of gloves is harmful to patients and is associated with adhesions and latex allergy and guidelines for standard principles states that powdered gloves should not be used (Pratt *et al.* 2001).

The cost of gloves varies considerably. In very general terms, non-sterile gloves are half the price of sterile gloves. However, this difference may be increased where sterile gloves are produced to a very high quality using expensive materials. The cost of gloves is an important consideration in an age of spiralling health care costs.

Learning outcome 3: Discuss when plastic aprons and gowns should be worn, stating the rationale

■ Activity | Make a list of those occasions when you have seen plastic aprons worn by nurses in practice settings and when you have seen gowns worn.

You might have seen aprons worn:

■ When handling body fluids and in other aspects of direct patient/client care, such as bathing, assisting with elimination and bed making.

- When food is being handled and when people are being helped with eating.
- When cytotoxic drugs are being prepared and administered.

You might have seen gowns worn:

- In operating theatres and maternity units.

The Department of Health guidelines for standard principles (Pratt *et al.* 2001, p. 32) state that: 'disposable plastic aprons should be worn when there is a risk that clothing or uniform may become exposed to blood, body fluids, secretions and excretions, with the exception of sweat. Full body, fluid repellent gowns should be worn where there is a risk of extensive splashing of blood, body fluids, secretions and excretions, with the exception of sweat, onto the skin of health care practitioners'. You may be able to relate this to your experience of when aprons and gowns are worn.

Plastic aprons provide an impermeable barrier between the nurse's clothes and the patient, and therefore help to protect both parties and reduce cross-infection. However, Callaghan (1998) examined the use of plastic aprons during direct patient contact and found no significant reduction in levels of uniform contamination. There were also serious misunderstandings among nurses concerning the ability of bacteria to cling to plastic aprons. The perception that bacteria do not adhere to plastic is not supported by the data. The study found that nurses rely on plastic aprons to keep their uniforms uncontaminated. Consequently uniforms were worn for more than one day and became heavily contaminated with a variety of bacteria. There have been suggestions that staff use full protective gowns for handling patients from their first onset of conditions such as diarrhoea, rather than just plastic aprons, to prevent transmission of infection (Weightman and Kirby 2000). However, Pratt *et al.* (2001) state that no studies support the routine use of gowns in general or specialist clinical settings.

In community settings, such as small staffed residences, there is an emphasis on social aspects of care and **normalisation** and therefore the use of plastic aprons is likely to be greatly reduced. However, when dealing with body fluids, they are still advisable.

Within hospital settings, Curran (1991) suggests that as plastic aprons are cheap, they should be used as intended by the manufacturers, and disposed of frequently. Callaghan (1998) explains how Curran's guidelines were expanded to form a colour-co-ordinated protocol:

- White plastic aprons for handling body fluids, for toileting, and for direct care. These must be used only for individual patients and then discarded.
- Blue for food-related activities. The apron should be discarded following the completion of the food handling.
- Green aprons for the operating theatre and maternity units, as single-use items and then discarded.
- Yellow for cytotoxic drug treatment, again for single use and then discarded.

Normalisation

Normalisation is a concept that has seen much development over the past 30 years. Currently it is viewed as a system that seeks to value positively devalued individuals and groups (see Emerson 1992, Swann 1997).

Using such a protocol may help to reduce contamination levels on aprons and the transmission of bacteria between nurses and patients. Some hospitals use different-coloured aprons when caring for people who are being source isolated in side rooms, to ensure that the same apron is not worn when caring for other patients. You will need to ensure that you become familiar with any local policies about wearing aprons. You should also note that plastic aprons should be worn as single-use items for one procedure or episode of patient care and then discarded and disposed of as clinical waste (NICE 2003; Pratt *et al.* 2001).

Finally, where there is a risk of blood, body fluids, secretions and excretions splashing into the face and eyes then facemasks and eye protections should be worn, and specialised respiratory protective equipment may be necessary, for example with patients who have TB (Pratt *et al.* 2001).

Summary

- The appropriate use of gloves and aprons is an important infection control measure. However, they must be removed with care, and disposed of appropriately. Hand decontamination should always follow.
- Nurses need to understand when to use gloves, aprons, gowns and masks and advise other staff and visitors accordingly.

NON-TOUCH TECHNIQUE

Non-touch technique involves avoiding direct contact between the skin of one person, normally the hands, and an 'at risk' site in another person. The idea is to avoid contamination through transferring bacteria from the nurse to the patient, or from the patient to the nurse. Non-touch technique acknowledges that even with effective handwashing, hands cannot be sterile. If a non-touch technique is used, then the nurse's hands will not come into contact with the patient or with sterile equipment. Non-touch technique is usually used in procedures that require asepsis, for example, catheterization, venepuncture, tracheal suction and wound care and is often referred to as 'aseptic technique'.

LEARNING OUTCOMES

By the end of this section you will be able to:

1. Assess when non-touch technique is required.
2. Prepare the patient and the appropriate equipment for non-touch technique, with special reference to wound dressings.
3. Outline how non-touch technique is performed and its underpinning rationale, with special reference to wound dressings.

Learning outcome 1: Assess when non-touch technique is required

 Activity

For the following list identify whether it is true or false that a non-touch technique is required:

1. Giving food to patients
2. Administering eye drops
3. Taking a patient's temperature
4. Assisting with teeth cleaning
5. Inserting urinary catheters
6. Wound dressings
7. Removal of sutures or clips.

You should have identified that the answers for 2, 5, 6 and 7 are true. Note that when instilling eye drops, it is possible to use a non-touch technique without using gloves (see Chapter 4 for details about instillation of eyedrops). For the three remaining procedures, 1, 3 and 4, hand hygiene is required but not a non-touch technique.

Procedures can vary widely between clinical settings but they should be rational and take account of relevant research. Generally, non-touch technique should be employed following surgery when skin integrity has been interrupted, following trauma to skin tissue, such as experienced by James, and during invasive procedures such as catheterisation. Mrs Lewis would require non-touch technique during her wound care, and her intravenous cannula would have been inserted using a non-touch technique. Nurses changing bags of intravenous fluids and administering her intravenous antibiotics would use a non-touch technique to reduce the risk of cross-infection. Any other invasive techniques that may be performed as part of her investigations and treatment would also require a non-touch technique. It has been suggested that a clean, rather than sterile, technique is sufficient in some wound care situations (e.g. chronic wounds) (Hollinworth and Kingston 1998). See Chapter 6 'Principles of wound care' for a discussion on clean versus sterile technique.

Learning outcomes 2 and 3 now explain the use of non-touch technique, as applied to wound dressings, as this is one of the most common reasons for using a non-touch technique.

Learning outcome 2: Prepare the patient and the appropriate equipment for non-touch technique, with special reference to wound dressings

Activity

Re-read the definition of non-touch technique. In order to maintain asepsis can you identify what might be the single most important action you can perform prior to performing non-touch technique?

The answer is hand hygiene. Take this opportunity to revisit the section concerned with hand hygiene. Non-touch technique is a prime example of when effective hand hygiene is of utmost importance.

Activity

To perform non-touch technique, a nurse can usually use gloves but can decide to use forceps. What do you think might be the advantages and disadvantages of each of these?

Because hands are not sterile, forceps were traditionally used to perform non-touch technique. However, forceps are awkward to use, and do not prevent the transfer of bacteria from wound to hands (Thomlinson 1987). When a patient moves suddenly they can also be dangerous. The relatively new use of disposable gloves has the advantage of greatly aiding dexterity, but can be more costly. Additionally, good gloving technique is required to prevent contamination of gloves. In some situations it may be helpful to use forceps as well, for example, when removing excess moisture from swabs, if used.

Activity

Discuss with a colleague how you would prepare James to have his wound dressed.

You would need to explain to James what you hope to achieve and gain his consent and co-operation. The whole experience of the accident that caused James's wound followed by undergoing wound dressings could be frightening for him, so nurses should be understanding and patient. The community nurse for learning disabilities should be involved in preparing James for the dressings and will be familiar with how to communicate with James effectively. It would be important to explain to James that dressings should be changed as soon as exudate is visible on the surface, as the dressing will no longer act as an impermeable barrier preventing bacteria from the outside reaching the open wound. If a wound is infected, then the moist exudate on the surface of the dressing will contaminate any surfaces it comes into contact with.

Activity

How might you prepare the environment before embarking upon a wound dressing, either in the community as for James, or in a hospital setting, as for Mrs Lewis?

In the community good lighting and James's comfort and privacy are factors that need to be taken into consideration. James has been having his dressing changed at his home near the farm and district nurses are used to adapting within the home environment. When James attends the local surgery for his dressings, facilities and preparation areas are likely to be superior to those at his home, with a clean treatment room and good handwashing equipment, giving James the best chance of his leg healing successfully.

Traditionally in hospital environments it was recommended that cleaning and bed making should cease before wound dressings are carried out, or invasive procedures undertaken. However, according to Ayliffe et al. (2001), even when substantial disturbance of bedlinen occurs, the increase in air-borne counts is unlikely to greatly increase the risk of infection. Cleaning, however, can raise dust, so you should avoid carrying out a wound dressing in the close vicinity of cleaning. Nurses should take this into account when planning when to carry out Mrs Lewis's dressing.

Next you need to consider what equipment is required.

Compare your list with that in Box 3.2.

Cleaning of dressing trolleys has been a source of debate. Traditionally they were cleaned between patients with alcohol wipes or spray. There is no evidence that bacteria on the trolley are transferred into the wound or vice versa, and the routine cleaning of trolleys between patients probably serves no useful purpose (Thomson and Bullock 1992). The trolley should be free from any visible soiling or dust, and the use of soap and water and disposable towels are sufficient for cleaning purposes. As with any cleaning of equipment it is the physical act of cleaning that is most important rather than the substance used.

Dressing packs vary in content with, for example, some containing forceps and some gloves. Commercially manufactured packs often state the content on the wrapper. Whatever the content you should check all packs for integrity. If the pack is damaged or torn it should be discarded as the contents can no longer be guaranteed sterile. You should also check that the pack has been sterilised and ensure that the expiry date has not elapsed.

A sterile solution such as normal saline can be used to clean and irrigate the wound, if indicated. See Chapter 6 'Principles of wound care' for a discussion on when and how wound cleansing should take place. As both James and Mrs Lewis have heavily exudating wounds due to their infections, cleansing will be necessary. Normal saline is available in sachets, but it is also produced in an aerosol can. Great care must be taken to avoid contamination of the aerosol when used, and in many settings it is advisable for each patient to have their

---

- A dressing trolley or surface that can be used for the equipment
- A sterile dressing pack
- Sterile cleansing solution (if cleansing required)
- Wound dressing appropriate for wound, based on assessment, as per patient's care plan (see Chapter 6 'Principles of wound care')
- Hypoallergenic tape and clean pair of scissors (if needed for the dressing)
- Clean disposable apron
- Receptacle for any equipment that will need to be resterilised in the Central Sterile Supplies Department (CSSD)
- Handwashing facilities and equipment and/or alcohol handrubs.

Box 3.2 Equipment for carrying out a wound dressing

own can, and certainly if the wound is known to be infected or contaminated (Williams 1996). When the district nurse was carrying out James's dressing at home, a can of saline could have been kept in his cottage. The choice of wound dressing depends on many factors. Wound assessment and choice of dressings is covered in detail in Chapter 6 'Principles of wound care'. The wound care for each patient, including type of dressing, frequency of dressing change and cleansing agent, should all be included in the care plan. If tape is to be used, it should be hypoallergenic tape, in good condition and clean, as should be the scissors. A clean apron to protect the nurse and the easy availability of a receptacle for used CSSD equipment completes the list.

Learning outcome 3: Outline how non-touch technique is performed and its underpinning rationale, with special reference to wound dressings

Activity

If you have access to a skills laboratory and equipment, collect a trolley, a dressing pack and a sachet of normal saline, and then wash your hands. If a fellow student is available, take it in turns to open the dressing pack without contaminating the equipment inside.

It is important not to touch and potentially contaminate the inner surface of the pack (which is your sterile field) other than at the corners, and with fingertips. Most dressing packs include either forceps or sterile gloves. If forceps are supplied, use a pair to arrange the equipment on your sterile field. If no forceps are supplied, you can use the sterile disposal bag over your hand to arrange the equipment. The disposal bag is then attached to the trolley. If forceps were used, they can now be discarded. Having done this, you can then practise pouring sterile fluid into a gallipot, but first clean the outside of the sachet with an alcohol swab. Try not to splash the fluid onto the sterile field as this provides a potential focus for bacterial transfer.

Activity

If gloves are not included in the dressing pack, add them now. Wash your hands again (or use the alcohol handrub) and put on the gloves.

You will need to put the gloves on without contaminating the outer surface of the glove or contaminating the dressing pack content. Peel open the glove pack and open up the inner glove pack carefully, handling corners only. Using the inner surface of the folded cuff, push your hand into the glove. If you line up your thumb with the thumb of the glove you will find the glove goes on more easily. Remember that 'practice makes perfect'. The second glove is easier to put on as you can use your other, gloved, hand to help.

Box 3.3 outlines a set of guidelines which you could use to change a wound dressing. These guidelines are intended for use when alone. If you have a second nurse available then this person can, after decontaminating hands, open the

Note: throughout the procedure continually observe patient's condition and take into account their comfort and privacy.

1. Decontaminate hands.
2. Explain the procedure, gain consent and co-operation.
3. Prepare the environment, including trolley.
4. Collect equipment and place on trolley. If CSSD items are to be used, ensure that a receptacle is available.
5. Position the patient and adjust clothing to expose required area.
6. Decontaminate hands and put on plastic apron.
7. Open the outer packaging of the pack and slip the inner package onto the trolley top.
8. If appropriate, loosen the dressing covering the wound.
9. Decontaminate hands.
10. Open the dressing pack using corners only, and avoiding sterile inner surfaces and content.
11. Open any additional equipment onto the sterile field.
12. If using **forceps**:
    - Use one pair to arrange the equipment on the sterile field, and then carefully place them back on the sterile field without contaminating it.
    - Attach the disposal bag to the trolley.
    - Then remove the dressing with the same pair of forceps and dispose of both the dressing and forceps into the bag.

    Or, if using **gloves**:
    - Use the disposal bag over one hand to arrange the equipment.
    - Then remove the dressing with your hand inside the bag, invert the bag and attach it to the trolley.

13. Pour solution (if using) into gallipot.
14. If appropriate, cover the exposed wound.
15. Decontaminate hands and pick up second pair of forceps, if using, or put on sterile gloves.
16. Discard wound cover and place sterile drapes around wound if required.
17. Cleanse the wound, if appropriate, by irrigating, or using swabs, working from the centre outwards.
18. Apply new dressing, or undertake required procedure.
19. Discard gloves or forceps, and if using gloves take care not to contaminate skin with outer surface of gloves.
20. Secure dressing and make patient comfortable.
21. Dispose of all equipment safely, remove apron and decontaminate hands.
22. Document the care, reporting any significant findings or effects on the patient.

Box 3.3 Guidelines for using non-touch technique, applied to a wound dressing

pack, be available to observe and support the patient throughout the procedure and open additional items onto the sterile field when required. Hollinworth and Kingston (1998) advise against excessive handwashing during wound dressings, suggesting that frequency with which handwashing is performed should be based on individual assessment. Using alcohol-based handrub instead, if available on the trolley, means that you will avoid leaving the patient during the procedure. When aseptic procedures are being performed with children, parents can provide support and encouragement.

The guidelines in Box 3.3 can be adapted as long as the underlying principles are maintained. The important principles of all aseptic/non-touch techniques when applied to wound dressings are that the open wound should not come into contact with any item that is not sterile and that any items that have been in contact with the wound should be discarded safely or decontaminated (Wilson 2001). This same principle applies to any other aseptic technique. For example, during catheterization (see Chapter 8) the sterile catheter, which will be inserted into the sterile urinary tract, must not be contaminated by anything that is non-sterile. Stacey's injection must also be carried out using aseptic technique. The needle will be piercing the skin (the protective barrier) and entering the sterile muscle. Therefore, the needle, syringe and drug must be sterile and should be prepared and administered using a non-touch technique (see Chapter 4).

Summary

- There are many situations where non-touch technique is necessary in order to prevent cross-infection during invasive procedures.
- Effective non-touch technique requires good hand hygiene, sterile equipment and the correct use of gloves or forceps as appropriate.
- Understanding the underlying principles of non-touch technique enables guidelines to be adapted safely to each individual situation.

SPECIMEN COLLECTION

Laboratory tests can assist with the diagnosis of an infection, and successful laboratory diagnosis depends on effective collection of a specimen. This requires appropriate and timely collection of specimens, the correct technique and equipment, along with rapid and safe transport (Meers *et al.* 1995). The sooner a specimen arrives at a laboratory the greater the chance of organisms surviving and being identified. In general, the greater the quantity of material sent for laboratory examination, the greater the chance of isolating causative organisms.

Specimens can be contaminated by poor technique giving rise to confusing or misleading results. Ideally samples should be collected before the beginning of treatments such as antibiotics or antiseptics, or the laboratory should be informed of which are being used. Both antiseptics and antibiotics affect the outcome of laboratory results.

LEARNING OUTCOMES

By the end of this section you will be able to:

1. Identify the general principles relating to the collection of any specimen.
2. Understand the principles of MRSA screening.
3. Show awareness of the general principles underpinning the collection of wound swabs and pus.

Note: The collection of urine and stool specimens is included in Chapter 8 'Meeting elimination needs', and collection of sputum specimens is included in Chapter 11 'Respiratory care: assessment and interventions'.

Learning outcome 1: Identify the general principles relating to the collection of any specimen

General principles of collecting any specimen include:

- Explaining the procedure to the person.
- Maintaining privacy while the procedure takes place.
- Ensuring that hands are washed before and after the procedure.
- Wearing non-sterile gloves if handling of body fluids is likely.
- Ensuring that tissue and fluid is collected from the suspected site of infection.
- Preserving any microorganisms collected in the relevant medium/container and preventing it becoming contaminated by other organisms.
- Placing the specimen in an appropriate and correctly labelled container and ensuring the request form is filled out correctly. The microbiology laboratory may be the provider of the correct specimen container. NB Do not label the container until after the specimen is collected, to prevent contamination of the label, and mistakes.

If specimens cannot be sent to a laboratory immediately they should be stored in a dedicated specimen refrigerator at 4°C. Blood cultures, however, go in an incubator at 37°C. Cottonwool swab sticks are used to take specimens from mucous membranes. The specimen stick is then inserted into a tube of soft agar which preserves any microorganisms for up to 24 hours. Bottles for transporting viruses are usually acquired from the laboratory and need prompt transport to the laboratory as soon as possible after the swab is taken.

Without full information it is impossible to examine a specimen adequately or to report it accurately. Also if specimens are not correctly labelled the laboratory cannot process the specimen and a further specimen will have to be obtained, thus delaying treatment.

Activity Can you make a list of the information that you think it would be essential to document and accompany the specimen? Why is full and correct information important?

You may have identified the following:

1. Patient's name and location (e.g. address, ward).
2. Hospital number and date of birth.
3. Consultant's/GP's name.
4. Date collected.
5. Time collected.
6. Clinical details of relevance to the specimen, for example signs of infection.
7. Date of onset of the illness.
8. Any antibiotic therapy being taken by the patient. Failure to provide this information could lead to a false report (Donovan 1998).
9. Type of specimen and site.
10. Name and telephone/bleep number of the doctor/nurse requesting the investigation, as it may be necessary to telephone the result before the report is despatched.

The specimen must be correctly labelled to ensure that it can be identified and matched with its corresponding request form. In this way the results of the tests are related to the correct patient. Nurses should ensure that specimens are sealed in appropriate containers (Wilson 2000). Collection of specimens is potentially hazardous as staff could be exposed to body fluids of people. It is the responsibility of managers to provide safe working conditions and ensure that rules are adhered to. However, all members of staff should be aware of the hazards to which they may be exposed and understand the relevance of the measures designed to protect them (Meers *et al.* 1995).

Learning outcome 2: Understand the principles of MRSA screening

MRSA screening is becoming increasingly prevalent (see later section 'Source isolation'). The Department of Health (2003) reports that the Netherlands have been highly successful in controlling MRSA by screening patients and isolating those found to be positive (colonised or infected), but the Dutch were able to set aside sufficient numbers of side rooms and provide a high staff–patient ratio.

In the UK, the circumstances under which MRSA screening is performed depends on local policy but may be:

■ Prior to transfer of patients to another hospital (particularly if to a specialist area such as a cardio-thoracic surgical unit where patients are extra vulnerable)
■ When admitting a patient from another hospital or a care home, particularly if MRSA is known to be prevalent there
■ When other patients in the environment have been found to be infected or colonised with MRSA.

The results will indicate whether or not source isolation is required. However it should be remembered that a negative MRSA screen does not guarantee the absence of MRSA, only that it was not found in those areas which were sampled.

■ **Activity**   Have you observed or been involved in MRSA screening in the practice setting? If so, what sites were swabbed and how was this performed?

After extensively reviewing the literature, the MRSA Working Party Report (1998) advises that choice of screening sites depends on clinical and epidemiological indications, and so local policy and individual patient features inform decisions about which sites are swabbed. Their recommendation is that initial screening should include the nose, the throat (if a denture wearer), the perineum/ groin, skin lesions such as wounds, ulcers, eczema and dermatitis, and invasive sites, for example intravenous and stoma sites. Additionally if the patient has an indwelling urinary catheter, a specimen of urine and a urethral swab may be taken, sputum if available may be sent for analysis, and sometimes the axilla is swabbed too.

You need to act in accordance with local policy when collecting specimens but the following procedures have been recommended for swabs. A transport (culture) medium is required and swabs taken from drier areas, like the nose and skin, should first be moistened by dipping them into saline or the culture medium.

■ **Nasal swabs**: The patient should sit facing a strong light source with the head tilted back. The moistened swab is inserted into the nostril and the swab taken from the anterior nares, directing the swab upwards in the tip of the nose and using a gentle rotating movement (Wilson 2000). Care must be taken when inserting the swab, especially in babies.
■ **Throat swabs**: A tongue depressor and a good light source are needed. The swab, taken quickly but gently, should be rubbed over the pharyngeal wall and/or the tonsillar fossa. This procedure is unpleasant and may cause the patient to gag.
■ **Perineal swabs**: The perineum is inconvenient to access for routine screening, but on normal skin, is the main carriage site. As an alternative,

the groin can be swabbed but it may be less sensitive (MRSA Working Party Report 1998).

Note that the MRSA Working party is reviewing its guidelines and updated recommendations can be expected in the near future.

Learning outcome 3: Show awareness of the general principles underpinning the collection of wound swabs and pus

Collection of a wound swab may be indicated when signs of infection (e.g. purulent discharge, swelling, redness, pain, pyrexia and delayed healing) are present. As you read in the scenarios, James has had a wound swab taken from his clinically infected wound. However, when a specimen is to be sent from a wound, if pus is present it should be withdrawn using a syringe and sent to the laboratory in a universal container, rather than on a swab; swabs taken from the pus are of little value (Ayliffe *et al.* 2001). Miller (1998) dismisses reliance on wound swabs for diagnosing wound infections, highlighting that many wounds are colonised rather than infected, and that microorganisms grown from the swab may not in fact be the causation of the infection. Wilson (2000) agrees and states that diagnosis of wound infection should be based on clinical signs of infection such as raised temperature, inflammation, redness, pus or swelling and pain.

Wound swabs or pus should be obtained at the beginning of the dressing procedure, after the dressing has been removed and prior to wound dressing. Donovan (1998) reviews the literature on how best to take a wound swab, and her recommendations can be found in Box 3.4. The swab should be taken from the infected site, avoiding surrounding skin and mucous membranes, and then placed in transport medium. The site of the wound must be stated on the request form so that the appropriate media can be set up. Different areas of the body have different natural flora, which can be pathogenic elsewhere (Donovan 1998). One swab only should be taken from a wound on any one occasion. If the wound is dry the swab should be moistened in the transport medium or sterile water as this will improve the efficiency of sampling (Wilson 2000).

- Irrigate the wound with a gentle stream of normal saline at body temperature (Lawrence 1997), to remove surface contamination.
- Moisten the wound swab with normal saline (Rudensky *et al.* 1992) or transport medium (Wound Care Society 1993).
- Move the swab across the whole wound surface, by using a zigzag movement across the wound while rotating the swab between the fingers (Cooper and Lawrence 1996).
- Sample the whole surface area (Gilchrist 1996) or 1 cm² if the surface is large (Levine *et al.* 1976).
- Place the swab straight into the transport medium.

Box 3.4 Wound swabbing technique (references cited by Donovan 1998)

Summary

■ Specimens can be important diagnostic aids and should be collected carefully, using recommended techniques, as the results of their analysis impact on the management of patients.

■ Prevention of cross-infection and contamination of the specimen are essential.

■ Specimens should be labelled accurately, and full accompanying information supplied.

SOURCE ISOLATION

The term source isolation is used to define the steps that are taken to prevent the spread of an infectious agent from an infected or colonised person – the source – to another person. Briefly, the precautions used for source isolation include protective barriers such as aprons and gloves, an emphasis on hand hygiene, and usually the use of a single room. Strict attention is paid to decontamination of equipment and to the disposal of contaminated linen and waste materials. In some instances, a group of patients with the same infection can be nursed together, for example in a bay, and this is termed **cohort nursing** (Wilson 2001). Local policy will guide on whether, and in what circumstances, cohort nursing is appropriate, but this might be used if, for example, there is a group of patients with MRSA, or on the children's ward, a group with **respiratory syncytial virus** (RSV). This is appropriate as long as they do not have another transmissible infection (Parker 1999). The MRSA Working Party Report (1998) advises that cohort nursing a group of MRSA patients together in one ward is preferable to having side rooms occupied by MRSA patients on many different wards.

The term source isolation therefore is used to indicate the management of a person who is a possible source of an infection, such as MRSA, that is readily spread to others. This distinguishes the management of the person from those patients who are extremely vulnerable to infectious disease because their immune system is compromised. This includes patients with prolonged neutropenia as a result of chemotherapy for leukaemia, lymphoma and bone marrow transplant (Gould and Brooker 2000). However, for these people because of the considerable risk of infection from their own body flora a 'germ-free' state is not possible and often simple protective isolation is recommended.

Protective isolation is considered to be a reversal of the precautions taken for source isolation (Parker 2000). It is used to protect patients from infection risks from themselves and others rather than to protect others from any risk that they pose. Protective isolation emphasises thorough handwashing, use of protective clothing such as gloves and aprons and single rooms as a reminder of special precautions needed, rather than the protective effect they confer. Management of these patients includes consideration of the food they eat. Most

Respiratory syncytial virus
This causes an acute viral infection, commonly affecting young children and leading to inflammation and obstruction of the bronchioles.

food contains microorganisms and these are not usually harmful in small numbers. However when people are highly susceptible, food such as salads are avoided and eggs should be thoroughly cooked because of the bacteria associated with them. Even ice cubes may have to be made with sterile water.

Invasive procedures are a major threat to immuno-suppressed patients and strict protocols must be followed when these are used (Gould and Brooker 2000).

In this section the focus is on source isolation because of its common occurrence in clinical practice.

LEARNING OUTCOMES

By the end of this section you will be able to:

1. Identify when source isolation is necessary and when routine precautions alone will be sufficient.
2. Discuss the implications of being infected, or colonised, with MRSA.
3. Consider the importance of communication and be aware of whom to inform when source isolation is required.
4. Outline the preferred requirements and equipment for isolation, and understand the principles underpinning care.
5. Explain the principles underlying the cleaning and disinfection of isolation rooms following discharge of patients.

Learning outcome 1: Identify when source isolation is necessary, and when routine precautions alone will be sufficient

Activity

In the practice scenarios you read that Mrs Lewis and Laura are being nursed in isolation. From what you have already read in this chapter why do you think this was considered necessary? Can you identify some of the infection control measures that would underpin their care?

Laura requires source isolation management and a single cubicle because of the highly infectious nature of chickenpox. While chickenpox is usually considered a mild childhood illness it poses a considerable risk to non-immune highly vulnerable people, which may apply to other children on the ward.

Mrs Lewis is known to have MRSA and the MRSA Working Party Report (1998) states that MRSA-infected patients, and where possible carriers, should be isolated in a single room (preferably with an air extraction unit), as air-borne particles containing staphylococci are released into the environment. For both Laura and Mrs Lewis routine precautions for dealing with body fluids, including emphasis on hand hygiene and use of protective clothing, are required and are discussed earlier in this chapter. Other routine measures that you should take, such as safe use of sharps, waste disposal and equipment, are discussed later in this chapter.

Generally when special precautions are used this depends on the type of infection, and care should be based on interpreting the specific route of transmission. Check back to Table 3.1, 'Routes of transmission', if you need to recap on these. It is normally advised that patients with air-borne infections, for example open TB, should be nursed in a side room (Parker 1999; Wilson 2001).

Patients, such as Stacey, with blood-borne infections (unless bleeding) can often be managed in the open ward using routine infection control precautions. This includes the safe management of sharps and the routine use of protective clothing where contact with body fluids or blood is likely (Wilson 2001). However, the circumstances of each individual and the environment will need to be taken into account when deciding whether to isolate in a side room, and advice from the local infection control team should be sought. Sometimes the person's clinical condition may prevent isolation or there may not be side rooms available (MacKenzie and Edwards 1997). In most cases, when a single room is necessary, the door should be kept shut. The infection control team can advise concerning individual cases, for example, when a patient is confused and their safety could be jeopardised by closing the door (MRSA Working Party Report 1998).

Managing outbreaks of diarrhoea and vomiting

Activity To prevent spread of infection to other people, what precautions should be taken if someone develops diarrhoea and vomiting in a small community-based unit?

You might have identified the following:

- Good personal hygiene is required, particularly handwashing before eating and after using the toilet.
- Normal crockery and cutlery are usually sufficient. Bacteria are easily removed by washing in hot water and detergent. However, cleaning of crockery and cutlery is best done at high temperatures in a dishwasher.
- If dishes are washed by hand, then clean hot water should be used with detergent. The items should be rinsed and left to drain, rather than being dried with a cloth, as these are easily contaminated (Wilson 2001). Dishcloths should be disposable.
- If possible the person should be allocated a toilet for their sole use.
- If there is a suspected outbreak of gastrointestinal illness, defined as when two or more clients or staff are affected by unexplained diarrhoea or vomiting, then further action may be needed, particularly if there are other vulnerable people within the residence. In small staffed units other residents' GPs and the infection control team would need to be informed. Stool specimens should be obtained from those affected even if they no longer have symptoms.

In a small community unit the above precautions should be enough to prevent cross-infection. However, if gastroenteritis occurs in an institutional setting, such as a hospital, affected patients must be transferred to single rooms where at all possible. Standard isolation procedures should then be put in place and the infection control department informed (Wilson 2001).

Learning outcome 2: Discuss the implications of being infected, or colonised, with MRSA

Mrs Lewis is an example of a person who is infected with MRSA and, as a potential source of infection to other hospital patients and staff, needs to be managed by source isolation. Since 1981, a particularly resistant strain of *Staphylococcus aureus* (MRSA) has been causing an increasing number of problems in hospitals throughout the world. *Staphylococcus aureus* is a microorganism commonly found on normal skin, particularly warmer parts such as the axillae, groins, perineum and nose. This carriage is termed colonisation, rather than infection; about 80 per cent of people with MRSA are colonised rather than infected with it (Public Health Medicine Environmental Group 1996). The organism referred to by the initials MRSA is a strain of *Staphylococcus aureus* that has become resistant to the antibiotic methicillin, hence the name methicillin-resistant *Staphylococcus aureus*. Strains of MRSA are usually resistant to all penicillins and all cephalosporins. In addition, they may be resistant to other first line antibiotics.

Activity — Why do you think it is important to try to prevent the spread of MRSA?

While, as stated above, many people are colonised rather than infected with MRSA, MRSA can result in a range of superficial infections of the skin and can cause hospital-acquired wound infections, as with Mrs Lewis. *Staphylococcus aureus* can also cause boils and abcesses and serious systemic infections, such as septicaemica and pneumonia (Wilson 2001). The MRSA Working Party Report (1998) presents substantial data to support the clinical importance of MRSA. Unfortunately, the few drugs currently available that have reliable activity against MRSA are very expensive and difficult to administer. They necessitate blood levels being monitored since they are highly toxic.

Serious staphylococcal infection usually occurs in people who are vulnerable because of underlying illness or medical interventions. Mrs Lewis, as a frail older person with diabetes and rheumatoid arthritis, fits into this category. Healthy people do not usually develop an infection though they can become colonised (Wilson 2001). *Staphlococcus aureus* and MRSA are usually carried 'silently'. The organism is most likely to be spread on the hands of staff as transient organisms. If staff have certain skin conditions, such as eczema or dermatitis, or have cuts on their skin, they are at increased risk of harbouring the organism and can spread it to other staff and patients. The organism can also be carried on skin scales from an infected patient or member of staff and may contaminate uniforms or clothing, especially if the clothing is damp. Handwashing, adequate cleaning and patient isolation are considered to be of particular importance in the control of MRSA (MRSA Working Party Report 1998).

Patients with MRSA are not usually considered to be a risk to the community at large, and MRSA is not a contraindication to living at home or being admitted to a care home (Public Health Medicine Environmental Group 1996). Indeed, infection control teams may recommend that patients with MRSA, such as Mrs Lewis, are discharged as soon as possible, to minimise risk to other susceptible hospitalised patients (Orchard 1998).

Learning outcome 3: Consider the importance of communication and be aware of who to inform when source isolation is required

Activity

List the key people who should be informed when a decision is made to isolate a patient. Try to link this to Mrs Lewis and Laura.

You may have identified the following: Mrs Lewis and Laura themselves, their families and friends, domestic staff, the infection control team, and possibly other departments e.g. X-ray. Further details about these will now be discussed.

Explanations to patients and relatives

Infections cause emotional as well as physical distress, and care should be taken to explain and reassure patients and their relatives as to the rationale underpinning isolation. Patient information leaflets are available for certain infections, such as chickenpox and MRSA, and these can back-up verbal explanations and should be available in different languages. It is essential that patients and relatives understand the rationale behind isolation so that they can fully co-operate with the restrictions. Providing information to patients about being isolated has been found to reduce the negative psychological effects (Gammon 1999a).

Some clinical areas ask that visitors only enter isolation rooms after permission and instruction from the nurse in charge. While children and susceptible visitors should be discouraged, for most infections the risk to visitors is minimal, as they do not have contact with body fluids (Wilson 2001). If a child such as Laura is isolated, visits from family members including young siblings usually pose no problem. But chickenpox is highly contagious and visits from other young children are inadvisable (Simpson 1998/9).

Explanations to domestic staff

The domestic supervisor should be informed of any patients who are being isolated. A dedicated mop, bucket and disposable cleaning cloths should be provided for the room. The domestic will need to wear apron and gloves when cleaning and these must be discarded into a yellow plastic bag before leaving the room. Most microorganisms are not able to survive on dry surfaces for long periods of time (Wilson 2001) and therefore the environment need not be a major factor in the transmission of infections. The normal standard of cleaning should be maintained and domestic staff should be reassured that the risks to their own health are minimal if protective clothing is worn and careful handwashing takes place. This is very important as otherwise the standard of cleaning may suffer (Wilson 2001). Additionally there is some evidence that increasing domestic cleaning time with emphasis on removal of dust by vacuum cleaning and allocation of responsibility for the routine cleaning of medical equipment can help to terminate prolonged outbreaks of MRSA (Rampling *et al.* 2001).

Infection control team

The clinical area will often have a list of communicable infections which indicates if isolation is necessary and highlights which material from the patient is potentially infectious. If in doubt, the infection control team can offer advice. The infection control team must be contacted if a patient has MRSA, or has been infected, colonised or transferred from a ward with MRSA cases in the recent past (usually defined as six months). Those patients isolated because of other infectious diseases should also be notified to the infection control team. As Laura developed chickenpox while on the children's ward, she could have infected other children before it was diagnosed, and therefore prior to her being isolated, so other contacts will need to be traced and immunity checked. Certain infectious diseases are notifiable to the Medical Officer for Environmental Health. It is the legal responsibility of the doctor in clinical charge of the patient to do this (Wilson 2001).

> **Activity**   When next in the practice setting find out who the members of the local infection control team are and where they are located.

The infection control team generally comprises an infection control nurse (ICN) and an infection control doctor. Their roles include planning, implementing and monitoring the infection prevention and control programme. They are available to offer advice on all matters relating to infection control and the patient. They also provide education to health care personnel and develop policy. An infection control committee from a variety of hospital departments provides advice and support for the infection control team (ICT).

Many community health care trusts also employ infection control nurses who work closely with the consultant for communicable disease control. The consultant is responsible for monitoring and controlling the spread of infection in the community (Wilson 2001). Many hospitals also use infection control link nurses to improve awareness of infection control in clinical areas. They receive basic training and help provide education, training, audit and surveillance in clinical areas. There should also be close liaison between the occupational health department and the ICT to ensure the health and safety of patients and staff alike (Wilson 2001).

Visits to departments

Staff in other departments and areas that the patient may need to visit should be informed so that any special arrangements can be made. They may be able to carry out the investigation immediately, to avoid the person waiting in receptions or corridors (Parker 1999), or at the end of the list if appropriate. This would be relevant to Mrs Lewis if she requires a hip X-ray or to Laura if she requires a chest X-ray. Porters need not wear protective clothing, but should be advised to wash their hands on completion of the journey (Wilson 2001). Any transporting staff with skin abrasions should wear gloves and the trolley or chair should be cleaned with detergent and hot water, or in accordance with local policy. Linen use should comply with local guidelines. Hot water and detergent should be used for handwashing at the conclusion of any contact (MRSA Working Party Report 1998).

Learning outcome 4: Outline the preferred requirements and equipment for isolation, and understand the principles underpinning care

Equipment for source isolation

Activity — Construct a list of equipment you think might be required for implementing source isolation, and subsequently for care of the patient.

Many of the items you might have listed relate to the general principles discussed earlier in this chapter: liquid soap or antimicrobial agent, alcohol-based handrub, non-sterile disposable gloves, plastic aprons and paper towels. You also need equipment for disposing of waste: yellow clinical waste bags, a red water-soluble bag and red linen bag, and a sharps box. Aprons and gloves worn by staff handling the patient or in contact with their immediate environment should be discarded into yellow plastic bags before leaving the room.

Masks are only recommended in situations such as highly infectious or potentially infectious multi-resistant TB (Lacey *et al.* 2001, Wilson 2001). The room should also have a good communication system and a television set (MRSA Working Party Report 1998).

As a general principle it is sensible to remove excess equipment from the room before patients are isolated. For children, such as Laura, toys need to be washable or disposable and preferably Laura's own toys should be used. Suviste (1996) investigated the role of communal toys in nosocomial infection on a children's ward. Hard plastic toys were identified as being heavily contaminated with normal bacterial flora. The study did not, however, test for viruses. Whenever possible a patient who is to be isolated should have their own designated equipment kept in that room. This might include instruments or equipment such as writing materials, sphygmomanometers, stethoscopes, and moving and handling equipment. If this is not possible, such items should be suitably disinfected before use on other patients (MRSA Working Party Report 1998). Some single rooms have their own adjoining bathroom but otherwise, as for Mrs Lewis, a commode is needed. Computer terminals have been surveyed and seem to pose a small risk of MRSA cross-infection but this risk can be further reduced if staff wash their hand before and after patient contact (Devine *et al.* 2001).

Additional points

Common concerns when caring for people in isolation are dealing with elimination, spillage of body fluids, use of non-designated equipment and crockery/cutlery. The use of the key principles discussed earlier – hand hygiene and the use of personal protective equipment – must be adhered to throughout all these aspects of care.

- **Elimination**: Body fluids and materials such as faeces, urine and vomit should be discarded directly into a bedpan washer, macerator or toilet.
- **Spillage of body fluids**: For any spillages of body fluids, gloves and apron must be worn and the fluid dealt with quickly. For a blood spillage, covering it with chlorine-releasing solution or granules may be recommended. Paper towels can be used for absorbing spilt fluids, and detergent and hot water used for cleaning the area. Paper towels used and all waste should then be discarded into a yellow waste bag. These precautions are the same in principle for all people in order to minimise the risk of cross-infection.
- **Using non-designated equipment**: As a general principle it is preferable that equipment is not taken out of the room during the period of isolation. However, if it is not possible to allocate a hoist, for example, solely for a patient's use, then the hoist frame should be disinfected before use by another patient. This in accordance with the general principle from the Department of Health, that where a piece of equipment such as a commode or hoist has to be used for more than one patient it must be cleaned following each and every episode of use (Pratt *et al.* 2001). This principle applies when sharing equipment regardless of whether or not the person is known to have an infection. Local policy will dictate precisely what is used for disinfection, but usually thorough washing with soap and hot water, followed by rinsing and drying, is advised. You should also check any special cleaning instructions from manufacturers.
- **Crockery/cutlery**: Crockery and cutlery rarely come into contact with infectious material. As such, they are unlikely to become contaminated and can be returned to the kitchen or catering department in the usual way (Wilson 2001).

Managing the psychological effects of isolation

■ Activity

Try to imagine:
- How might Mrs Lewis feel, being isolated in a side room?
- How might Mr Cox feel being isolated in the cubicle with Laura?
- What might nurses do to reduce the effects of isolation?

Gammon (1999a) states that source isolation can be an extremely frightening and anxiety-provoking experience for both patients and relatives. He goes on to suggest that the psychological effects of source isolation are not well understood and that more research is needed. He does, however, describe how patients may feel confined, imprisoned and shut in. Moreover, depression, irregular sleep patterns, and even hallucinations, disorientation and regression are described. A small qualitative study by Oldham (1998) cites patients saying 'There are times when I am completely forgotten'; 'I feel very shut out at the moment'. Additionally there is some evidence that patients do not understand the reasons for isolation and need to receive explanations about this in order to support treatment (Myatt and Langley 2003).

The literature concerning isolation of children is greater in volume (Gammon 1999b), and indicates that children and their parents suffer high levels of anxiety and depression as a consequence of isolation. Laura needs to be isolated to protect others from her infection, and the door to her room should be kept closed. Laura is old enough to be aware of this and might be concerned or even frightened by this. Additionally, being in the cubicle, Mr Cox would probably feel isolated, and at a time when he is separated from his wife and baby who are at home. Nurses should be prepared to sit with Laura to give him breaks when needed. Laura's parents will want to know how long Laura is likely to be isolated which, depending on local policy, might be until the spots are dry and crusted. Alternatively, once Laura's chest infection is sufficiently improved she may be discharged home.

Nurses should be sensitive to the psychological implications of being labelled infectious and of being isolated. Patients who are isolated may receive less attention and contact from nurses as they are not in immediate view, and because nurses must put on gloves and apron before entering, quick casual contact is reduced. It is important for nurses to try to reduce patients' fears and problems of isolation and ensure that they approach people in an understanding manner (see Chapter 2: The nurse's approach: self-awareness and communication).

Learning outcome 5: Explain the principles underlying the cleaning and disinfection of isolation rooms following discharge of patients

■   *Activity*   Using the discussion above and any experience you have from clinical practice, make a list of the actions that need to be taken when patients are discharged from isolation rooms.

Patients and their relatives need to be kept informed and the usual discharge procedures should be adhered too. Patients who are known to be infected or colonised with MRSA may be subject to additional guidelines, for example, policy may state that if the patient is to be discharged home, the GP and the district nurse must be informed in advance. Similarly, if the patient is discharged to another hospital, or a care home, then their medical and nursing staff should be informed in advance. Local policy may also dictate that the medical records of patients known to be infected or colonised with MRSA should carry a clear mark of identification or are electronically tagged on the computer patient activity system.

In terms of cleaning the room, you may have considered the following, but as always, do check local policy:

■ **Equipment**: Used or soiled disposable equipment must be placed into a yellow plastic bag for incineration. It is not usually necessary to discard unopened packets of disposable equipment. Non-disposable ward equipment, like commodes or hoists which have been kept in the room during the patient's stay, need to be cleaned before being removed from the room. The local disinfection policy will indicate precisely how this is achieved, or the infection control nurse can advise. Any equipment that has not been in contact with infected material does not need special cleaning (Wilson 2001). However, Blythe *et al.* (1998), in a study concerned with MRSA and the environment, highlighted the importance of not overlooking electrical equipment such as call bells and television sets, and pointed out that carpets may become more easily contaminated than hard flooring.

■ **Bedlinen**: This should be placed in an alginate bag and then into a red nylon outer bag to prevent dissemination of microorganisms to laundry staff.

■ **Furniture**: All furniture and surfaces, including bed frames and mattresses, should be cleaned with hot water and soap. Mattresses and bed frames can be a source of cross-contamination even though they are not visibly soiled (Barnett *et al.* 1999). Mattresses and plastic-covered pillows should be checked for permeability and tears. Local policy should be adhered to and may indicate that these items should be condemned if damaged. Curtains may need to be sent for laundering.

■ **Room cleaning**: When the equipment has been dealt with, domestic staff, wearing plastic aprons and gloves, should clean the floors and surfaces in the usual way with detergent and hot water. The plastic apron, gloves and any disposable wipes should be discarded into a yellow plastic clinical waste bag and the mop head, if not disposable, placed into a plastic bag for laundering. The mop bucket and handle should be washed and left to dry. Room cleaning must be meticulous and all traces of dust should be removed. Once the room has been thoroughly cleaned, it can be reused immediately (Wilson 2001), but ensure that all surfaces are dry before reuse.

Summary

■ While routine precautions are sufficient to prevent cross-infection in many circumstances, in some situations additional measures are necessary in the form of source isolation.

■ Source isolation requires correct use of hand hygiene, gloves, aprons and waste disposal, and usually a single room for the person who is identified as a source of infection, with, if possible, equipment for their sole use.

- The psychological effects of source isolation have been documented; it is important for nurses to be aware of these and provide psychological support and information.
- Discharge of patients from isolation and terminal cleaning of the room and its equipment should be carried out in accordance with sound infection control principles and local policy.

SHARPS DISPOSAL

Safe disposal of sharps, such as needles, blood glucose lancets, intravenous cannulae and catheter stylets, is important not only in relation to maintaining a safe environment, but also in preventing cross-infection. In a critical review of the literature, Hanrahan and Reutter (1997) indicated that sharps injuries are the most common cause of blood-borne cross-infection in health care professionals.

LEARNING OUTCOMES

By the end of this section you will be able to:

1. Understand the need and reasons for the safe disposal of sharps.
2. Explain the principles for the safe use and disposal of sharps.
3. Identify the actions required following needle stick injury.

Learning outcome 1: Understand the need and reasons for the safe disposal of sharps

Activity

Identify with a colleague two possible reasons for the importance of disposing of sharps safely.

The main reason for the need to dispose of sharps safely is the physical prevention of cross-infection through needle stick injuries. In the UK it is estimated that 16 per cent of occupational injuries that occur in hospitals are due to needle stick injury (Pratt *et al.* 2001). The most common infections arising from blood-borne transmission are bacterial infections and viral infections, such as hepatitis B, hepatitis C and HIV (Hanrahan and Reutter 1997; Russell 1997). The staff who are caring for Stacey know that she is a hepatitis B carrier and therefore if they sustained a needle stick injury from her used injection needle they would be at risk of acquiring hepatitis B, if they are not immune. However this information is not always available, and patients themselves may not know that they are carrying a blood-borne disease. This is why sharps disposal should be carried out in the same way for all patients. The average risk of transmission of blood-borne pathogens following a single percutaneous exposure has been estimated to be (Pratt *et al.* 2001):

- Hepatitis B virus (HBV) 33.3 per cent (1 in 3)
- Hepatitis C virus (HBC) 3.3 per cent (1 in 30)
- Human immunodeficiency virus (HIV) 0.31 per cent (1 in 319).

In the first instance, it is the injured health care professional who is at risk of contamination from a patient source. However, the professional may then pass the infection back to other patients if the correct procedures are not followed.

A second important reason for ensuring the safe disposal of sharps is the professional and moral responsibility of nurses to protect patients and colleagues from risk (Nursing and Midwifery Council 2002). The distress that almost invariably occurs following sharps injuries is concerned with individuals' understandable fear of the blood-to-blood transmission of bacteria and viruses.

Activity

Discuss with a colleague how you would feel if you sustained a needle stick injury where the patient source was suspected of having a blood-borne infection.

Learning outcome 2: Explain the principles for the safe use and disposal of sharps

Activity

Make a list of the key safety factors you think you should take into account when using and disposing of sharps.

There are many factors to take into account and you may have been able to identify some of the following, which were taken from the Department of Health guidelines for 'Standard principles for the safe use and disposal of sharps' (Pratt *et al.* 2001, p. 35):

- Sharps must not be passed directly from hand to hand and handling should be kept to a minimum.
- Needles must not be bent or broken prior to use or disposal.
- Needles and syringes must not be disassembled by hand prior to disposal.
- Needles should not be recapped.
- Used sharps must be discarded into a sharps container (conforming to UN3291 and BS 7320 standards) at the point of use.
- The sharps container must not be filled above the mark indicating that they are full.
- Containers in public areas must not be placed on the floor and should be located in a safe position.

Other important points

Preferably take a sharps bin to the patient. Always place sharps carefully into the container and never drop or throw them from a distance. Never put fingers into the sharps container, nor kick or shake the container in order to make more room. Do not attempt to clean the sharps container, particularly around the lip. If there is concern regarding the container, it should be disposed of regardless of how full it is. The responsibility for the disposal of sharps lies with the individual who has been using them.

Community trusts should have clear policies on the disposal of sharps used in clients' homes. Kiernan (1997) suggests that sharps containers should be located in the individual's home and that they should be removed when two-thirds full by the local clinical waste disposal collection service. The National Institute for Clinical Excellence (2003, p. 7) states that the licensed route in accordance with local policy must be used to dispose of containers. Therefore policies for community trusts, residential and nursing homes may vary and you will need to ensure that you are familiar with the relevant policies for the areas that you study and work in.

Activity	What should you do when a sharps box is full (i.e. once it is two-thirds full or the contents have reached the 'full' mark on the box)?

Containers should be sealed according to the manufacturer's instructions, which are often found on the outside of the box. In addition, organisations may request extra precautions, for example sealing over the lid with tape marked 'hazard'. Sealed containers should be left at identified collection points in the manner prescribed by the local policy, and labelled with date and source. It is usual for portering staff to remove the boxes and take them to a central point for transport to the incinerator. If you observe that a sharps box is full, be proactive about taking these steps and don't leave them for someone else to deal with as an overfilled sharps bin is very hazardous.

Activity	List the people who may be harmed if the local trust policy on the disposal of sharps containers is not followed correctly.

You may have thought of the following:

- Patients and their visitors
- Nurses
- Doctors and other health professionals
- Porters
- Transport drivers
- Staff at the incinerator.

Sharps boxes placed more than 1.2 m (4 feet) above the ground are associated with increased risk of sharps injuries (Weltman *et al.* 1995). On children's wards and other areas where children may be present, sharps boxes must always be positioned where they cannot gain access to them.

Learning outcome 3: Identify the actions required following needle stick injury

Activity	With a colleague, discuss what you think should be done following a needle stick injury.

All health care employers are required to develop mechanisms for dealing with sharps injuries. These include identifying the employee's responsibility to report the injury and their subsequent entitlement to be provided with counselling and testing services. However, before this stage is reached, emergency action should be taken. Now check your ideas with Table 3.2.

Table 3.2 Action after a needlestick injury. Note that you should consult and follow your local policy throughout. It is the responsibility of the member of staff involved and their manager to see that all procedures are carried out

Emergency action	1. Encourage bleeding at the site by squeezing
	2. Wash wound with soap and water
	3. For splashes to eyes, mouth or into broken skin, rinse thoroughly with plenty of running water
	4. Call for assistance
	5. Cover wound with waterproof dressing
Reporting	1. Inform your manager immediately
	2. Complete accident/incident form
	3. Identify patient source if possible
	4. Report to the occupational health department immediately
	5. If the occupational health department is closed attend the Accident and Emergency department for further advice
Follow-up	1. Make use of counselling if required
	2. Attend for testing if indicated
	3. Follow medical advice

The policies outlined above are also used if blood or body fluid is splashed into the eyes or mouth, or onto broken skin.

Activity

When you are next in the practice setting, seek out and read the local clinical policy on the action to be taken following a sharps injury.

Summary

- Sharps pose a potential hazard to nurses, other staff and the public.
- All nurses must follow national and local policy and handle and dispose of sharps safely in order to prevent the risk of needle stick injury to themselves and colleagues.
- All Trusts have agreed procedures to follow in the event of a needle stick injury and these should be adhered to carefully.

CLINICAL WASTE DISPOSAL

Clinical waste includes human or animal tissue such as blood or other body excretions. It also includes drugs and other pharmaceutical products, soiled surgical dressings, swabs and instruments, discarded syringes, needles, cartridges, broken glass and other sharp surgical instruments in contact with the items mentioned above. Other waste arising from medical, nursing, dental, veterinary, pharmaceutical or other similar practice, that may cause infection to persons coming into contact with it, is also considered to be clinical waste (Wilson 2001).

Nurses have a responsibility, along with other employees, to dispose of waste safely. The responsibilities of those who produce waste such as hospital trusts are described in the Environmental Protection Act 1990 and the Environmental Protection (Duty of Care) Regulations 1991. These Regulations require the producers of waste to manage it safely and transfer it only to an authorised person (Wilson 2001).

LEARNING OUTCOMES

By the end of this section you will be able to:

1. Identify the importance of the correct disposal of clinical waste for the environment and for individuals, including health care workers.
2. State the colour-coding system for waste bags and the recommended process for their disposal.
3. Discuss the storage of clinical waste.

Learning outcome 1: Identify the importance of the correct disposal of clinical waste for the environment and for individuals, including health care workers

Activity

Discuss with a colleague the issues you believe are of greatest importance concerning the safe disposal of clinical waste, with respect to both the environment and to individuals within health care settings.

Issues that you may have considered are:

■ Increasing amounts of waste material are being generated globally and the disposal of this is becoming ever more difficult and expensive.
■ Landfill sites are less available than formerly, and environmentally safe incinerators are expensive. If not well maintained they can produce toxic emissions.
■ Clinical waste is more expensive to dispose of than domestic waste. It is therefore a source of potential unnecessary expenditure for the health care provider if not correctly labelled and dispatched.
■ For individuals within health care settings there exists the potential to be harmed by exposure to toxic, hazardous or infected material, and the possibility of transmitting infection to other health care workers or patients.

Using the definition at the beginning of this section make a list of the materials that might be considered clinical waste in each of the four practice scenarios.

Material contaminated with blood or body fluids, such as the paper towels used for cleaning up Stacey's vomit or soiled wound dressings from James or Mrs Lewis, are examples of clinical waste. Other clinical waste includes excretions, secretions, unwanted specimens, sharps, used disposable medical and nursing equipment (like Mrs Lewis's intravenous fluid administration set) and aids to care, such as gloves and aprons. Just thinking about the four people in the scenarios and their care highlights how much clinical waste is generated in health care.

Learning outcome 2: State the colour-coding system for waste bags and the recommended process for their disposal

■ □   **Activity**

Drawing on practice experience, try to answer the following questions:

1. What colour bag should be used for uncontaminated paper and other household waste and what is the recommended process, or method, to dispose of this bag?
2. What colour bag should be used for material contaminated with blood or body fluid, human or animal tissue and what is the recommended process or method to dispose of this bag?
3. What colour should a sharps bin be? What is the recommended process, or method for its disposal?

Now check your answers. A colour coding system for waste bags has been adopted nationally to segregate waste (Health Services Advisory Committee of the Health and Safety Executive 1992).

Uncontaminated material

Uncontaminated paper and other household waste should be placed in **black** bags and the recommended process for disposal is landfill.

Contaminated material

Material contaminated with blood or body fluid, human or animal tissue should be discarded into **yellow** bags and treated as if infected. The bags should be separated from other waste. If leakage of body fluids is likely to happen then a second bag or impervious container should be used to prevent exposure to, and possible contamination of, those who handle waste products. In common with sharps containers, waste bags should be properly sealed when approximately two-thirds full. If overfilled, waste bags tend to break open. They should be labelled with the point of origin, in order to identify the source if problems arise during disposal (Wilson 2001).

Incineration is the process recommended for the disposal of this type of waste. When incinerators are in good working order, this method is suitable for most types of clinical waste, but very wet or dense loads may affect the efficacy of the process. Certain categories of non-infected human clinical waste such as sanitary towels, urine containers, incontinence pads and stoma bags can be placed in **yellow bags with a black stripe** and disposed of in landfill if a site is licensed for this use (Wilson 2001).

Some forms of clinical waste such as pathology specimens can be autoclaved then placed in **blue or transparent with blue** inscription bags. These can then, having been autoclaved, be disposed of in landfill sites.

Sharps bins

A sharps bin should be **yellow** and incineration is the recommended method of disposal. Incineration reduces the mass and volume of waste and renders it unrecognisable prior to landfill. Design and performance of incinerators is regulated by the Environment Agency (see www.environment-agency.gov.uk). Incinerator emission standards were established in October 1995 (84/360/EEC). Alternative methods for plants that do not meet the specifications include: autoclaving, chemical methods, gasification, irradiation, microwaving and disinfection by continuous feed auger. The aim of all methods is to render waste unrecognisable, non-hazardous and acceptable for landfill.

Meers *et al.* (1995) state that much money could be saved if it were possible to separate the 90 per cent of waste that can be disposed of in the same way as domestic waste, from the remaining 10 per cent of clinical waste that requires special provision. In practice, this has been difficult to achieve and it appears that many trusts have taken the safe though expensive and environmentally unsound decision, to treat all their waste as clinical waste.

Linen

Although linen is not clinical waste it still requires careful handling, bagging and disposal. Used hospital linen can become contaminated with microorganisms from patients' body fluids or the infections they have. The laundry process decontaminates linen through the mechanical process of washing, the detergent used and the temperature of the water. The process must include sufficient time for all parts of the load to be washed at an adequate temperature. Any microorganisms that remain after washing can be destroyed by tumble drying and ironing (Wilson 2001).

■ **Activity**	Can you name three different types of linen bag and the category of linen that should be placed in each? Why are the different categories needed?

The categories are needed to protect laundry staff from cross-infection. Additionally the categories protect other staff and patients by ensuring that linen is adequately decontaminated during the laundering process. The categories can also help to prevent damage to the fabric being washed. There are three main types of linen bag. The first is white linen or clear plastic and is used for used, soiled and foul linen. It is recommended that this is washed at 65°C for 10 minutes or 71°C for 3 minutes for thermal disinfection. Duvets should withstand washing at 71°C and comply with Department of Health standards of retardancy (Wilson 2001). For infected linen a water-soluble bag with a red outer bag is required. This is used for infectious diseases or at other times as advised by the infection control team. The laundry staff do not open and sort the linen in the inner bag and the linen is washed and thermally disinfected, as for used linen. A third type of bag with an orange stripe is used for fabric likely to be damaged by thermal disinfection, for example wool. These items are washed at 40°C and hypochlorite added to the penultimate wash.

Learning outcome 3: Discuss the storage of clinical waste

Activity Find out where clinical waste is stored prior to collection in your local hospital and community setting.

There should be a local policy available to all staff and an overall risk management policy in place. Additionally a waste manager should be designated to monitor, evaluate and review the policy (Health Service Advisory Committee 1999; NHS Executive 1999).

Each Trust has its own arrangements, but the following points apply everywhere. In the hospital setting, clinical waste is often stored adjacent to the main buildings and for considerable periods of time prior to collection. It is therefore important that the storage area is dry and secure and that different coloured bags are kept separately. To prevent cross-infection, the area should not be accessible to animals, insects or rodents. Children in particular must be denied access. Staff handling the waste should be trained to do so, wear protective clothing, and handle bags by the neck only, to avoid the risk of injury from protruding items.

In the community setting, waste produced and handled by clients and their families can usually be discarded with normal household waste where the duty of care is exempt. Thus the district nurse when carrying out James's dressing at home would have been able to simply discard the used dressing into his household rubbish. The clinical waste then becomes mixed with large amounts of ordinary waste and is not regarded as a hazard (Wilson 2001). However, the increasing trend towards discharging patients early from hospital settings and ventures such as 'hospital at home' schemes may alter this view. In the community setting sharps generated by people such as those taking insulin for diabetes should be placed in sharps bins and some local authorities arrange for the collection of these from chemists. If sharps bins are not available, then other forms of rigid containers are sometimes used and/or the needles are blunted with needle clippers.

Local authorities have a legal obligation to provide a collection service for infectious waste if requested, but this often applies only to patients known to be infected with blood-borne viruses or those undergoing kidney dialysis. Some patients feel that collection infringes on their right to confidentiality and for this reason prefer to transport waste to their local GP or health centre for subsequent disposal.

Summary

- The different categories of waste must be disposed of safely and appropriately to prevent hazards to NHS staff and the public.
- Nurses are highly involved in the generation of clinical waste and must, therefore, show understanding of, and responsibility towards, the correct disposal of clinical waste.

CHAPTER SUMMARY

This chapter started by explaining standard principles and precautions that are recommended to prevent cross-infection. Each section of the chapter has focused on the practical skills involved and how they can be applied in different situations. Having worked your way through this chapter you should now be aware of the fundamental principles that underpin the prevention of cross-infection. The principles are relevant to all other practical nursing skills, and this chapter will, therefore, be referred to within many other chapters in this book.

Health care-associated infections are very costly. They cause patient distress and anxiety and increase the length of hospital stay. There is also the additional cost of specific treatments such as antibiotics as well as increased cleaning agents. Other costs include the extra materials needed to care for a person with an infection, ranging from protective clothing to dressings and many other disposable items. Additionally the cost of the multidisciplinary team including nurses is increased. A longer term cost is the delay in returning to work, which can have negative financial implications both for patients and for the state. Finally there is the cost related to the delayed admission to hospital of other people needing treatment.

The Code of Professional Conduct (Nursing and Midwifery Council 2002) demands that nurses protect and support the health of individual patients and clients and the health of the wider community whilst at the same time being personally accountable for their practice. Therefore there is a professional as well as moral imperative to aid the prevention of cross-infection. This is of fundamental importance to the health, safety and well-being of patients, nurses and other health care practitioners alike.

REFERENCES

Ayliffe, G.A.J., Babb, J.R. and Taylor, L.J. 2001. *Hospital-acquired Infection: Principles and prevention*, third edition. London: Arnold.

Barnett, J., Thomlinson, D., Perry, C. *et al.* 1999. An audit of the use of manual handling equipment and their microbiological flora – implications for infection control. *Journal of Hospital Infection* **43**, 309–13.

Blythe, D., Keenlyside, D., Dawson, S.J. and Galloway, A. 1998. Environmental contamination due to methicillin-resistant staphylococcus aureus (MRSA). *Journal of Hospital Infection* **38**, 67–70.

Callaghan, I. 1998. Bacterial contamination of nurses' uniforms: a study. *Nursing Standard* **13**(1), 37–42.

Carr, J. and Wilson, B. 1987. Self-help skills: washing, dressing and feeding. In Yule, W. and Carr, J. (eds) *Behaviour Modification for People with Mental Handicaps*. London: Croom Helm, 143–60.

Cochrane, J. 2000. Moral precepts of hand washing in a community healthcare setting. *Journal of Community Nursing* **14**, 19–20.

Curran, E. 1991. Protecting with plastic aprons. *Nursing Times* **87**(38), 64, 66, 68.

Dancer, S.J. 2002. Handwashing hazard? *Journal of Hospital Infection* **52**, 76.

Department of Health 2001. *Valuing People: A new strategy for learning disability for the 21st century*. London: DH.

Department of Health 2003. *Winning Ways: Working together to reduce healthcare associated infection in England*. London: DH.

Devine, J., Cooke, R.P.D. and Wright, E.P. 2001. Is methicillin-resistant staphylo-coccus aureus (MRSA) contamination of ward-based computer terminals a surrogate marker for nosocomial MRSA transmission and handwashing compliance? *Journal of Hospital Infection* **48**, 72–5.

Donovan, S. 1998. Wound infection and swabbing. *Professional Nurse* **13**, 757–9.

Emerson, E. 1992. What is normalisation? In Brown, H. and Smith, H. (eds) *Normalisation: A reader for the nineties*. London: Routledge, 1–15.

Emmerson, A.M., Enstone, J.E., Griffin, M. *et al.* 1996. The second national preva-lence survey of infection in hospitals. *Journal of Hospital Infection* **32**(3), 175–90.

Fletcher, L. and Buka, P. 1999. *A Legal Framework for Caring: An introduction to law and ethics in health care*. London: Macmillan.

Gammon, J. 1999a. Isolated instance. *Nursing Times* **95**(2), 57–60.

Gammon, J. 1999b. The psychological consequences of source isolation: a review of the literature. *Journal of Clinical Nursing* **8**, 13–21.

Gould, D. 1994. The significance of hand drying in the prevention of infection. *Nursing Times* **90**(47), 33–5.

Gould, D. and Brooker, C. 2000. *Applied Microbiology for Nurses*. London: Macmillan.

Hanrahan, A. and Reutter, L. 1997. A critical review of the literature on sharps injuries: epidemiology, management of exposures and prevention. *Journal of Advanced Nursing* **25**, 144–54.

Health Services Advisory Committee of the Health and Safety Executive 1992. *Safe Disposal of Clinical Waste*. Sheffield: HMSO.

Health Service Advisory Committee 1999. *Safe Disposal of Clinical Waste*. Sudbury: HSE Books.

Hollinworth, H. and Kingston, J. 1998. Using a non-sterile technique in wound care. *Professional Nurse* **13**, 226–9.

Kiernan, M. 1997. Disposing of sharps at home. *Community Nurse* **3**(1), 34.

Lacey, S., Flaxman, D., Scales, J. and Wilson, A. 2001. The usefulness of masks in preventing transient carriage of epidemic methicillin-resistant staphylococcus aureus by healthcare workers. *Journal of Hospital Infection* **48**, 308–11.

Lowbury, E.J. 1991. Special problems in hospital antisepsis. In Russell, A.D., Hugo, W.B. and Ayliffe, G.A.J. (eds) *Principles and Practice of Disinfection, Preservation and Sterilisation.* Oxford: Blackwell Science, 310–29.

MacKenzie, D. and Edwards, A. 1997. MRSA: the psychological effects. *Nursing Standard* **12**(11), 49–51.

Meers, P., Sedgwick, J. and Worsley, M. 1995. *The Microbiology and Epidemiology of Infection for Health Science Students.* London: Chapman and Hall.

Miller, M. 1998. How do I diagnose and treat wound infection? *British Journal of Nursing* **7**, 335–8.

MRSA Working Party Report 1998. Revised guidelines for the control of methicillin-resistant staphylococcus aureus infection in hospitals. *Journal of Hospital Infection* **39**, 253–90.

Myatt, R. and Langley, S. 2003. Changes in infection control practice to reduce MRSA infection. *British Journal of Nursing* **12**, 675–81.

Naikoba, S. and Hayward, A. 2001. The effectiveness of interventions aimed at increasing handwashing in healthcare workers – a systematic review. *Journal of Hospital Infection* **47**, 173–80.

National Institute for Clinical Excellence (NICE) 2003. *Infection Control. Prevention of healthcare-associated infection in primary and community care.* London: NICE. Available from http://www.nice.org.uk. Accessed 2 January 2004.

NHS Executive 1999. *Controls Assurance Standard. Waste Management.* Wetherby: Department of Health.

Nursing and Midwifery Council 2002. *Code for Professional Conduct.* London: NMC.

Oldham, T. 1998. Isolated cases. *Nursing Times* **94**(11), 67–9.

Orchard, H. 1998. Infection with MRSA: why it is still a growing problem. *Nurse Prescriber/Community Nurse* **4**(9), 46–8.

O'Toole, S. 1997. Disposable gloves. *Professional Nurse* **13**, 184–7, 189, 190.

Parker, L.J. 1999. Current recommendations for isolation practices in nursing. *British Journal of Nursing* **8**, 881–7.

Parker, L. 2000. Is protective isolation necessary? *Nursing Times NT Plus* **96**(46), 10–12.

Pratt, R.J., Pellowe, C., Loveday, H.P. *et al.* 2001. The epic project: developing national evidence-based guidelines for preventing healthcare associated infections. Phase 1: Guidelines for preventing hospital-acquired infections. *Journal of Hospital Infection* **47** Suppl: S1–82.

Price, P.B. 1938. The classification of transient and resident microbes. *Journal of Infectious Disease* **63**, 301–8.

Public Health Medicine Environmental Group 1996. *Guidelines on control of infection in residential and nursing homes.* London: Department of Health.

Rampling, A., Wiseman, S., Davis, L. *et al.* 2001. Evidence that hospital hygiene is important in the control of methicillin-resistant *Staphylococcus aureus*. *Journal of Hospital Infection* **49**, 109–6.

Russell, P. 1997. Reducing the incidence of needlestick incidents. *Professional Nurse* **12**, 275, 276, 278.

Simpson, C. 1998/9. Infection control. *Paediatric Nursing* **10**(10), 30–3.

Suviste, J. 1996. The toy trap uncovered. *Nursing Times* **92**(10), 56–9.

Swann, C. 1997. Development of Services. In Gates, B. (ed.) *Learning Disabilities*, third edition. London: Churchill Livingstone, 39–54.

Thomlinson, D. 1987. To clean or not to clean? … cleaning discharging surgical wounds. *Nursing Times* **83**(9), 71, 73, 75.

Thomson, G. and Bullock, D. 1992. To clean or not to clean? … cleaning trolleys before dressings. *Nursing Times* **88**(34), 66, 68.

Tortora, G.J., Funke, B.R. and Case, C.L. 1998. *Microbiology: An introduction*, sixth edition. California: Benjamin Cummings.

Weightman, N.C. and Kirby, P.J.G. 2000. Nosocomial *Escherichia coli* 0157 infection. *Journal of Hospital Infection* **44**, 107–11.

Weltman, A.C., Short, L.J., Mendelson, M.H. *et al.* 1995. Disposal-related sharps injuries at a New York city teaching hospital. *Infection Control and Hospital Epidemiology* **16**, 268–74.

Williams, C. 1996. Irriclens: a sterile wound cleanser in an aerosol can. *British Journal of Nursing* **5**, 1008–10.

Wilson, J. 2000. *Clinical Microbiology and Introduction for Health Care Professionals*, eighth edition. London: Baillière Tindall.

Wilson, J. 2001. *Infection Control in Clinical Practice*, second edition. London: Baillière Tindall.

Administration of medicines

Veronica Corben

In almost every practice setting, nurses administer medicines or supervise their administration. In order to do this safely, nurses require a breadth of knowledge including pharmacology, legal and policy issues, how to administer medicines via a variety of routes and how to do calculations. Only a registered nurse can administer drugs unsupervised, but to develop competence requires considerable experience and practice. Therefore students need to take every opportunity to build up their knowledge and skills during the pre-registration nursing programme.

This chapter includes:
- Legal and professional issues in medicine administration
- Safety, storage and general principles of medicine administration
- Administration of oral medication
- Application of topical medication
- Administration of medication by injection routes
- How to calculate drug doses.

Note that administration of inhaled and nebulised medication is included in Chapter 11 'Respiratory care: assessment and interventions' and administration of rectal medication (via suppositories or enemas) is included in Chapter 8 'Meeting elimination needs'.

> **Recommended biology reading:**
> It is important that you have an understanding of how drugs are absorbed, and how they reach the site where their action is required. The following questions will help you to focus on the biology underpinning this chapter's skills. Use your recommended text book to find out:
>
> - What are drugs? What do they do? How do they know where to act?
> - How do they achieve their effects?
> - What are placebos? When might they be used?

- What do the terms bioavailability, agonist and antagonist mean?
- Which routes of administration would be described as enteral and which as parenteral?
- What factors will affect the absorption rate of orally administered drugs?
- What is the first pass effect?
- Drugs often have unwanted side effects. What do the terms nephrotoxic and hepatotoxic mean?
- In order to be effective, levels of the drugs must be within the therapeutic range. What could happen following the administration of a wrong dose?
- Drugs must be metabolized in order to be eliminated from the body. Where does drug metabolism occur?
- How are drugs excreted from the body?
- What factors will affect the absorption, distribution, metabolism and elimination of drugs?
- What do the terms drug interactions, drug toxicity, drug tolerance, drug dependence and drug addiction mean?

It will also be useful to revise the structure of the skin.

Note that the introductory chapters in the following books are helpful:

Hopkins, S.J. 1999. *Drugs and Pharmacology for Nurses*, thirteenth edition. Edinburgh: Churchill Livingstone.

Prosser S., Worster B., MacGregor J. *et al.* 2000. *Applied Pharmacology: An introduction to pathophysiology and drug management for nurses and healthcare professionals*. London: Harcourt Publishers.

Trounce, J. 2000. *Clinical Pharmacology for Nurses*, sixteenth edition. New York: Churchill Livingstone.

PRACTICE SCENARIOS

The following practice scenarios illustrate situations where medicines are being administered via several different routes, and where nurses require knowledge of these drugs' actions and side effects, as well as how to store and administer them safely. They will be referred back to throughout the text.

Adult

Mercy Makumbe is 68 years old. She has recently had a below-knee amputation of her leg, has a long history of cardiovascular disease, and has now been transferred to her local community hospital, where she is currently receiving subcutaneous heparin, as well as oral morphine solution for pain. For years she has taken diuretics and other medication for her cardiac problems and she is concerned about having to take regular strong pain-relieving medicines too. She has also been prescribed fucidin cream for a small infected area behind one ear. A recent urinalysis showed blood in her urine.

EMLA cream

EMLA (eutectic mixture of local anaesthetics) contains local anaesthetic and when applied to the skin enables an intravenous cannula to be inserted or blood to be taken (venepuncture) without causing pain. It is used extensively with children but can also be used for adults with needle phobia. At least 45 minutes must be allowed post application to produce adequate analgesia.

Down's syndrome

This is a congenital condition caused by an extra chromosome, often leading to a characteristic physical appearance and a low IQ. Other physical effects (e.g. heart disease) are often associated with it. There is an increased risk of dementia at a younger age.

Dementia

This is chronic and progressive in nature, has many causes and commonly presents with memory and language impairment, decline in self-care ability, and behavioural and personality changes (Jacques and Jackson 2000).

Health facilitator

A member of the community learning disabilities team (often a nurse) who supports a person with learning disabilities to access the health care they need. See 'Valuing people' (Department of Health 2001a).

Child

Daisy Wheeler is 17 months old. She has been unwell for several days, and her GP prescribed oral amoxicillin 2 days ago for a suspected urinary tract infection. Daisy remains unwell, being hot, lethargic and irritable, and so she has been referred to the children's ward for further investigations. On the ward, Daisy has **EMLA cream** applied to the back of her hands, as she is to have blood tests. She is pyrexial, and receiving regular paracetamol to control this – her mother says she is sometimes reluctant to take it.

Learning disability

Sheila Payne, a 56-year-old woman, has **Down's syndrome** and has been diagnosed with **dementia**. She lives in a large group home. Every day from about 2 pm she becomes very distressed and starts shouting and screaming; these are considered to be symptoms of her dementia. She has been prescribed promazine on an 'as required' basis, but the support workers are reluctant to administer the drug, as they are unused to giving drugs on this basis and are concerned about whether it might have side effects. Her **health facilitator** is the community nurse for learning disabilities and she is visiting regularly at present to give support.

Mental health

Malcolm Barber is 49 years old and has a long history of schizophrenia. His main carer is his wife. His condition was stabilised on oral medication, until he experienced side effects of weight gain and akathesia (an inability to sit still). Because of these side effects, he stopped taking the medication, began to neglect himself and developed symptoms of psychosis. This deterioration led to his admission to an acute mental health unit as a voluntary patient. On admission he was given a test dose of a depot, which is a slow-release injection of an anti-pyschotic drug. This led to an improvement in his mental state, with minimal side effects. The plan is for him to continue with these injections two weekly at his local surgery.

LEGAL AND PROFESSIONAL ISSUES IN MEDICINE ADMINISTRATION

There are a number of legal and professional issues relating to managing safety of drugs which must be adhered to by nurses.

LEARNING OUTCOMES

By the end of this section you will be able to:

1. Identify key aspects of legislation, policies and professional issues governing drug administration.
2. Understand important professional issues for nurses who are administering medicines.

Learning outcome 1: Identify key aspects of legislation, policies and professional issues governing drug administration

Activity

Who do you think might provide rules about drug administration? Discuss this with one of your colleagues. It may help to consider abuse of drugs, and who regulates this. What have you seen about drug safety in magazines and on television?

All major issues related to managing the prescribing and safety of medicines are regulated by Government legislation. This means that all issues connected with medicines management involve legal as well as professional issues (Griffith and Griffiths 2003).

This is different to most activities nurses undertake. Traditionally medicines were prescribed by doctors. However legislation has recently been passed to permit specially trained nurses to prescribe certain medicines in specific circumstances without requiring a doctor to do so (Griffith and Griffiths 2003). This is known as nurse prescribing. In the future, more nurses will be able to prescribe a wider range of drugs.

Activity

See if you can find a nurse who is able to prescribe and ask him/her about what this involves. You will probably be doing it one day!

You are probably aware that there is government legislation that covers abuse of drugs, sale of medicines over the counter, labelling of medicines, and pharmacies in supermarkets. There are two important acts of parliament that provide this public protection, and infringement of these is a criminal offence. They are:

- The **Misuse of Drugs Act, 1971**, which controls the storage, sale and administration of controlled (addictive) drugs (see below).
- The **Medicines Act, 1968**, which controls the labelling, sale and distribution of all medicines, and established a licensing system.

Useful categories of medicines defined in the Medicines Act (Hopkins 1999) are:

1. **Prescription only medicines (POM)**: These can only be obtained on a prescription. In hospitals almost all medicines are POM, and therefore each patient has a prescription chart. If you have any medicines prescribed by your GP take a look at the label; you will see that POM is clearly written on it.
2. **General Sale List (GSL)**: This is a restricted list of simple medicines that can be freely sold through almost any outlet, for example garages and supermarkets. However there is control over these too, in hospital settings.
3. **Pharmacy only medicines (P)**: These can only be sold in the presence of a pharmacist, but do not require a prescription.

Activity

Can you think of an example for each of the above three categories of medicines?

Appropriate examples would be: POM – antibiotics; GSL – aspirin; and P – cough mixtures. There are many other examples of course.

Controlled drugs

Activity

'Controlled drugs' were briefly mentioned above. Can you think why a drug should need to be controlled in some special way? What might make a drug particularly dangerous if people could access it easily?

A controlled drug is addictive, because of the probable dependency that could result from it. These drugs may not be as toxic to the body as others that are more easily available. For example, taking an overdose of just ten paracetamol tablets can be fatal but these are not controlled. However, access to pethidine, morphine or any other drugs of the family that we call 'opiates' (because they are derived from opium), can cause addiction, with all its consequences, very quickly if taken for non-therapeutic reasons. These drugs are therefore dangerous and their sales need to be controlled because of their addictiveness, not their toxicity. They are controlled under the Misuse of Drugs Act, 1971, already mentioned. Mercy, like many other patients, may be anxious about taking morphine because of this view of potentially addictive drugs. This issue is considered in Chapter 12, in a discussion about analgesics.

Since 1985, controlled drugs have been subject to different levels of restriction (Nursing and Midwifery Council 2002), and are divided into five separate 'schedules', for example temazepam, a form of night sedation, is a schedule 4 drug, whereas pethidine is a schedule 2 drug. Scheduled drugs need to be kept in even more safe conditions than others. In in-patient settings, schedule 2 drugs have to be kept within two locked cupboards, and local policy may require drugs from other schedules to be kept in these conditions too. In people's homes, schedule drugs must also be kept very securely, but the level of safety has to be negotiated with the people concerned, because it is within their property (Hopkins 1999).

Controlled drugs can only be ordered by a registered nurse, and must be administered by a registered nurse with a second checker, who fits the criteria for a checker for the local drug policy. This may vary in community settings and where people may be self-medicating. You will need to check these details in every setting you work in, and try to access the appropriate drug policy. Checking administration of controlled drugs requires an understanding of the gravity of the issue, as detailed above. For this reason, student nurses may be able to check these drugs, but in some areas this may not be permitted. It might be that local policy is that you can be a checker once you enter the branch. Your local drug policy, referred to later, will inform you. Checking during administration involves the whole procedure from preparing the drug with each checker individually calculating the dose, administration of the drug and disposal of any remaining drug and equipment. This means that if you were the second checker when Mercy receives her morphine, you would have to accompany the staff nurse throughout the procedure. As a student nurse, you need to feel confident to check and give such drugs. You may decide that you need more observational practice and knowledge before being prepared to take on such a role.

Registers of controlled drugs must include details of stock and drugs administered, and must be signed by both persons providing such detail. They should be kept for at least 2 years (Hopkins 1999).

Activity	As you are now aware, there are laws that govern administration of medicines. Can you think of other organisations that may be involved in drug regulation too?

You should have included professional bodies and employers.

Professional bodies

Professional bodies involved in drug regulation in the UK include the British Medical Association, the Royal Pharmaceutical Society of Great Britain and the Nursing and Midwifery Council (NMC). Pharmacists provide expert knowledge about drugs, and often have an information adviser who can provide instant and accurate advice. Initiatives to expand the role of community pharmacists and to improve GP collaboration continue to be developed (Pilling *et al.* 1998). The NMC issues guidance via statements of principles on many issues, including administration of medicines, to all its registered nurses in all branches. It is vital that nurses read these and abide by them, to protect patients/clients and themselves professionally. The booklet *Guidelines for the Administration of Medicines* (Nursing and Midwifery Council 2002) makes it clear that drug administration is about thought and judgement as well as a task, and that registered nurses must take personal accountability for their actions.

Activity	You may have been provided with a copy of the above-mentioned NMC booklet, but if not look at a copy in the library or ask a registered nurse to show you their copy. You can also download it from the NMC's website (www.nmc-uk.org).

In relation to Sheila's medication, the care staff have responsibility for administering her medication, which will be prescribed by Sheila's GP and supplied by the local pharmacy. However, the community nurse for learning disabilities has a duty of care to Sheila and her role is to educate the staff about how to give 'as required' medication. She can also support them in monitoring the effect of the medicine, observing for any side effects, and supporting Sheila to access her GP if alternative medication would be more appropriate. The nurse has accountability for this educational and supportive role. Although as a student you are not professionally accountable you need to be thinking about these issues in preparation for becoming a registered nurse. The nurse could also involve other members

Health Action Plan
A personal action plan developed for each individual with a learning disability, containing details of their health interventions, medication taken, screening tests etc. See *Valuing People* (Department of Health 2001a).

of the community team concerning ways of helping Sheila. All these elements relating to Sheila's medication will be documented in her **Health Action Plan**.

Employers

Employers, both private health care employers and NHS Trusts, also produce drug policies for their individual organisations. Group homes, such as the one where Sheila lives, will have a policy about medicine administration. These policies contain useful information in a usually easily read form, and they refer to the student role and other issues too. They should always be accessible in practice areas, even if you do not have your own copy. It is one of the most important documents in all areas of practice! Staff must work to the regulations set out in their particular employer's policy.

Activity

Find out where the drug policy is kept in your current, or next, practice placement.

Learning outcome 2: Understand important professional issues for nurses who are administering medicines

Professional issues of particular relevance are personal accountability, knowledge and honesty.

Personal accountability

As with all interventions carried out by registered nurses, when administering medicines a registered nurse takes personal accountability for his or her actions. This means that if you as a student give out medication under supervision, the registered nurse is accountable for what you do, as well as for what they do themselves.

Knowledge

Nurses need to have a working understanding of medicines administered, therapeutic dosages and side effects (Watt 2003). As a student, you need to have a basic knowledge of the medicines you are involved in administering and continue to develop this throughout your pre-registration programme, and after registration. New medicines are constantly being developed and knowledge about existing medicines is expanding.

Activity

Look back at the scenarios and identify any examples where there could be particular issues about side effects of medicines. Why do you think nurses need to know about side effects of the drugs they are administering, and where do you think you could find out about these?

The side effects from Malcolm's oral medication were so unpleasant that he stopped taking these drugs, leading to a recurrence of his mental health symptoms.

A urinalysis has shown blood in Mercy's urine (haematuria). Nurses caring for her would need to be aware that this could be a side effect of the heparin she is prescribed as heparin is an anticoagulant. Morphine has a number of unpleasant side effects including constipation, and these might cause Mercy to be reluctant to take them. Promazine, which Sheila is taking, is a phenothiazine, and this group of medicines have a number of possible side effects. It is also worth noting that people with learning disabilities may be hypersensitive to medication or may experience side effects different to those commonly expected. Medicines have generally not been trialled with this client group. Therefore staff should be extra vigilant for any unusual effects when medication is prescribed for a person with learning disabilities.

There is a compendium called the *British National Formulary* (BNF) which provides up-to-date information about all aspects of drugs, including side effects. This book should be available in all clinical settings but the BNF can also be accessed at www.bnf.org. This would help you understand why Malcolm's medication has been changed. This compendium would also be useful in Mercy's case, where she is taking a variety of medicines together, and you may want to know about their interactions. If a person is taking four or more medicines this is referred to as polypharmacy and it is known to be associated with problems such as falls (Department of Health 2001b).

Honesty

If you have reason to suspect an error in the administration of a medicine, always report it immediately to the nurse in charge. Similarly if you do not agree with a dosage or any other aspect of a prescription, always have the courage to say. Errors cannot be retracted, and the patient is the one who ultimately suffers. When administering medicines to children, incorrect administration is even more serious, as they have less physiological reserve to cope with errors (Woodrow 1998). An atmosphere of openness and honesty is now being positively encouraged in this respect at all times (Nursing and Midwifery Council 2002).

Summary

- Administration of medicines by a student must be under direct supervision of a registered nurse.
- Administration of medicines must comply with both legal and professional requirements, therefore nurses must be familiar with the relevant legislation and written guidance from the NMC and work within their employers' policies.
- Nurses must take responsibility for developing their knowledge about the medicines they are administering, and recognise their personal accountability in relation to the administration of medicines.

SAFETY, STORAGE AND GENERAL PRINCIPLES OF MEDICINE ADMINISTRATION

LEARNING OUTCOMES

By the end of this section you will be able to:

1. Discuss issues concerning the safety and storage of medicines.
2. Understand the general principles of medicine administration.

Learning outcome 1: Discuss issues concerning the safety and storage of medicines

The Duthie report (1988) recommended safety procedures for storing and handling drugs.

Activity

When you are next in practice, ask a practitioner what these safety procedures are and check them with the points below.

You should have found out about the following:

- **A safe place**: This will be different depending on the setting, for example in hospital, this will be in a locked cupboard or immobilised medicine trolley, but in a person's home it could be the kitchen table, if a patient is immobile and lives alone. Remember: even lotions and cleaning agents need to be stored like medicines, in a locked or safe place, especially where there are children around, as in Daisy's family. In some settings, for example community hospitals, where Mercy is a patient, patients may have their own locked cupboards where they can access their medication themselves (Nursing and Midwifery Council 2002). It is important that continuous assessment of patients' competency to self-medicate is performed, and appropriate documentation completed. As discussed earlier, controlled (addictive) drugs, like morphine, should be kept within two locked cupboards.
- **A cool place**: Medicines are often quite unstable chemically, and may even be manufactured with a stabiliser included in the chemical compound. They generally become more unstable if warm, hence a cool dark place, away from direct sunlight is most suitable for storage. This is why medicines are usually stored in dark bottles. Some drugs need to be stored in a refrigerator, for example insulin and some antibiotics, sedatives and atypical depot injections. Daisy's antibiotics will be in liquid form and need to be kept in a fridge. In residential settings of any kind, a separate locked drugs fridge should be used which has a visible temperature gauge on the outside, and the temperature is regulated to 8°C (Hopkins 1999).

■ **Stock rotation**: As with food storage, medicines need to be kept in chronological order, with new items put to the back, and the older ones used first. The unqualified staff working in Sheila's group home would need to be aware of this. Remember: where the expiry date is given as a month and year, the medicine can be used until the last day of that month.

■ **Labelling of medicines**: Most UK medicines have an approved (non-proprietary) name and a brand (proprietary) name. The approved name is the chemical name, and is used by all prescribers. The brand name may be different, depending on the company who has produced it. For example, cold remedies may contain the same constituents, but be marketed under different names. This could cause confusion, so all prescriptions should display the approved name, especially in hospital settings (Sexton and Braidwood 1999) and this is strictly controlled under the Medicines Act (1968). European law now requires use of the Recommended International Non-proprietary Name (rINN) for medicines (BNF 2004). Most British approved names (BANs) are the same as the rINNs but a few BANs have had to be altered, and are listed in the BNF. For example, frusemide, a commonly prescribed diuretic, will be known as furosemide. Medicine containers are labelled with a number specific to a batch of medicines produced at the same time. For this reason medicines should never be transferred from one container to another. Labels could also be misread and different medicines be mixed in the same container.

■ **Holding drugs keys**: These should always be held by a registered nurse, preferably the nurse in charge. As a student therefore, you should never hold keys.

In areas where there is no registered nurse, as in some settings for people with learning disabilities like Sheila's group home, you may be advised not to be involved in drug administration. This is because staff will be unable to comply with professional regulations (Nursing and Midwifery Council 2002) although, as discussed earlier, there will be a different policy in place. Talk to your lecturers about this.

Learning outcome 2: Understand the general principles of medicine administration

Remember that the administration of drugs must be under direct supervision of a registered nurse until you qualify. Good patient/client assessment is vital before administering a drug of any kind.

■ **Activity**

> What precautions and preparations would you need to consider before giving medication to patients/clients by any route? A prescription chart may help you with your answer.

Box 4.1 outlines the points you should have considered and these are discussed in more detail below.

- Patient/client identity
- Allergies
- Consent
- Time
- Route
- Prescription
- Dose.

Box 4.1 Medicine administration: checks that should be made

- **Patient/client identity**: How do you know that this is the correct person for the drug? The use of identity bands in residential settings may provide the answer. However, the person may not have a name band, for example in out-patient settings, when a patient is newly admitted, or long-term residents in settings for older people or people with a learning disability, like Sheila. You will need to ask the person, or a friend or relative to tell you their name and date of birth, where possible. If you merely ask the person to acknowledge what you think their name is, they may agree regardless, because of their developmental level of functioning or if they are too unwell to think clearly.
- **Allergies**: Does the person have any allergies, for example to antibiotics? An allergic reaction to a drug could produce a serious local or systemic reaction – anaphylaxis. Anaphylaxis is a potentially life-threatening condition, and is discussed in detail by Henderson (1998).
- **Consent**: Does the person understand what the drug is for, and agree to it being given? Only in rare circumstances does consent not need to be given. Can you think what these situations might be? A situation where it might be acceptable to administer drugs without consent would be if the medication is considered essential (e.g. life saving) and the person is unconscious, very unwell, or unable to understand for developmental reasons. People who are detained under section 3 of the Mental Health Act (1983) (Department of Health and Welsh Office 1993) may be administered drugs to treat their mental health condition without consent, even if they have declined this treatment, for up to three months. However it is important to note that it is only the drug(s) required for their mental health condition, as specified on their section papers, that can be given without consent. Any other drugs prescribed (e.g. for a physical condition) can only be given with their consent. Appropriate presentation of the drug, for example in user-friendly containers, will increase the likelihood of it being taken (Ling 1999). A clear explanation about the drug and rationale for its prescription is also essential. The explanation should take into account level of understanding and developmental stage, as in Sheila's case. Parental consent must be gained when administering medicines to children (Watt 2003). Many packets of paediatric medicines contain leaflets particularly useful for parents.

- **Time**: Is the medicine due now or is it prescribed only if required by the person? Staff caring for Sheila need to understand about medicines prescribed only when necessary and how to assess whether they are needed. An inability to assess Sheila's condition could lead to her prescribed medication not being administered when needed, causing her distress, or to the medicine being prescribed unnecessarily on a regular basis. Malcolm and his wife need to understand the importance of him receiving his depot injection on exactly the correct day. Some drugs need to be taken with food if they need an acid medium in which to be metabolised, whereas others, for example flucloxacillin, should be taken on an empty stomach because an acid medium would break the drug down before it can be absorbed in its useful form (Caldwell 1999). Mercy is taking diuretics, which are usually prescribed in the morning, to prevent a diuresis late in the day or at night. She needs to understand that it is preferable to take morphine at regular intervals, instead of waiting until the pain is already severe. It is now known that paracetamol can be as effective as stronger painkillers when taken regularly rather than only when necessary. This is a good example of the importance of keeping up-to-date with evidence-based knowledge.

- **Route**: How is the drug to be given, and is this the most appropriate route? For example an oral route may not be appropriate if the person is feeling nauseated. Some drugs are only given by injection because they are destroyed by the gut. Heparin, as prescribed for Mercy, is one such example.

- **Prescription**: Is this written clearly throughout, including the drug itself (using the approved name), the date and signature of the doctor, and the route and time of administration? Is the person's name, and any special instructions, for example 30 minutes before food, clearly written? If any of this information is unclear or missing, the registered nurse must not give the drug (Henry 1998). Any alteration to a prescription must be signed and dated by the doctor. In an emergency, verbal messages may be taken over the phone by a registered nurse (Nursing and Midwifery Council 2002), and the prescription chart signed by the prescribing doctor within 24 hours. Many employers request that the drug is repeated to two nurses over the phone. Student nurses should not become involved in verbal messages. Again, always check local drug policy on these issues. You may find that abbreviations are used on prescription charts. The *British National Formulary* states that while generally directions on prescriptions should be written in English without abbreviations, it is recognised that some Latin abbreviations are used (www.bnf.org).

Activity	The following abbreviations are all recognised by the *British National Formulary*. What do they mean? (Answers are at the end of the chapter.) b.d., o.d., o.m., o.n., q.d.s., t.d.s., stat, e/c, i/m, m/r, mL, p.r.n.

■ **Dose**: Nurses have to decide or advise how much of a drug to give to a patient if the prescription gives a varied dose, for example 5–10 mg. This means exercising professional judgement. The nurse needs to consider if the dose appears correct for the person. Oral doses will often be larger than intravenous doses. This is because drugs have to pass through the gut and liver before entering the circulation, and some of the drug may be lost here, rather than entering the circulation directly. This is called the **first pass effect** (check up on your reading if necessary). This is why enteral drugs take longer to work than parenteral drugs, which do not have to pass via the liver first. You will also need to consider whether the dose involves a complex calculation or whether it is to be given to a child. In both these cases two nurses will be needed (Sexton and Braidwood 1999). At home, however, Daisy's mother will administer her medicines unsupervised. Remember, if a calculation has to be done both nurses need to work it out separately and then compare the answer, as otherwise it is really only one calculation. In children especially, the answer will usually be a small amount (Woodrow 1998).

 Activity   Check with your local drugs policy about your role as a student in being a checker for drug calculations and for administering drugs to children.

Summary

■ Nurses need to be familiar with legislation and local policies concerning storage of drugs and be aware of issues that could affect their safety.
■ It is crucial that drugs are stored safely, whether in hospital or in the community, and in appropriate conditions, thus maintaining their effectiveness.
■ There are a number of key safety principles that apply to drug administration by any route to any individual, and it is very important to adhere to these, to uphold safety of patients/clients.

ADMINISTRATION OF ORAL MEDICATION

LEARNING OUTCOMES

By the end of this section you will be able to:

1. Identify the different types of oral medication available.
2. Outline how to administer oral medication safely.

Learning outcome 1: Identify the different types of oral medication available

What types of oral medication have you seen? Devise a list with a colleague.

You may have considered:

- **Tablets**: These are convenient, are accurately dosed and relatively cheap. They often contain additives to prevent disintegration in the gastrointestinal tract.
- **Capsules**: These are oval-shaped, with a coat of hard gelatin. They are useful for bitter drugs, and for unpleasant liquid like chlormethiazole. Remember: never open capsules as they are made to be swallowed whole (Trounce 2000).
- **Elixirs and syrups**: These flavoured and sweetened liquids are particularly useful for children, as in Daisy's case. Many are sugar-free, especially those for children.
- **Emulsions**: These are a mixture of two liquids, one dispersed through the other (Trounce 2000), for example oil and water. They need to be shaken well to mix the contents.
- **Linctus**: This is a sweet syrupy preparation, for example cough linctus (Trounce 2000).

Note that there are two other forms of medicines which, although taken into the mouth, are not swallowed:

- **Sublingual medications**: These are produced as sprays or as tablets, and are absorbed through the mucosa under the tongue. As the sublingual area is very vascular, absorption and effect of the drug occur rapidly.
- **Buccal medications**: These medicines are usually produced as tablets, and are put onto the gum under the lip. Again, the effect of the drug is rapid.

When these routes are used, very careful instructions should be given so that the person fully understands that sublingual and buccal tablets should not be swallowed.

Learning outcome 2: Outline how to administer oral medication safely

Before administering any drug, you should know:

- What the drug is
- How it works
- The normal dosage, which in children is often calculated according to their weight (Woodrow 1998)

- Any side effects
- Any extra precautions you may need to tell the person.

We are now going to look at how you would actually give oral medication to a patient. What should you always do before any intervention with patients? You should, of course, wash your hands thoroughly (see Chapter 3) and gain consent, as discussed earlier. You should identify the appropriate bottle or packet of medicine that corresponds with the prescription. Check all the prescription details with the bottle label, and also the expiry date and any special instructions. Think also about the positioning of the person before administering. A baby or young child like Daisy will need holding, and an adult might also require effective support, as sitting up well (if not contraindicated) will make swallowing much easier and safer.

Liquids

For children, like Daisy, and people with swallowing difficulties, which includes some people with learning disabilities, most oral medicines prescribed will be in liquid form. Liquids are much more quickly absorbed than tablets because the gastrointestinal transit time is reduced (Caldwell 1999). Many paediatric suspensions are sold with a double-ended spoon, which can measure 2.5 and 5 mL volumes but 5 mL medicine syringes can be bought from chemists.

First shake the bottle for even distribution, then hold the bottle with the label uppermost, so that the medicine cannot flow over the label and deface it. Now carefully pour into a measuring glass, at eye level for accuracy. If the dose is 1 mL or less, use a 1 mL syringe and aspirate it directly from the bottle or via a quill, and then put the lid back on the bottle. It may be useful to use a syringe for withdrawing larger quantities too, as they are more accurate than medicine pots. This would be appropriate for measuring Mercy's morphine. The *British National Formulary* recommends that for any oral medication prescribed in doses other than multiples of 5 mL, an oral syringe should be used (www.bnf.org). Oral syringes have a different appearance from usual syringes and they should always be used for oral drugs, if available, to reduce risk of mistakes. For example if an oral medication is given intravenously in error, this would have serious or even fatal, consequences.

Tablets

If the tablets are in a bottle, tip the correct amount into the lid, and then tip into a medicine glass or spoon. The lid is as clean as the inside of the medicine bottle. Many tablets are now supplied in blister packs, so that they can be individually sealed and then pushed out through a foil backing into a medicine pot without being touched (Hopkins 1999). If a liquid form of a medicine is unavailable, and the person concerned cannot swallow tablets, it may be necessary to crush tablets in food. They might be more acceptable to a child if put in jam or ice cream etc. However tablets should only be crushed as a last resort (Wright 2002) and if medication (crushed tablets or liquid) is mixed with food this must be with the person's permission and not done with the intention of giving medicine without consent, which has significant legal, professional and ethical dimensions.

The UK Central Council for Nursing, Midwifery and Health Visiting (2001) released a statement looking in detail at this issue advising that such action can only be justified in exceptional circumstances, emphasising that mentally competent adults have a legal right to refuse treatment. Smith (2002) reviews the issue of covert administration of medicines in relation to older people, highlighting concerns from many quarters, including Action on Elder Abuse.

Some tablets should not be crushed as their action is damaged by the crushing action. These include long-acting or enteric-coated tablets, for example prednisolone (Sexton and Braidwood 1999).

Administering the medicine

You next need to decide how to administer the drug. Can the person self-administer or do you need to administer it on a spoon? Is the medicine best put into the mouth from a syringe? Parents will usually be the best people to administer medication to their child. Sheila's carers might wonder how they can give medication to her when she is so distressed. The nurse can educate them in recognising early signs that the medicine is needed to prevent this situation. For obvious reasons (prevention of cross-infection) never touch medication with your hand. If the person cannot self-administer, put it into their mouth using some form of utensil. Gentle downward stroking motions over the larynx may help with swallowing (Wong 1993). Always provide adequate fluids, about 50 mL for an adult, to ensure medication has been swallowed, and allow a choice of fluid, particularly with children. Ensure that the person has swallowed all the medication before documenting. A patient may pocket tablets, spit them out when you have gone or be unable to totally clear them from the mouth. Reward a child, at least verbally, if the medicine is taken well, but avoid negative behaviour if the reverse occurs.

■ **Activity**

For this exercise you need a tube of Smarties, a small cup, a bottle of water and a syringe. You should be able to access a syringe in the skills laboratory, but you may need permission – do check. Practise tipping a Smartie out into the lid and then into the cup without touching it. Then try drawing water up from the bottle with a syringe. Now try feeding Smarties on a spoon from a cup to a willing volunteer, taking care not to touch the sweet.

When documenting drug administration, the registered nurse must countersign the signature of any student they are supervising (Nursing and Midwifery Council 2002). If you are the second checker for a controlled drug you should sign the register, along with the registered nurse. If any prescribed drug is not given for some reason (e.g. refusal) this must also be documented and further action taken as necessary. After drug administration, clear away all equipment, and wash your hands again.

Consider how you would dispose of unwanted medicines. Tick below those methods you think should be used:

1. Return to chemist or pharmacy.
2. Put into a waste bin.
3. Put down a sink.
4. Flush down the toilet or sluice.
5. Kept safe for another time.

You should have ticked numbers one, three and four, and five in some circumstances (Duthie 1988). Medicines can always be returned to a chemist or the hospital pharmacy for disposal. Small quantities of medicine that have been either dropped or taken out of the container and then not required can be disposed of via the domestic waste, a sink or toilet, providing it is not contraindicated as being harmful even in small quantities, as with cytotoxic drugs. Medicines should never be put as they are into a waste bin, where someone else could have access to them. Unused medicines can be kept safe for another time, provided they are kept in the original container and are not part of a course, for example antibiotics, when the course should always be completed. When Daisy is discharged her parents will need to be aware of this.

Have a look at your local drugs policy and see what it says about disposal of drugs.

Remember: Nurses/carers need to evaluate whether the medication has been effective and whether side effects have occurred, as in Mercy's case. In children responses may be very different from those in adults (Watt 2003).

Summary

■ Both preparation and administration of oral medicines should be performed systematically, ensuring that drug policy is adhered to, promoting safety and prevention of cross-infection.
■ Careful assessment should ensure that the administration of oral medication is performed in an acceptable and appropriate manner for each individual, taking into account factors such as age and swallowing ability.

APPLICATION OF TOPICAL MEDICATION

The topical route consists of drug administration via the epidermis (outer layer of the skin) and external mucous membranes. It therefore includes administration into eyes and ears.

Remember: The same controls as described earlier for oral medicines apply to topical administration (Marsden 1998). Often these medicines are kept on bedside lockers and are not given at such precise times as other forms of medicines.

LEARNING OUTCOMES

By the end of this section you will be able to:

1. Understand the indications and preparations used for the topical route.
2. Show awareness of how topical medication is administered and the particular precautions that are necessary.

Learning outcome 1: Understand the indications and preparations used for the topical route

Activity

Mercy is prescribed fucidin cream for the small infected area behind her ear. Why might a topical antibiotic cream have been prescribed for her?

The topical route permits local rather than systemic absorption of the drug, and reduces its side effects on the body generally. In Mercy's case it would have been considered appropriate as the lesion is small and superficial. You read earlier that Daisy has had local anaesthesia (EMLA cream) applied to her skin and this is another example of topical medication applied to act on a local area. For children over one year, when the epidermis is fully developed, topical medication provides an effective and painless route (Choonera 1994).

Medications are increasingly becoming available in topical form. Common examples are patches applied to the skin being used for pain relief (fentanyl) or angina (glyceryl trinitrate). Many topical medications are designed to give a 24-hours slow release of the drug and therefore continuous action. Topical preparations also include drops into eyes and ears, where absorption occurs through the mucous membranes. Topical preparations reduce, but do not eliminate, unwanted systemic side effects (Marsden and Shaw 2003). There must be enough absorption from the site of application to be effective.

Topical preparations come in several forms:

- **Pastes**: These contain a large amount of powder and a little water in their composition, and are therefore fairly stiff, and may be difficult to spread (Hopkins 1999). Lids need to be carefully secured to prevent drying when exposed to the air, which would make them even drier in texture.
- **Creams**: These are easier to spread and less prone to solidification, as they are emulsions – either oil dispersed in water (e.g. aqueous cream), or water dispersed in oil.
- **Ointments**: These may be water- or oil-based, are semi-solid and are usually available in a tube. They are more occlusive and therefore better for dry lesions (Selli 1995). Creams and ointments should be applied exactly as prescribed, for example steroid creams are always applied very sparingly (Sexton and Braidwood 1999). Sometimes directions are given as a weight in grams and, as a rough guide, 2 g is a 10 cm length from a standard nozzle (Trounce 2000).

- **Patches**: Medication in this form comes sealed in a small patch, with a peel-off sheet, which exposes the adherent part to be placed on the skin. You need to follow the instructions for where it should be placed, but most are applied to the abdomen or chest, in a relatively hairless region if possible, and the site is alternated each time the patch is changed, usually every 24 hours. The skin needs to be sufficiently permeable to allow absorption, so areas with good vascularity, like the trunk, are preferable (Trounce 2000).

- **Drops**: Drops are presented in solution in either single-use containers called minims, or in a larger bottle with a pipette-type end or dropper. Care must be taken to ensure that they are used for one person only, that the expiry time once opened is observed, usually 28 days (Kelly 1994), and that they are refrigerated if indicated. Patients need to be aware of these instructions, never to stop drops without consulting a doctor, and to use one minim for each eye each time unless a bottle has been provided. Drops facilitate relatively rapid absorption compared with ointment, which provides a more sustained drug action, and less systemic toxicity (Kelly 1994).

- **Sprays**: These are produced in containers under pressure and enable a fine spray to be directed onto the area requiring it, for example nasally.

■ *Activity*	If you have access to a dropper, you may want to practise this skill onto a target on a piece of paper.

Learning outcome 2: Show awareness of how topical medication is administered, and the particular precautions that are necessary

■ *Activity*	Many of the principles which we have already discussed, for example explanation and consent, infection control and safety issues etc., apply to topical medication as well. Can you think of any extra precautions that might be necessary when administering topical medications?

While infection control is necessary when administering medication by any route, there are specific aspects relating to topical medication. Eyes in particular are highly susceptible to infection, which can have a devastating effect on sight. Creams and ointments must be applied to skin without risk to nurses or patients. Attention to hand decontamination is therefore essential, before and after application of topical medication. In addition you might have identified that the patient's position when topical medication is applied needs careful consideration.

Applying medication to eyes, ears and noses

Eyedrops and eye ointments should be applied with the face horizontal, the person preferably lying flat. Looking up reduces the blink reflex (Kelly 1994), as well

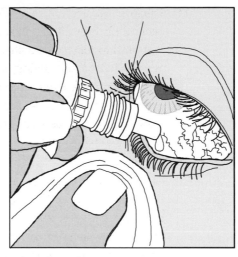

Figure 4.1 Administration of eyedrops.

as making it easier to get the drops or ointment into the correct place. Slowly squeeze the bulb when applying drops, and drop vertically, from as near to the patient as possible, without actually touching the eye. Always put the drop inside the lower lid (Fig. 4.1) (Marsden 1998). This holds the drops for approximately three times longer than the globe of the eye (Kelly 1994). Children need extra help to keep the eye still while instilling drops. Eyedrops can sting and some leave an aftertaste at the back of the throat (Marsden 1998).

Ensure the eye is kept shut for 60 seconds after application, and always instill drops before ointment, if both are being used, as the ointment leaves a film over the eye, preventing the drops being absorbed. Eye ointment should be applied to the inside of the lower lid (Fig. 4.2), and the eye held closed afterwards for a short time, where possible. This enables the ointment to settle. Applications of ointment to the eye are therefore usually applied at night. Vision may be blurred afterwards for a while. Excess medication should be wiped away with a clean tissue.

If eye medication is being applied to both eyes, use separate products for each eye, and apply it to the least affected one first, to reduce the risk of spreading the infection.

For application into ears, lying with the ear to be treated uppermost is most effective, and for nasal sprays, the person should be upright. Nasal medication should be administered 20 minutes before food so that the nasal passages are clear, which makes eating easier. A useful tip is to ensure the patient has blown their nose or cleared their mouth or throat before administration and to follow closely any special instructions accompanying the spray.

Applying topical medication to the skin

For application of ointment or cream to the skin, gloves should be worn if someone other than the patient is applying the medication. This is partly to prevent

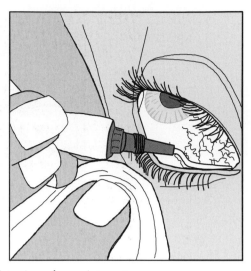

Figure 4.2 Administration of eye ointment.

cross-infection from you to the patient and vice versa, but also to prevent you absorbing any of the medication you are applying into your own skin. Encourage people to apply topical medication themselves to promote independence and reduce the risk of cross-infection, although this will not always be possible. For example, in Mercy's case it might be difficult with the sore area being behind her ear. Often a certain level of manual dexterity is required to apply topical medication and people need to be assessed for their ability to manage this treatment themselves. All stages of the skill will need to be taught, with handwashing explained carefully so that the medicine is not inadvertently transferred to other parts of the body. Young children may need coaxing from parents to co-operate.

Creams and ointments should be gently massaged in the direction of the hair flow (Selli 1995). Following application, it may be best for the patient to remain still for several minutes and the type of covering to be applied, if any, must be considered. People may require advice about clothing and instructions about possible staining or soiling. Remember: Always evaluate the effectiveness of the treatment and report and document progress or deterioration to the doctor or nurse in charge.

Summary

- Topical drugs are prepared in many different formats, and have a number of advantages, such as direct action on the affected area, and slow absorption through the skin.
- Specific instructions should be followed carefully.
- Measures to prevent cross-infection when administering topical medication are particularly important.

ADMINISTRATION OF MEDICATION BY INJECTION ROUTES

Nurses in most settings give injections on occasions, and it is therefore a practical skill that you will want to acquire during your pre-registration programme. However, injections, especially intramuscular ones, are being used less and less these days, so you need to make the most of any opportunity to give them (Hemsworth 2000). Intravenous injections are used more commonly in children than intramuscular ones now.

Note that **parenteral** means the administration of medication by a route other than via the gastrointestinal tract. This route includes all drug administration by injection and topical routes too. **Enteral** means absorption via the gastrointestinal tract only. This then includes all forms of oral administration. It may help you to review again the first pass effect and parenteral routes.

LEARNING OUTCOMES

By the end of this section you will be able to:

1. Appreciate the rationale for using the injection route.
2. Outline the principles of, and issues relating to, administering a drug by injection.
3. Discuss health and safety issues, especially for nurses, when giving injections.
4. Identify the key principles of practice for administering intramuscular and subcutaneous injections.

Learning outcome 1: Appreciate the rationale for using the injection route

Activity

What injection routes have you seen used and where do you think the point of the needle rested on administration? Why do you think these routes were chosen?

You may have seen injections into muscle (intramuscular), into the fat layer under the skin (subcutaneous), into veins through a cannula (intravenous) or under the skin (intradermal). Injections can also be given into joints, into the epidural space or directly into the heart. Note that as a student nurse you can only give intramuscular and subcutaneous injections, and this must be under direct supervision. That is why only these routes are discussed in this chapter.

To use the intravenous route you will require further training, and supervised practice as a registered nurse. The intradermal route is used mainly for local anaesthetic prior to invasive procedures. It is also used for some vaccines, for example the BCG against tuberculosis (Department of Health 1996). Registered nurses in some specialities undergo preparation to give intradermal injections. The other injection routes mentioned are mainly used by medical staff.

Note: Evidence-based literature related to injection technique is very limited, so you need to keep your reading up to date and abide by local policies. The Vaccination Administration Taskforce (VAT) (2001), when investigating all aspects of vaccine administration, thoroughly reviewed the literature relating to injection administration, and will be referred to where appropriate in this section.

Rationale for injections

Here are some of the situations in which an injection will be used rather than any other route for the administration of drugs:

- When speed of effect is required. The drug is more rapidly absorbed into the circulation when it avoids the gastrointestinal tract completely (Rodger and King 2000).
- When patients are nil by mouth.
- When the drug is destroyed by digestive enzymes in the gut, for example insulin.
- When long-term release of a drug is required, for example depot injections in mental health clients, as in Malcolm's case.

Key features of the intramuscular (I/M) route:

- The effects are more rapid than the subcutaneous route because of the good blood supply to skeletal muscles, so it takes approximately 10 minutes for the effect to begin (Rodger and King 2000).
- Skeletal muscle has relatively few pain receptors (Campbell 1995) so it should be fairly painless. However, not everyone would agree with this!
- Absorption can last for 2–5 weeks if desired, using oil-based, slow-release preparations, as in Malcolm's scenario.

Key features of the subcutaneous (S/C) route

- A large variety of sites are available as any subcutaneous tissue can be used (Campbell 1995).
- The injections are relatively painfree (Workman 1999).
- The speed of action is slower than the I/M route because of the poorer blood supply. The medication administered therefore has a longer duration, which can be useful.
- The person's ability to absorb needs to be considered. If peripheral circulation is poor, the drug may stay in the subcutaneous region and not be absorbed.

Learning outcome 2: Outline the principles of, and issues relating to, administering a drug by injection

Remember, all safety procedures for the oral route apply to injections too.

Activity

Consider the following issues in relation to I/M and S/C injections. What have you seen in practice?
- Skin cleaning
- Injection sites
- Syringe and needle selection.

Compare what you have observed with the points below.

Skin cleaning

Views vary considerably about this (Hemsworth 2000). Lawrence *et al.*'s study (1994) indicated that a 5-second disinfection time using alcohol-based swabs results in a 97 per cent reduction in all bacteria except spore-forming bacteria. Other studies have suggested that social cleanliness is sufficient (Koivisto and Felig 1978, Royal College of Paediatrics and Child Health 2002). Mallett and Dougherty (2000), while recognising the inconsistencies in the evidence, recommend skin cleaning prior to injections for patients who are immunocompromised and thus susceptible to infection.

The Vaccination Administration Taskforce (VAT) (2001) advises that skin cleansing is unnecessary in socially clean patients and that if cleansing is required soap and water is adequate. They warn that if spirit swabs are used, the site must be left to dry as vaccines can be inactivated by alcohol. The Royal College of Paediatrics and Child Health (2002) estimate the rate of abscess formation to be 1 per 1–2 million injections. They comment that skin preparation has been largely abandoned with no sudden increase in abscess occurrence and that formal skin preparation is not necessary prior to injection administration. Thus in practice, alcohol swabs are now rarely used prior to injections, with apparently no adverse effects, but you should check your local policy on this issue. Alcohol swabs are always contraindicated when subcutaneous insulin and heparin are administered, as alcohol interferes with the drug action and hardens the skin (Workman 1999).

Injection sites

The site used is influenced by such factors as age, medication to be injected and general client condition.

Intramuscular sites are shown in Fig. 4.3. In adults, up to 4–5 mL can be given into most sites, but only 1–2 mL in deltoid muscle. In children, much smaller amounts are acceptable.

The gluteus maximus muscle has the slowest uptake of medication, whereas the deltoid has the fastest (Trounce 2000). The deltoid is excellent for small volumes as the site area is small, and minimal undressing is required. The Vaccination Administration Taskforce (2001) recommended this site for vaccines in children over one year and adults. For children less than one year the deltoid muscle is insufficiently developed and the antero-lateral aspect of the thigh, the vastus lateralis, is recommended (VAT 2001). This muscle is easy to access, has few major blood vessels in the area and is suitable for all age groups. The rectus femoris muscle is useful for self-administration, but can leave considerable discomfort (Rodger

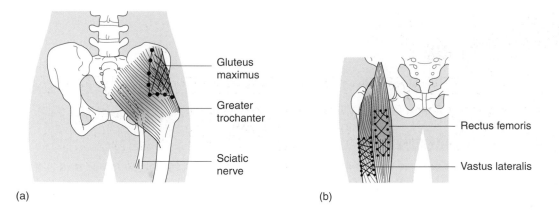

(a)

(b)

Gluteus maximus

Greater trochanter

Sciatic nerve

Rectus femoris

Vastus lateralis

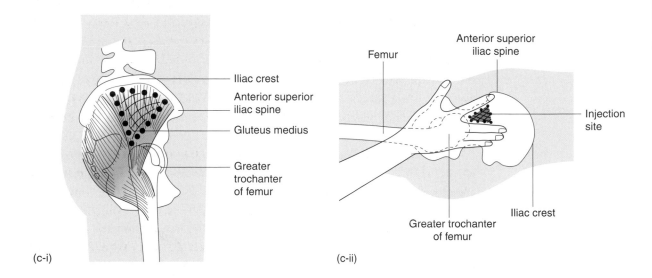

(c-i)

(c-ii)

Iliac crest

Anterior superior iliac spine

Gluteus medius

Greater trochanter of femur

Femur

Anterior superior iliac spine

Injection site

Greater trochanter of femur

Iliac crest

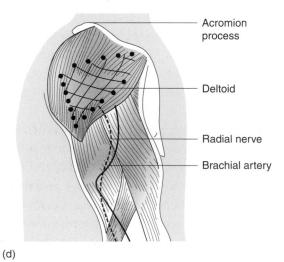

(d)

Acromion process

Deltoid

Radial nerve

Brachial artery

Figure 4.3 Intramuscular injection sites. (a) Gluteus maximus site (upper outer quadrant of buttock); (b) Quadriceps sites: vastus lateralis (outer middle third of thigh), rectus femoris (anterior middle third of thigh); (c-i) Ventrogluteal site (hip); (c-ii) Locating the ventrogluteal site; (d) Deltoid site (upper arm).

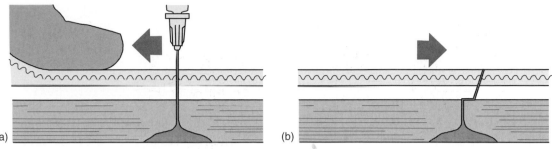

Figure 4.4 The Z-track technique. (a) Skin spread to the left on administration of intramuscular medication, (b) Skin released afterwards, showing formation of Z-track as a result.

and King 2000). The ventrogluteal site is a fairly new area to be used for injections, but is free of penetrating blood vessels and nerves and contains a large muscle mass, making it a good site to use for adults (Rodger and King 2000). However, though seen as the site of choice, it is rarely used by nurses in the UK, currently.

If the gluteus maximus muscle in the buttock is used, it is important to quarter the buttock first and then to administer in the upper outer quarter, thus avoiding the sciatic nerve totally. Any other quarter could cause nerve injury. This site is not recommended for infants and children (Royal College of Paediatrics and Child Health 2002).

Studies have indicated that when injecting intramuscularly it is beneficial to spread the skin 2–3 cm sideways (Fig. 4.4) to provide a Z-track, which reduces the chance of leakage and pain (Rodger and King 2000). Once the needle has entered the skin, it need not be stretched, as the exit point is now Z-shaped. This method will be advantageous when giving Malcolm his injection, as depot injections can cause discomfort. Some suggest that this technique should always be used (Keen 1990).

Subcutaneous sites are numerous, but the main ones are shown in Fig. 4.5. When administering by this route, ensure a skin fold is gently pinched to free the adipose tissue from the underlying muscle (Workman 1999). Patients should always be encouraged to give their own injections when possible. This is particularly applicable to people with diabetes who take insulin and have been admitted to hospital.

Syringe and needle selection

Syringes are selected according to the volume to be given. Volumes of 1 mL and under must be given in a 1 mL syringe, because of the smaller units of graduation, usually 0.1 mL. Some drugs require a special syringe. For example insulin needs a syringe that is marked off in units, which is how insulin is prescribed. Insulin syringes incorporate a needle as well. Some injections (e.g. low molecular weight heparin) are pre-prepared and these also have a needle attached. Otherwise needles are selected according to the route and sometimes according to the body adipose of the person. For example, for an I/M injection, if there is a large amount of adipose a longer needle will be required to ensure the drug

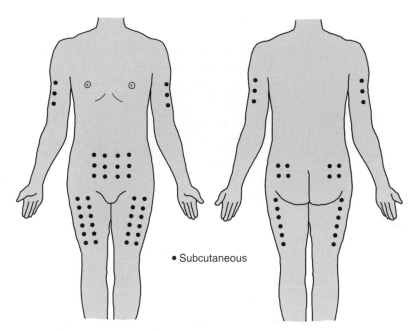

Figure 4.5 Subcutaneous sites for injection.

enters the muscle. Nurses sometimes underestimate the required needle length by trying to be kind to patients, but using too short a needle means that the drug does not enter the muscle (Newton *et al.* 1992).

Needles are colour coded according to their gauge (G); the higher the gauge the narrower the lumen of the needle. The Vaccination Administration Taskforce (2001) identifies standard UK sizes as:

- Green: 21 G and 38 mm (1½ in) long
- Blue: 23 G and 25 mm (1 in) long
- Orange: 25 G and 10 mm (⅜ in), 16 mm (⅝ in) or 25 mm (1 in) long.

In general, green needles are used for adult I/M injections and blue needles for child I/M injections. Orange needles are used for S/C injections, although as stated earlier, the most commonly given S/C injections have a short thin needle already attached to the syringe (insulin or low molecular weight heparin). As you can see, nurses should use a green needle for Malcolm's depot injection.

Learning outcome 3: Discuss health and safety issues, especially for nurses, when giving injections

Activity   What hazards might nurses encounter when administering injections?

Drug contamination

There can be a danger of contact dermatitis, particularly if there is frequent exposure to a certain drug. For example, a nurse making up a penicillin solution for injection could contaminate their hands with the drug. Repeated contact can cause skin sensitisation and, in these instances, gloves should be worn.

Needlestick injury

Apparently 3.4 per cent of recorded sharps injuries happen to student nurses (Infection Control Nurses Association (ICNA) 2003). The first thing to remember is that you should never re-sheath used needles. These are contaminated and should be left uncovered on the injection tray and disposed of immediately into a designated sharps container. A study by the Royal College of Nursing in 2000 revealed that 3.3 per cent of all sharps injuries occurred when used needles were re-capped (cited by ICNA 2003). Also put all syringes, needles and glass ampoules into the sharps container, first separating needles and syringes using the tapered slot on the top of the box (Campbell 1995). Never overfill the sharps box.

Despite these precautions, needlestick injuries can still occur (particularly when sharps boxes are overloaded), so what should you do if this happens?

- Remove the needle quickly.
- Encourage the wound to bleed by applying indirect pressure.
- Then place the injured area under cold running water.
- Cover with a dressing or plaster if required.
- Complete an incident form.

The Occupational Health Department policy will advise you as to whether further action is necessary. Chapter 3 'Preventing cross-infection' covers all these issues in detail. Further guidance can be found in your local Infection Control Policy, and the Infection Control Nurses' Association (2003) guidelines.

Note that unless the injection is prepared beside the person, you will need to re-sheath the **unused** needle carefully after drawing up the drug, to prevent the needle becoming contaminated on exposure to air.

Learning outcome 4: Identify key principles of practice for administering intramuscular and subcutaneous injections

Activity   Discuss with a colleague or lecturer any anxieties you may have about giving injections, and how this could affect your ability to administer safely. Remember that although injections can be uncomfortable, they have been prescribed to enhance recovery or relieve symptoms.

The steps when giving an I/M or S/C injection are discussed in points 1–18 below:

1. Ensure that the drug is due to be given, written up correctly, and that the patient has given consent. Look back to where consent was discussed earlier in this chapter if necessary. Appropriate explanation needs to be given taking into account ability to understand.
2. Wash your hands properly.

3. Assemble equipment: Injection tray or equivalent, appropriate syringe and needle, cottonwool swab (or alcohol swab if local policy), medication and diluent if required.

4. Check details of the medication, then draw it up either directly from the vial or, if powder, by mixing according to the manufacturer's instructions. When drawing up from a glass ampoule the Vaccination Administration Taskforce (2001) recommends using a needle no larger than 21 G to eliminate the risk of drawing up glass fragments. Some injections are supplied with a separate diluent and very specific instructions for preparation so always check carefully.

   ■ Always use the exact volume and diluent recommended to provide the most therapeutic concentration, and hold the syringe at eye level to achieve this.

   ■ Remember to check the vial for cracks, precipitation or cloudiness.

   ■ With multi-dose vials that have already been used, clean the rubber bung with an alcohol swab and allow it to dry before piercing.

   ■ Single-dose vials that have been newly opened do not need to be cleaned.

   Note: It is not always necessary to change needles after drawing up the liquid as the needles are made of steel and cannot be blunted easily and the more you tamper with the equipment, the more the risk of contamination. However the Vaccination Administration Taskforce (2001) recommends the needle is changed if it has had to pierce a rubber bung to draw up the medication.

5. Recheck the person's details and medication, consent and name band if appropriate. The approach you take to the person is very important in developing rapport and reducing anxiety about the injection. It is better not to state, nervously, that this is your first injection! With children, some form of simple distraction is very important (Watt 2003). This is also appropriate for people of other ages, including those with a learning disability.

6. Position the person comfortably, supporting the limbs if necessary. Depot injections like Malcolm's can be very uncomfortable. Babies and children should be held firmly. It is rare these days, however, for the I/M route to be used for children of any age, except when administering immunisations.

7. Identify the site. For I/M sites look again at Fig. 4.3. Take into account the volume of drug to be administered and convenience to the person when choosing the site. Some large injections need to be divided and given into two sites. An example is pabrinex, given to people undergoing alcohol detoxification, which is 7 mL – too large for any site. You should also rotate sites if repeated injections are being given. It helps to look at the muscle itself, especially in children, and check if it is of a large enough size to take the volume. Make sure a child has the ability to maintain the required position throughout the procedure. Young children are best held firmly on a parent's lap (Vaccination Administration Taskforce 2001).

What would be the I/M site of choice for:

(a) A fully dressed woman who is prescribed an I/M tetanus injection (0.5 mL)?
(b) A patient lying on his back in bed, who has abdominal pain which is worse on movement, and is prescribed an I/M injection of 100 mg of pethidine (2 mL) and 10 mg of metoclopramide (2 mL)?

The obvious sites would seem to be:

(a) The deltoid muscle, as this can take an injection of 1–2 mL and is less intrusive for this woman, who need only roll her sleeve up. You will remember from earlier that this is the preferred site for vaccinations (VAT 2001).

(b) This volume injection is too great for the deltoid. As this man has pain on movement, it would be better to inject into his thigh (vastus lateralis) so that he does not have to move.

8. Check the skin is socially clean and clean the skin if required to do so by local policy.

9. Intramuscular injections: spread the skin. Subcutaneous injections: bunch the skin, to release the subcutaneous tissue from the muscle. A study by Polak *et al.* (1999) showed that many subcutaneous injections in children in fact go into the muscle.

10. Hold the needle at approximately 90 degrees for all I/M and most S/C injections (as for insulin or low molecular weight heparin) (Katsma and Katsma 2000). If an S/C injection is being given with a longer needle the angle traditionally used is 45 degrees (Workman 1999) (Fig. 4.6).

11. Having first warned the patient, gently insert two-thirds of the needle into the skin.

12. With I/M injections, pull back on the plunger. If blood appears in the syringe, support the skin, withdraw the needle and try again (Hemsworth 2000). This is because the needle must have entered a capillary, and the route would then be intravenous rather than I/M. If no blood appears,

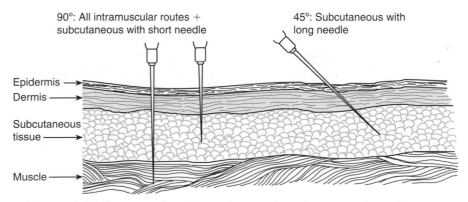

Figure 4.6 Subcutaneous and intramuscular injections: diagram to show skin, subcutaneous and muscle layers, and needle insertion.

administer the drug slowly, (especially when giving a depot as with Malcolm), at the recommended rate (if one is prescribed) or at 1 mL per 10 seconds (Keen 1990). Note that drawing back on the plunger is unnecessary with S/C injections, which are entering much less deeply and so are very unlikely to enter a capillary.

13. Observe the person carefully throughout the procedure, providing reassurance as necessary.

14. Quickly withdraw the needle, supporting the skin with the cottonwool swab and apply gentle pressure over the site. Do not rub the skin (Rodger and King 2000). Can you think why not? You will cause local irritation and may alter the drug absorption rate by doing so.

15. Ensure the person is comfortable. Check that there is no untoward form of reaction, either systemic or local. All nurses should be aware of signs of anaphylaxis (a severe allergic reaction) (see Henderson 1998 for further reading). Some drugs are known to be more likely to cause a severe allergic reaction, for example pabrinex (Trounce 2000).

16. Dispose of equipment according to local policy (see Chapter 3, sections on 'Sharps disposal' and 'Waste disposal').

17. Document on the prescription chart, in the person's notes or wherever is required.

18. Return to the patient about 15 minutes later to check the effectiveness of the drug. The site itself should be checked 2–4 hours after administration (Rodger and King 2000).

Activity	You may have the opportunity to access equipment in the skills laboratory so that you can practise drawing up an injection. There may be an artificial injection pad (showing the layers of the skin, the subcutaneous tissue and muscle) available which you can practise injecting into. This can help you to become familiar with the equipment and technical aspects of the skill, and thus increase your confidence.

Injections are an invasive procedure and there can be untoward effects.

Activity	You yourself will have experienced injections. What do you think are the main problems associated with them?

You may have identified:

■ **Pain**: This may be unavoidable, but can be reduced by distraction techniques, especially when administering to children – think about what form this could take. However, as stated earlier, injections, especially I/M, are avoided with children whenever possible as they can be traumatic, and might lead to needle phobia. Other routes will be used whenever possible. Applying the local anaesthetic cream (EMLA) (Lander *et al.* 1996), preferably an hour in advance, will reduce the pain, in the same way it has been applied in preparation for Daisy's blood tests. However, the Vaccination Administration Taskforce (2001) advises that generally using local anaesthetic cream prior to vaccinations is impractical but can be used if needle phobia is preventing vaccination. Keeping the skin taut also helps to reduce pain as it stretches the small nerves and reduces sensitivity (Stilwell 1995). Ice packs may be similarly useful. With an I/M injection, try to encourage the person to relax by choosing a comfortable position for them, as injecting into a tense muscle will be more painful.

- **Tissue damage**: Again a degree of this is probably unavoidable but damage due to the needle may be reduced by good technique. Damage can be caused by the drug being administered. This can be avoided by ensuring correct dilution according to manufacturer's instructions, and by using the appropriate technique, for example always use the Z-track technique for depot injections like Malcolm's. Bruising may sometimes be unavoidable as when giving subcutaneous anticoagulants because of the anticoagulant nature of the drug. The nurses administering Mercy's injections should rotate the site to prevent local damage. You should never inject into an already bruised area.

- **Infection**: Using non-touch technique (see Chapter 3) in the preparation and administration of an injection should render this very rare. Occasionally a local abscess may develop in a very vulnerable patient (Hemsworth 2000) and this could become more generalised if untreated. Making sure the skin is socially clean, as discussed earlier, will help reduce the risk.

- **Hypersensitivity**: It is important to obtain a clear allergic history from patients before giving a drug for the first time. Ensure that you observe the patient/client carefully during administration and after, especially during the first few doses. Because of the first pass effect, the action and therefore reaction to the drug will be faster than when given orally.

- **Staining of the skin**: This may occur with pigmented drugs like iron. Using the Z-track method should leave intact tissue above the injected material in an indirect line, thereby preventing leakage to the surface tissue (Campbell 1995).

Summary

- Student nurses can give intramuscular and subcutaneous injections under supervision. It is advisable to take opportunities to observe and then practise injection administration, so that skill and confidence develops.
- It is important to understand the sites, equipment and hazards involved in I/M and S/C injections, and to be aware of how complications can be avoided.

HOW TO CALCULATE DRUG DOSES

Nurses often worry about their ability to calculate drug doses (Woodrow 1998). However, if you follow the simple rules and standard formulae you cannot go wrong! One of the commonest issues concerns the ability of nurses to do basic maths like understanding decimals, rather than using the formulae. Therefore if you think you have a problem with basic maths, talk to a friend or family member, and ask them to help you solve it. The application of the formulae is for most people the easy part. Computer-assisted learning packages are also available and are of great value to some students (Wong 1990). With increasing technology, the mathematics required is often more complex and critical (Weeks 2000).

Tip: Try to be involved in doing calculations in the clinical setting whenever possible. Many nurses find this easier than doing calculations from a book or in the classroom (Wilson 2003).

This section covers key areas in drug calculations, and includes some exercises and answers. For further study and more practice exercises you are referred to: Gatford, J.D. and Phillips, N. 2000. *Nursing Calculations*, sixth edition. London: Churchill Livingstone. This book also includes basic maths like decimals and fractions.

LEARNING OUTCOMES

By the end of this section you will be able to:

1. Show insight into the need for effective numeracy skills in practice.
2. Handle fractions and decimals in calculations.
3. Understand conversion of units within drug calculations.
4. Use a formula to calculate medication.

Learning outcome 1: Show insight into the need for effective numeracy skills in practice

Activity

Consider what the outcome of occasionally getting a calculation slightly wrong would be. Can you ever be justified in giving a person an inaccurate dose?

The answer must always be no. You have to be 100 per cent accurate all the time. Even a small discrepancy will mean that the patient will not receive the prescribed dose, and this could be very harmful. Also, not understanding the full implications of decimals could mean that a patient receives ten times more or less than the prescribed dose if the decimal point is one place wrong.

Activity

Discuss with your colleagues the advantages and disadvantages of using calculators to calculate drug doses. Should these be allowed? They are now commonplace in schools and are freely available to all.

There is great debate about this. They can increase accuracy and are certainly useful for complex calculations (Woodrow 1998). However, there may be occasions when a calculator is unavailable or not working. It is also only as good as its operator, hence if the wrong numbers are put in by mistake, the answer will be wrong. Also, if you are totally unable to work without a calculator, you cannot estimate easily what the right answer will be, and therefore have no way of checking that the calculator answer is about right (Lumsden and Doodson 2003). The Nursing and Midwifery Council (2002) states that using calculators should not 'act as a substitute for arithmetical knowledge and skill' (p. 7).

It would seem sensible, therefore, to be able to calculate drug doses manually and by calculator, to prevent any chance of error.

Learning outcome 2: Handle fractions and decimals in calculations

Converting fractions to decimals

In a fraction, for example ⅜, the lower figure tells you how many times the whole has been divided, in this case into eighths. If the lower figure was 4, this would tell you that the whole had been divided in quarters. The top number tells us how many of that division there are, so in this fraction there are three eighths.

Try to think of the line between the two numbers as a dividing line. To convert the fraction into a decimal, you need to divide the top number by the bottom number. Thus: ⅜ = 3 divided by 8. This obviously will not result in a whole number, so the answer is going to be 0. something.

The figures after the decimal point indicate a different type of fraction, this time expressed in tenths or decimals. These are the units we use in fractions of drug doses. Most calculations will divide into relatively easy numbers, because the nurse has to be able to give that proportion of the drug without dividing into complicated amounts, for example a dose of ⅕ tablet or 0.0065 mL etc. would, of course, be unrealistic and unsafe. In the fraction we have been looking at – ⅜: 3 divided by 8 = 0.375. This answer has three figures past the decimal point and may be rounded up to 0.38.

Calculation exercise 1

Try the following conversions into decimals, to two figures past the decimal point only (round up if 5 or above or down if below 5): (Answers are at the end of the chapter.)

(a) 3/9 =
(b) 6/12 =
(c) 25/75 =
(d) 4/20 =
(e) 7/10 =
(f) 6/30 =

To divide and multiply decimals

Your calculations will always involve multiplying and dividing by units of 10 (see next section). Because decimals represent fractions in tenths, this makes these processes very easy:

- To multiply by 10, move the decimal point one place to the right. For example, $0.05 \times 10 = 0.5$; $5.8 \times 10 = 58$.
- If you want to multiply by a different unit of ten, e.g. 1000, move the decimal point to the right by the number of 0s. In the case of 1000, three places, in the case of 100, two places. For example, $0.06 \times 1000 = 60$; $5 \times 1000 = 5000$; $0.67 \times 100 = 67$.
- If there are no more figures to move the point over, add 0 to fill the spaces. For example, $5.8 \times 100 = 580$.
- To divide by 10, or multiples of, do the reverse. For example, $500/10 = 50$; $6.3/100 = 0.063$; $25/1000 = 0.025$.

Calculation exercise 2

(Answers are at the end of the chapter.)

(a) $2.5 \times 100 =$

(b) $0.3 \times 1000 =$

(c) $54 \times 10 =$

(d) $36/100 =$

(e) $125/1000 =$

(f) $5.5/1000 =$

Learning outcome 3: Understand conversion of units within drug calculations

It is essential to use the same units throughout a drug calculation – you cannot work with both micrograms and milligrams, or millilitres and litres. Therefore you need to convert the drug doses in the calculation into the same units. It does not matter which unit you change them into. However most people find whole numbers easier to work with, even if they are very large (Lumsden and Doodson 2003). There is a simple rule for conversion which is the rule of thousands: Everything that needs converting is achieved by either dividing or multiplying by a thousand. This is because:

$$1000 \text{ micrograms} = 1 \text{ milligram}$$
$$1000 \text{ milligrams} = 1 \text{ gram}$$
$$1000 \text{ grams} = 1 \text{ kilogram}$$
$$1000 \text{ millilitres} = 1 \text{ litre.}$$

With a few exceptions, these are the units used in drug prescriptions. So, to convert 5 milligrams (mg) into micrograms (µg), you need to multiply by $1000 = 5000$ micrograms.

To convert the other way, you need to divide by 1000, e.g. 50 micrograms to milligrams = 0.05 mg.

In essence, to convert to a larger unit, you need to divide the figure, so there will be less of them. To convert to a smaller unit you need to multiply so there will be more of them.

Calculation exercise 3

(Answers are at the end of the chapter.)

(a) 2000 μg = __ mg
(b) 2 litres = __ mL
(c) 50 mg = __ g
(d) 3 mg = __ μg
(e) 3500 mL = __ litres
(f) 125 μg = __ mg

Learning outcome 4: Use a formula to calculate medication

Remember: There is one magic formula for all calculations! There are no exceptions and it can be used for tablets and liquids for oral doses or injections. The formula is:

Dose prescribed/stock dose × Stock volume (if a fluid) = dose to be given.

For example, 80 mg of frusemide (a diuretic) is needed for Mercy, and the stock dose is 40 mg tablets. Thus, to follow the formula:

$$\text{Dose prescribed} = 80\,\text{mg}$$
$$\text{Stock dose} = 40\,\text{mg}$$
$$80/40 = 2 \text{ tablets}$$

For example, Daisy is prescribed amoxicillin and her dose might be (depending on her weight) 250 mg. She would require the medicine as a liquid, a suspension, and the stock bottle may be 125 mg per 5 mL. Thus the calculation would be: 250/125 × 5 = 10 mL.

Now try Exercise 4. Remember that in each calculation you must ensure that the drugs are in the same units before you apply the formula.

Calculation exercise 4

(Answers are at the end of the chapter.)

(a) 200 mg trimethoprin required. Stock dose = 100 mg tablets
(b) 100 mg chlorpromazine required. Stock dose = 25 mg tablets
(c) 10 mg diazepam elixir required. Stock dose = 5 mg per 5 mL
(d) 1.2 g augmentin required. Stock dose = 600 mg tablets
(e) 240 mg paracetamol elixir required. Stock dose = 120 mg per 5 mL

(f) 50 mg morphine elixir required. Stock dose = 10 mg per 5 mL
(g) 40 mg pethidine required. Stock ampoule = 50 mg per mL
(h) 6 mg morphine is required. Stock ampoule = 10 mg per mL
(i) Heparin 2000 units required. Stock ampoule = 5000 units per mL

Most paediatric drugs are calculated on the child's weight. It is very important therefore that their weight is measured and recorded accurately (usually checked by two people – check local policy), and that this is monitored constantly in a sick child. This may result in the drug dosage changing rapidly.

Summary

- All nurses must be able to calculate drug doses accurately, and for this a basic understanding of fractions and decimals is needed.
- There are formulae that can be used when a calculation is required, and it is important to develop skill in their application.
- Students do not carry out drug calculations unsupervised, but it is advisable to start working on this skill at an early stage, in preparation for registration, and as students may be asked to be second checkers for a calculation at some stage during the pre-registration programme.

CHAPTER SUMMARY

This chapter has explained the importance of having a basic understanding of the laws concerning drug administration, and of ensuring that local drugs policies are adhered to in practice. You should now be able to understand the need for a working knowledge of the drugs you are giving, and be able to calculate doses accurately. The chapter has stressed the importance of safe practice with regard to drug administration and the student role, and should have helped you to understand the reasons for different routes of administration. It should have prepared you to administer drugs safely in a variety of clinical settings.

Remember: The golden rule in drug administration is to be honest to yourself. If you do not understand or agree with what is being given for any reason, you must challenge the situation you find yourself in.

ANSWERS TO EXERCISES

ABBREVIATIONS (SOURCE: www.bnf.org)

b.d. = twice daily; o.d. = daily; o.m. = every morning; o.n. = every night; q.d.s. = to be taken 4 times daily; t.d.s. = to be taken 3 times daily; stat = immediately; e/c = enteric coated; i/m = intramuscular; m/r = modified release; mL = millilitre; p.r.n. = when required.

DRUG CALCULATIONS EXERCISES

Exercise 1

(a) 3/9 = 0.33
(b) 6/12 = 0.5
(c) 25/75 = 0.33
(d) 4/20 = 0.2
(e) 7/10 = 0.7
(f) 6/30 = 0.2

Exercise 2

(a) $2.5 \times 100 = 250$
(b) $0.3 \times 1000 = 300$
(c) $54 \times 10 = 540$
(d) 36/100 − 0.36
(e) 125/1000 = 0.125
(f) 5.5/1000 = 0.0055

Exercise 3

(a) 2000 µg = 2 mg
(b) 2 litres = 2000 mL
(c) 50 mg = 0.05 g
(d) 3 mg = 3000 µg
(e) 3500 mL = 3.5 litres
(f) 125 µg = 0.125 mg

Exercise 4

(a) 2 tablets
(b) 4 tablets
(c) 10 mL
(d) 2 tablets
(e) 10 mL
(f) 25 mL
(g) 0.8 mL
(h) 0.6 mL
(i) 0.4 mL

REFERENCES

British National Formulary on-line at www.bnf.org. Accessed 7 July 2004.

Caldwell, N.A. 1999. Drug absorption, distribution, metabolism and elimination. In Luker, K.A. and Wolfson D.J. (eds) *Medicines Management for Clinical Nurses*. Oxford: Blackwell Science, 31–50.

Campbell, J. 1995. Injections. *Professional Nurse* **10**, 455–8.

Choonera, I. 1994. Percutaneous drug absorption and administration. *Archives of Diseases of Childhood* **71**, 73–4.

Department of Health and Welsh Office 1993. *Code of Practice: Mental Health Act 1983*. London: HMSO.

Department of Health 1996. *Immunisation against Infectious Disease*. London: HMSO.

Department of Health 2001a. *Valuing People: A new strategy for learning disability for the 21st century*. London: DH.

Department of Health 2001b. *Medicines and Older People: Implementing medicines-related aspects of the NSF for older people*. London: DH.

Duthie, R.B. 1988. *Guidelines for the Safe and Secure Handling of Medicines: A Report to the Secretary of State for Social Services by the Joint Committee of the Standing Medical Nursing and Midwifery and Pharmaceutical Advisory Committees*. London: HMSO.

Gatford, J.D. and Phillips, N. 2000. *Nursing Calculations*, sixth edition. Edinburgh: Churchill Livingstone.

Griffith, R. and Griffiths, H. 2003. Administration of medicines Part 1: the law. *Nursing Standard* **18**(2), 47–53.

Hemsworth, S. 2000. Injection technique. *Paediatric Nursing* **12**(9), 17–20.

Henderson, N. 1998. Anaphylaxis. *Nursing Standard* **12**(47), 49–55.

Henry, J.N. 1998. *BMA New Guide to Medicines and Drugs*. London: Dorling Kindersley.

Hopkins, S.J. 1999. *Drugs and Pharmacology for Nurses*, thirteenth edition. Edinburgh: Churchill Livingstone.

Infection Control Nurses Association. 2003. *Reducing Sharps Injuries by Prevention and Risk Management*. Bathgate: Infection Control Nurses Association.

Jacques, A. and Jackson, G.A. 2000. *Understanding Dementia*, third edition. Edinburgh: Churchill Livingstone.

Katsma, D.L. and Katsma, R.P.E. 2000. The myth of the 90 degree angle – intramuscular injection. *Nurse Educator* **25**(1), 34–7.

Keen, M.F. 1990. Get on the right track with Z track injections. *Nursing* **20**, 59.

Kelly, J.S. 1994. Topical ophthalmic drug administration: a practical guide. *British Journal of Nursing* **3**(10), 518–20.

Koivisto, V.A. and Felig, P. 1978. Is skin preparation necessary before insulin injection? *Lancet* **1**, 1072–3.

Lander, J., Nazarali, S., Hodgins, M. *et al.* 1996. Evaluation of a new topical anaesthetic agent: a pilot study. *Nursing Research* **45**(1), 50–3.

Lawrence, J.C., Lilly, H.A. and Kidson, A. 1994. The use of alcoholic wipes for disinfection of injection sites. *Journal of Wound Care* **3**(1), 11–14.

Ling, M. 1999. The patient's role in optimising treatment. In Luker, K.A. and Wolfson, D.J. (eds) *Medicines Management for Clinical Nurses*. Oxford: Blackwell Science, 104–29.

Lumsden, H. and Doodson, M. 2003. Neonatal Drug Calculations: a practical approach. *Journal of Neonatal Nursing* **9**(1), 14–18.

Mallett, J. and Dougherty, L. 2000. *The Royal Marsden Hospital Manual of Clinical Nursing Practices*, fifth edition. Oxford: Blackwell Science.

Marsden, J. 1998. Use of eye drops and ointments in A and E. *Emergency Nurse* **6**(8), 17–22.

Marsden, J. and Shaw, M. 2003. Correct administration of topical eye ointment. *Nursing Standard* **17**(30), 42–4.

Medicines Act 1968. London: HMSO.

Misuse of Drugs Act 1971. London: HMSO.

Newton, M., Newton, D. and Fudin, J. 1992. Reviewing the three big injection routes. *Nursing* **2**(9), 34–42.

Nursing and Midwifery Council 2002. *Guidelines for the Administration of Medicines*. London: NMC.

Pilling, M., Geoghegan, M., Wolfson, D.J. and Holden, J.D. 1998. The St Helens and Knowsley Prescribing Initiative: a model for pharmacists-led meetings with GPs. *Pharmacy Journal* **260**, 100–2.

Polak, M., Kakou, B., Leridon, L. *et al.* 1999. Short needles (8 mm) reduce the risk of IM injections in children with type 1 diabetes. *Diabetes Care* **22**, 161–5.

Prosser, S., Worster, B., MacGregor, J. *et al.* 2000. *Applied Pharmacology: An introduction to pathophysiology and drug management for nurses and healthcare professionals*. London: Harcourt Publishers.

Rodger, M.A. and King, L. 2000. Drawing up and administering intramuscular injections: a review of the literature. *Journal of Advanced Nursing* **31**, 574–82.

Royal College of Paediatrics and Child Health 2002. *Position Statement on Injection Technique*. London: Royal College of Paediatrics and Child Health.

Selli, R. 1995. Which topical steroid? *Community Nurse* **1**(3), 36–8.

Sexton, J.A. and Braidwood, C.C. 1999. The nurse's role in medicines administration – operational and practical consideration. In Luker, K.A. and Wolfson, D.J. (eds) *Medicines Management for Clinical Nurses*. Oxford: Blackwell Science, 237–57.

Smith, J. 2002. A bitter pill to swallow. *Nursing Older People* **14**(8), 33–4.

Stilwell, B. 1995. Injections. *Community Outlook* **1**(1), 21–2.

Trounce, J. 2000. *Clinical Pharmacology for Nurses*, sixteenth edition. New York: Churchill Livingstone.

Vaccination Administration Taskforce 2001. *UK Guidance on Best Practice in Vaccine Administration*. London: Shirehall Communications.

UK Central Council for Nursing, Midwifery and Health Visiting 2001. *UKCC Position Statement on the Covert Administration of Medicines: Disguising medicine in food and drink*. London: UKCC (available from www.nmc-uk.org).

Watt, S. 2003. Safe administration of medicines to children Part 1. *Paediatric Nursing* **15**(4), 40–3.

Weeks, K. 2000. Written drug dosage errors made by students: the threat to clinical effectiveness and the need for a new approach. *Clinical Effectiveness in Nursing* **4**(4), 20–9.

Wilson, A. 2003. Nurses' maths: researching a practical approach. *Nursing Standard* **17**(47), 33–6.

Wong, T.K. 1990. Drug Calculations for nurses – a computer assisted learning application. *Nurse Education Today* **10**, 274–80.

Wong, D.L. 1993. *Whaley and Wong's Essentials of Paediatric Nursing*, fourth edition. St Louis: Mosby.

Woodrow, P. 1998. Numeracy skills. *Paediatric Nursing* **10**(6), 26–32.

Workman, B. 1999. Safe injection technique. *Nursing Standard* **13**(39), 47–53.

Wright, D. 2002. Medication administration in nursing homes. *Nursing Standard* **16**(42), 33–8.

Caring for people with impaired mobility

Glynis Pellatt

Mobility is a multidimensional concept, encompassing physical, cognitive, emotional and social dimensions. A change or deficit in any one aspect impacts on all the other dimensions, affecting ability to interact with the environment and move from one environment to another (Rush and Ouellet 1993). Nurses in many settings encounter patients and clients who have impaired mobility and are therefore at risk of a number of complications. Nurses have an important role, therefore, in actively preventing these complications as well as aiming to promote mobility safely whenever possible. Correct moving and handling techniques are necessary when caring for people with impaired mobility and some key principles of safe moving and handling are referred to during this chapter. It is essential that you remain up-to-date with these techniques, and attend organised classroom sessions. As a registered nurse, you will also need yearly updates.

This chapter includes:
- Pressure ulcer risk assessment
- Pressure ulcer prevention
- Prevention of other complications of immobility
- Assisting with mobilisation and preventing falls.

Recommended biology reading:
The following questions will help you to focus on the biology underpinning this chapter's skills. Use your recommended text book to find out:

- What systems are involved in movement and posture? Don't forget that individual cells need oxygen and nutrients.
- Which cells actually shorten and lengthen? What controls their activity?
- What are joints?
- What are the different types of joints?
- Are all joints moveable?

- What are tendons and ligaments?
- Why does damage to these tissues take so long to heal?
- How do we maintain flexibility?
- What are the functions of our muscles and bones?
- What happens to them if we are immobile?
- What other body systems would be affected by immobility?
- How would immobility affect metabolic rate and energy balance?
- How would you feel if you were unable to move about?

Note: it will also be useful to revise the layers of the skin.

PRACTICE SCENARIOS

The following scenarios illustrate situations where nurses need to assist with and promote mobility, and implement measures to prevent complications of impaired mobility.

Adult

Mr Jack Jones is a 78-year-old man who has been admitted to a medical ward from the Accident and Emergency (A&E) department with a right-sided hemi-plegia following a **cerebrovascular accident** (CVA). He is well nourished and his general condition is good. He is conscious but his speech has been affected.

Child

Tracey Livingstone is 12 years old. She has fallen off her horse and fractured her sixth cervical vertebra. She has no sensation below the level of the injury, has some arm and hand function but no movement in her legs. She has a neuro-genic bladder, which is managed by a supra-pubic catheter, and a **neurogenic bowel**, which is emptied daily, so she is usually continent. She is up in a wheel-chair undergoing her rehabilitation programme.

Learning disability

Marion Pearce is a 42-year-old woman with a severe learning disability who lives in a community unit. Due to accompanying physical disabilities she uses a wheelchair for mobilising. She is underweight and incontinent of urine and faeces; her skin tends to be dry. Joint deformities make it very difficult to position her comfortably in the wheelchair. She has a poor appetite and is unable to feed herself or manage her own hygiene needs. Marion's **health facilitator** is the community nurse for learning disabilities. Her **Health Action Plan** includes input from a number of different health professionals including the occupational therapist and the physiotherapist.

Cerebrovascular accident

This is cerebral damage caused either by decreased blood flow or haemorrhage. Effects vary but it often causes paralysis down one side of the body (hemiplegia), and speech and swallowing difficulty. Commonly termed a 'stroke'.

Neurogenic bladder and bowel

This is damage to the neurological pathways that regulate bladder and bowel function.

Health facilitator

A member of the community learning disabilities team (often a nurse) who supports a person with learning dis-abilities to access the health care they need. See *Valuing People* (Department of Health 2001a).

Health Action Plan

A personal action plan developed for each individual with a learning disability, containing details of their health interventions, medication taken, screening tests etc. See *Valuing People* (Department of Health 2001a).

Mental health

John Barnes, aged 52 years, is a client on an acute mental health admission ward. He has severe depression and also has a history of limited mobility and chronic pain following an accident 10 years ago. He needs a walking frame for support but unfortunately fell on the ward recently and sustained a fractured wrist which is now in a plaster cast.

PRESSURE ULCER RISK ASSESSMENT

A **pressure ulcer** (sometimes referred to as a bedsore, pressure sore or decubitus ulcer) is defined by the European Pressure Ulcer Advisory Panel (EPUAP) as 'an area of localised damage to the skin and underlying tissue caused by pressure or shear and/or a combination of these' (EPUAP 2003). Pressure ulcers most commonly occur over bony prominences (Collins 2001; Cowan and Woollons 1998; James 1998) but pressure damage can occur in other areas in some circumstances. *The Essence of Care* (Department of Health 2001b) identified benchmarks of best practice for eight fundamental aspects of care and one of the sections focuses on pressure ulcer risk assessment and prevention. The document recommends that screening for pressure ulcer risk should take place at first contact with further assessment being carried out for people identified as at risk, by staff who have the necessary expertise.

LEARNING OUTCOMES

By the end of this section you will be able to:

1. Identify how pressure ulcers are formed and the areas of the body which are most at risk.
2. Discuss why some people are more likely to develop pressure ulcers.
3. Use a pressure ulcer risk calculator to identify people at risk of pressure ulcers.
4. Discuss the importance of accurate documentation of pressure ulcer risk assessment.

Learning outcome 1: Identify how pressure ulcers are formed and the areas of the body that are most at risk

Activity

Hold a clear plastic tumbler in your hand using your fingertips. Press with your fingers and notice how your fingertips have gone very pale. Now release the pressure and look at your fingertips: they will have a red flush.

The red flush is called **reactive hyperaemia**.

Pressure damage occurs when skin and other tissues are compressed between bone and another surface. Body cells will die if the flow of blood in the capillary bed is not sufficient to supply oxygen, carbohydrates and amino acids for metabolism and to remove carbon dioxide and the products of catabolism (James 1998). The presence of reactive hyperaemia is a strong indicator of potential damage (Wiechula 1997). Capillary closing pressure is the degree of external pressure required to occlude the blood vessels. It is suggested that external pressures above the mean capillary blood pressure will cause capillary closure. The average mean capillary blood pressure in healthy people is 20 mmHg, but this can be much lower in ill health (Simpson *et al.* 1996).

The time taken for irreversible changes to take place leading to tissue death varies. If pressure is relieved while the capillary and lymphatic circulation are intact, this results in a sudden increase in blood flow to the area as the build-up of metabolites acts on the arteriole sphincters. However, if the capillaries and lymphatic circulation have been irreversibly damaged the hyperaemia will be non-blanching. The reddening is caused by blood leaking from damaged capillaries. The term 'non-blanching' means that when you apply light finger pressure to the red area it remains red rather than whitening as it does in blanching hyperaemia where the micro-circulation is still intact. The damage present in non-blanching hyperaemia will progress to deeper layers if the pressure is not relieved.

There is an inverse relationship between time and pressure. A person can endure a large amount of pressure during a short amount of time or a low amount of pressure over a longer time without sustaining tissue damage (Armstrong and Bortz 2001).

■ *Activity*	What areas of the body are most at risk of developing pressure ulcers? Which of these sites are risk areas for the people in the scenarios?

As stated earlier, the skin over bony prominences is particularly at risk of pressure ulcers and these areas are shown in Fig. 5.1.

■ The sacrum, hips, heels, elbows, knees and malleoli are a particular problem for patients who are confined to bed, visiting X-ray, or being operated on in theatre. When Mr Jones was first admitted to A&E he would have been at risk if lying immobile on a trolley for some time during initial assessment and investigations. Lying on a trolley, X-ray table or operating theatre table adds to the risk to vulnerable areas due to immobility, and people who are being operated on in theatre will be unable to feel the pain caused by pressure and shearing forces (Schoonhoven *et al.* 2002). Anaesthetic agents lower blood pressure and alter tissue perfusion, which also increases the likelihood of tissue damage (Armstrong and Bortz 2001).

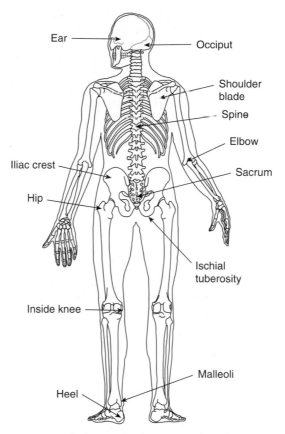

Ear

Occiput

Shoulder blade

Spine

Elbow

Iliac crest

Sacrum

Hip

Ischial tuberosity

Inside knee

Malleoli

Heel

Figure 5.1 Skin areas particularly at risk of pressure ulcer formation.

■ In the seated position nearly half the body weight is supported by only 8 per cent of the areas at or near the ischial tuberosities (Collins 1999). Tracey and Marion both use a wheelchair and Mr Jones has limited mobility and will be seated in a chair quite a lot, therefore the skin areas over their ischial tuberosities and the inner aspects of their knees are vulnerable. Patients who are immobile in the seated position have a more rounded shape that allows them to rock backward on to the sacrum, creating friction and shear forces (Collins 1999).

■ Babies and children have an uneven distribution of body weight: their heads comprise a disproportionately large amount of the total body weight compared with adults. This is why the occipital region is at risk of pressure (Olding and Patterson 1998).

You may also have identified the shoulder blades, iliac crests, sides of feet, ears and spine. However it has to be remembered that pressure ulcers can occur anywhere, particularly if there are tight clothes, splints, ill-fitting plaster casts or appliances such as oxygen masks that cause pressure (Butcher 1999). Nurses caring for Mr Barnes should be aware that his plaster cast could rub, particularly

- Persistent erythema
- Non-blanching hyperaemia
- Blisters
- Discoloration (purplish/bluish localised areas of skin in people with darkly pigmented skin)
- Localised heat (replaced by coolness if the tissue becomes damaged)
- Localised oedema
- Localised induration

Box 5.1 Signs of early pressure ulcer development (from NICE 2003, p. 7)

if it becomes too loose or too tight, and so should advise him to report any discomfort. Skin covered by antiembolic stockings is also vulnerable (National Institute of Clinical Excellence 2003).

Inspection of vulnerable areas

Areas of the body at risk of pressure ulcers are usually termed **pressure areas** and nurses should be vigilant about checking these areas for early signs of pressure. The vulnerable areas of risk for each patient, as discussed above, should be inspected regularly but people can also be taught to inspect their own skin, using a mirror where necessary, and this would be part of Tracey's rehabilitation. Signs of early pressure ulcers can be found in Box 5.1.

Learning outcome 2: Discuss why some people are more likely to develop pressure ulcers

 Activity   Sit in a straight-backed chair. Now see how long you can sit there without moving.

How long did you manage: 5 minutes, 10 minutes or longer? What was it that made you move? You probably found that your pressure areas became very uncomfortable and eventually you had to move position. Reduced mobility is considered to be the most important factor in the development of pressure ulcers (Fletcher 1996; Simpson *et al.* 1996). The body's defence against pressure is to shift weight frequently, whether asleep or awake, as a response to sensory stimulation. Therefore anyone with reduced mobility, including people with impaired consciousness, have an increased risk of developing pressure ulcers.

Some people have reduced sensation to pressure and pain neurologically induced by medical conditions such as **multiple sclerosis**, **spinal cord injury** (Tracey) or cerebrovascular accident (Mr Jones). Some medication, such as sedatives, may cause a chemically induced reduction in sensitivity to pressure

Multiple sclerosis
Progressive destruction of myelin sheaths of neurones in the central nervous system. Can cause loss of movement and sensation.

Spinal cord injury
Damage to the spinal cord, which causes paralysis and loss of sensation below the injury.

Extrinsic

- Pressure
- Shearing
- Friction.

Intrinsic

- Reduced mobility
- Reduced sensation
- Moisture
- Acute illness: pyrexia, infection
- Ageing
- Body weight: emaciation, obesity
- Poor nutrition
- Pain
- Poor oxygen perfusion.

Box 5.2 Factors contributing to pressure ulcer formation

and pain. Sedation can also cause people to be too drowsy to move around (Fletcher 1996). Mr Barnes is depressed and could lack the motivation to move, or pain may prevent him moving. Some people, such as those with dementia, are unable to respond to pressure stimuli and spontaneously alter their position (Fletcher 1996). In recent years it has been noted that pressure damage can occur in women who have received epidural analgesia to control pain during labour by blocking sensation in the lower trunk and legs (Butcher 1999).

Factors that render people at increased risk of pressure ulcers are often classified as **extrinsic** (outside the person, e.g. environmental) or **intrinsic** (to do with individuals themselves). Reduced mobility and sensation are therefore intrinsic factors.

Activity

Think about factors other than reduced sensation and mobility that may make people susceptible to pressure ulcers. Try to think of some extrinsic factors and some other intrinsic factors.

Box 5.2 lists the main factors contributing to pressure ulcer formation, and these are now discussed.

Extrinsic factors

We have already discussed the role of pressure in causing pressure ulcers. Shear occurs when a person begins to move or slide due to gravity but the skin under pressure remains stationary. Tissues are then wrenched in opposite directions, resulting in disruption or angulation of capillary blood vessels causing ischaemia. Shear can be very destructive to deep tissues (Simpson *et al.* 1996). Friction damage is caused by the surface of the skin sliding along the support surface when the tissue is under compression. Shear and friction could be a problem for Tracey, Marion and Mr Jones, because they may slide if not properly positioned in their chairs.

Intrinsic factors

- **Moisture**: Moisture makes skin more vulnerable as it may stick to the support surface. Too much moisture can macerate the skin (Wiechula 1997), and contamination by urine and faeces adds to the vulnerability. Marion is incontinent of urine, making her particularly at risk. The risk of pressure ulcer development can be increased fivefold by the presence of even small amounts of moisture (Dealey 1997). See Chapter 8 for a detailed discussion of how incontinence affects skin integrity.

- **Acute illness**: Acutely ill people are especially vulnerable to pressure ulcer formation for a number of reasons. Pyrexia increases the **metabolic rate**, particularly the demand for oxygen, which endangers ischaemic areas. Severe infection can also cause nutritional disturbances and local bacteria increase the demand on local metabolism by both their own requirements and the response of the body's defence mechanism (Simpson *et al.* 1996). In children a sudden rise in temperature and rapid spread of infection affects the wound-healing process due to the system's inability to counteract such a significant attack (Pickersgill 1997).

- **Ageing**: Pressure ulcers are more common in people over 65 years old, like Mr Jones. The skin contains collagen, which gives it its tensile strength. Collagen contains thin strands of elastin that provide flexibility. As people age the strength of the collagen and the elasticity of the elastin decrease. This leads to sagging and wrinkling of the skin as well as greater risk of damage due to trauma (Penzer and Finch 2001).

- **Bodyweight**: Weight status and weight loss are associated with pressure ulcer development and poor healing of pressure ulcers (Ferguson *et al.* 2000). People who are underweight have less cushioning over bony prominences (Fletcher 1996) therefore this is a risk factor for Marion who is underweight. Obese people may not be able to lift clear and therefore drag themselves up the bed (Russell 1998), thus exerting a greater load on pressure points (Fletcher 1996).

- **Poor nutrition**: Malnutrition and dehydration are recognised risk factors for pressure ulcers (NICE 2003), and many people are already malnourished on admission to hospital (Strachan-Bennett 2003). Marion has a poor appetite, and nutrition, including adequate hydration, plays an important part in pressure ulcer prevention (Ferguson *et al.* 2000). Lewis (1998) suggests that protein, zinc, vitamin C and iron have a role in preventing pressure ulcers. In older people who have a fractured neck of femur, the

Metabolic rate
The overall rate at which heat is produced in the body

fracture increases nutritional requirements as well as reducing mobility, which may lead to pressure damage.

- **Pain**: Pain prevents patients from repositioning themselves, particularly at night. Jack may experience pain in his affected shoulder due to poor recovery of arm function (Gibbon 2002), making it even more difficult to move himself when in bed. Mr Barnes has chronic pain and could have difficulty moving, especially now he has an arm in a plaster cast.

- **Poor oxygen perfusion**: Patients that have poor oxygen perfusion due to conditions such as heart disease, respiratory disease, **anaemia** and **diabetes** have a lower peripheral capillary pressure. Smoking exacerbates poor oxygen perfusion in all these conditions (Young 1997).

Anaemia
Reduced haemoglobin concentration in the blood, or abnormal haemoglobin, resulting in reduced oxygen-carrying capacity.

Diabetes (mellitus)
A disease caused by deficient insulin release leading to inability of the body cells to use carbohydrates, and an elevated blood glucose.

Learning outcome 3: Use a pressure ulcer risk calculator to identify people at risk of pressure ulcers

The National Institute for Clinical Excellence (NICE 2003) recommends that patients should be assessed for pressure ulcer risk using both formal and informal procedures and that assessment should take place within 6 hours of admission to a care episode. Pressure ulcer risk calculators are systems that have been developed to help to identify people at risk of developing pressure ulcers. They use scoring systems based on the risk factors for pressure ulcers discussed earlier.

Activity

Have you seen any pressure ulcer risk calculators used in the practice setting? If so, which ones have you seen?

There are many pressure ulcer risk calculators in use including those listed below. The calculator used should be appropriate to the clinical setting and research among a similar care group should be available to support the calculator's accuracy.

- **The Norton Score**: This was developed in 1962 (Norton *et al.* 1962) in a unit for the care of older people. It consists of five headings, each giving a numerical score. A score under fourteen indicates a patient is at risk of developing a pressure ulcer. The predictive value of the scale is said to be derived from the fact that it is based on factors known to predispose patients to pressure ulcers (Smith *et al.* 1995).

- **The Waterlow Scale**: The Waterlow risk assessment card was developed for use with general adult populations (Waterlow 1985, 1988). It identifies three degrees of risk status: 'at risk', 'high risk' and 'very high risk'. The tool also aims to provide guidelines on the selection of preventive aids and equipment and to promote the user's awareness of the causes of pressure ulcer development (Simpson *et al.* 1996). It is widely used in the UK (sometimes in adapted forms) and the revised 1995 version

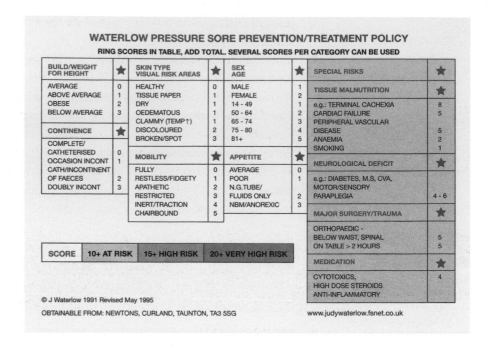

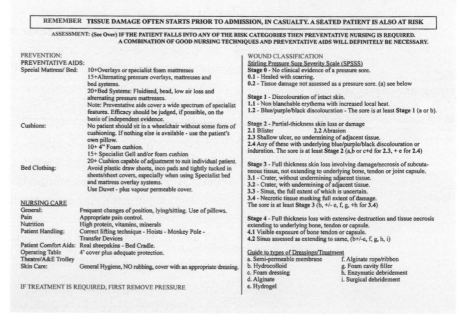

Figure 5.2 The Waterlow card (revised version 1995). (Reproduced with kind permission of Judy Waterlow.)

can be seen in Fig. 5.2. The developer of this tool emphasises that education to accompany its use is essential and has set up a web page (www.judywaterlow.fsnet.co.uk) and developed a manual 'Pressure Sore Prevention Manual' for this purpose.

■ **Pressure sore prediction score**: This was developed at the Royal National Orthopaedic Hospital for orthopaedic, trauma and spinal-injured patients

(Lowthian 1987). The scale consists of six questions with 'yes', 'yes but', 'no', 'no but' answers.

- **The Pattoid System**: This was developed as a risk assessment tool for paediatric patients (Olding and Patterson 1998). It identifies three levels of risk- 'low risk', 'medium risk' and 'high risk'.
- **The Braden Scale**: This was developed to predict pressure ulcer risk due to intrinsic factors (Bergstrom *et al.* 1987). It consists of six subscales, the first three subscales reflect primary factors (sensory perception, activity, mobility) contributing to pressure. The other three subscales (moisture, nutritional status, friction and shear) reflect factors contributing to diminished tissue tolerance.

Activity

Either use the Waterlow score in Fig. 5.2 or use the pressure ulcer risk assessment tool in use in your practice setting to assess the people in the scenarios for pressure ulcer risk. Ask a colleague to undertake the same exercise. Now compare your answers with those of your colleague. Did you both arrive at the same score for each of the people?

By carrying out the above activity you were assessing reliability of the tool, which relates to whether different people using the tool arrive at the same score. There are many different scales to choose from but all risk calculators are based on factors that are known to predispose people to pressure ulcer formation. However the variety of risk assessment scales in use today reflects the lack of consensus regarding the relative importance of each group of predisposing factors (Pang and Wong 1998). To be accurate, risk calculators need to demonstrate **sensitivity** (the ability to predict patients who will develop pressure ulcers) and **specificity** (the ability to predict patients who will not develop pressure ulcers) (Butcher 1999). Some calculators may overpredict the risk of pressure ulcers, which has cost implications when pressure-relieving equipment is being provided. On the other hand if a scale underpredicts, then this has cost implications both in financial terms if a patient's stay in hospital is prolonged, as well as the human cost of pain and suffering from a pressure ulcer.

Simpson *et al.* (1996) offer some recommendations to optimise risk assessment tools:

1. Select a tool that is appropriate to the patient/client group.
2. Ensure all members of the nursing team are familiar with the tool.
3. Ensure risk assessment is undertaken at appropriate times during a patient's hospital stay, especially when a major change in health status has occurred.
4. Regularly review the cut-off point used to describe risk threshold by reviewing pressure ulcer incidence data in conjunction with published literature on the application of the tool.

The National Institute for Clinical Excellence (NICE 2003) advises that pressure ulcer risk calculators should be used only as an *aide memoire* and that they should not be a substitute for clinical judgement.

Learning outcome 4: Discuss the importance of accurate documentation of pressure ulcer risk assessment

Activity

Consider why it is important to record information relating to pressure ulcer risk in nursing documentation.

The care plan is the principal means of communication between the nurses caring for a patient. Tingle (1997) pointed out the medico-legal problems existing in pressure ulcer care. There are regular cases and complaints involving poor standards of communication which include inadequate documentation and non-reflective practice (Stephens and Bick 2002). It is vital that there is evidence of risk assessment and pressure ulcer prevention in patient records. The National Institute for Clinical Excellence (NICE 2003) emphasises that all formal risk assessments should be documented and readily available to all members of the multidisciplinary team.

Summary

- There are many factors which can render a person vulnerable to pressure ulcer formation.
- Pressure ulcer risk calculators can help nurses to identify accurately those at risk but should not replace clinical judgement.
- There are a range of pressure ulcer risk calculators available. Nurses need to choose one suitable for their patient/client group after considering available evidence.
- Documentation of pressure ulcer risk assessment is essential for medico-legal reasons and to promote good communication.

PRESSURE ULCER PREVENTION

Incidence rate of pressure ulcers

The number of new patients with pressure ulcers in a population during a specified timespan. Usually expressed per 1000 population per year.

Prevalence rate of pressure ulcers

The total number of patients with pressure ulcers occurring at a specific time (e.g. on a certain day) in a particular population. Expressed per 1000 population.

It is estimated that 95 per cent of pressure ulcers are preventable; the 5 per cent that are not preventable are due to pre-admission problems such as lying on the floor for a long period of time following a fall (Hampton 1998). However it has been argued that the drive towards early discharge, expansion in day care and technologies that lengthen the survival of patients who until recent years would not have survived, has resulted in more very ill hospital patients (Gould *et al.* 2000). Therefore comparisons between the **incidence rate** and **prevalence rate** of pressure ulcers made several years apart are no longer valid.

LEARNING OUTCOMES

By the end of this section you will be able to:

1. Discuss why pressure ulcer prevention is an important aspect of the nurse's role.
2. Identify ways of preventing pressure ulcers in people at risk.

Learning outcome 1: Discuss why pressure ulcer prevention is an important aspect of the nurse's role

Activity

Why is it important that a pressure ulcer prevention plan is implemented for people identified at risk of pressure ulcers?

You may have thought of some or all of the following points.

- Pressure ulcers can have serious physical effects. They can lead to infections including osteomyelitis (infection of bone) (Culley 1998), which can result in amputation, and they can be instrumental in a patient's death (Young 1997). The scar tissue resulting from a pressure ulcer will predispose the patient to a further pressure ulcer due to the reduced tissue strength.
- Pressure ulcers are likely to have a marked effect on health-related quality of life (Clark 2002). They can cause pain, loss of independence and social isolation (Arblaster 1998). They are chronic wounds (see Chapter 6) and can adversely affect body image and self-esteem (Culley 1998).
- Patients with pressure ulcers remain in acute settings five days longer than patients without pressure ulcers (Hampton 1998).
- Pressure ulcers are a financial drain on the National Health Service with an estimated financial cost in the UK of at least £750 million per year (Stephens and Bick 2002). There has been considerable pressure from Government to reduce the incidence of pressure ulcers (Gould *et al.* 2000).
- Pressure ulcers have been identified as a key indicator of quality care (Department of Health 1993). Most provider units collate data on the number of pressure ulcers sustained by their patients, and purchasers use this data as a means of assessing quality of care (James 1998).

There are therefore many reasons why pressure ulcers must be prevented. Prevention of pressure ulcers has always been a nursing role; Florence Nightingale believed that good nursing care could prevent pressure ulcers (Russell 1998). However there is a growing opinion that a multidisciplinary approach must be taken towards the prevention of pressure ulcers (Dealey 1997), and this view is supported by *The Essence of Care* (Department of Health 2001b). Nevertheless, as nurses assess, plan implement and evaluate care to meet all aspects of patients/clients' needs, they are in a key position to deliver care to prevent pressure ulcers.

Learning outcome 2: Identify ways of preventing pressure ulcers in people at risk

Activity

List some methods of pressure relief that you have observed in practice and consider which might be suitable for the four patients/clients in the scenarios.

Pressure ulcer prevention can take several forms. It includes maintaining and improving tissue tolerance to pressure, protection against pressure, shear and friction forces and education of staff, patients/clients and carers.

Pain control

If pain is not properly controlled this will prevent patients from moving, so adequate pain control is essential. Correct handling of Mr Jones's hemiplegic arm will help to prevent shoulder pain (Gibbon 2002). Mr Barnes has chronic pain from his previous injury, and acute pain from his newly fractured wrist. The nurses caring for him, in conjunction with the multidisciplinary team, must implement appropriate pain management strategies and promote his comfort (see Chapter 12 'Managing pain and promoting comfort').

Nutrition

Dietary intake may need to be supplemented, particularly to increase protein, vitamin C and zinc intake (Dunford 1998), and it is appropriate to refer at-risk patients to the dietician. This may be necessary for Marion, and the staff who are caring for her need to understand the importance of nutrition in maintaining her skin integrity. This will be included in Marion's Health Action Plan. Working through Chapter 9 will assist you in developing your skills in assessing and meeting nutritional needs.

Promotion of continence and skin care

Marion is incontinent and skin that is in contact with urine or faeces for a long period of time is at risk of maceration and breakdown. Her skin must be kept clean and dry, but constant washing removes the body's natural oils by drying the skin (Russell 1998). Washing with skin cleanser that contains emollient is preferable to soap. If pads are used to contain incontinence, super-absorbent pads are preferable as they keep skin dry. Faeces are very excoriating to the skin, so should be dealt with promptly. Chapter 8, in the section on promoting continence and managing incontinence, explains in detail how incontinence threatens skin integrity and how skin can be cared for after incontinence to prevent problems. It will also help you to develop your skills in promoting continence, which may include bladder and bowel training programmes.

Moving and handling techniques and repositioning

You will be attending moving and handling sessions throughout your pre-registration nursing programme and these will prepare you to employ good moving and handling techniques to prevent people being dragged up the bed, thus avoiding friction and shear. You will be able to practise these techniques under supervision in the classroom. The aim is to teach the principles of good practice so that you have the flexibility to apply, modify and adapt the principles to different situations (Cook and Nendick 1999). The use of slide sheets, low friction fabric rollers and hoists makes moving and repositioning safer for both patients and staff and these are more comfortable for patients (Hawkins *et al.* 1999). Both Marion's and Tracey's carers need educating about correct moving and handling techniques and how to use the necessary equipment.

Pressure damage can be avoided by repositioning patients regularly to ensure tissue perfusion. This will be necessary for Mr Jones, Marion and Tracey, who all have a high risk of pressure ulcers. However the exact time limits for particular point pressures in most patient situations and, therefore, the required frequency for patient repositioning, are unknown (Lowthian 1997). The National Institute of Clinical Excellence (2003) advises that turning schedules should be devised on an individual basis rather than ritualistically. *The Essence of Care* benchmark for best practice recommends that patients/clients' needs for repositioning should be assessed and documented, and that there should be ongoing reassessment (Department of Health 2001b). Regular turning of patients also helps to reduce the incidence of pulmonary infection and the development of sepsis (Hawkins *et al.* 1999).

Support systems

A wide range of support systems have been developed to assist in the protection of the skin against pressure damage. *The Essence of Care* benchmark for best practice states that 'Patients at risk of developing pressure ulcers are cared for on pressure redistributing support surfaces that meet their individual needs (including comfort)' (Department of Health 2001b, p. 129). Support systems are available as mattresses, bed systems, overlays and seat cushions. They are designed either to reduce or relieve pressure.

Seat cushions

Tracey and Marion spend a lot of time in their wheelchairs and will need appropriate wheelchair cushions that will relieve pressure. Sitting time in wheelchairs may need to be restricted to less than 2 hours for people with a high risk of pressure ulcers (NICE 2003). Wheelchair cushions should fit the seat and the user, should be at the right height, be stable, promote symmetrical posture and positioning and be comfortable for patients. No particular seat cushions have been shown to perform better than others (NICE 2003). The **interface pressure** readings should be acceptable and the patient or carer should be able to maintain the cushion (Collins 2001). An alternative means of positioning is to use a moulded chair to fit the person's body shape. Beanbags or wedges are often used for people with disabilities (Harris 2000).

Mr Jones needs to be correctly positioned in his chair. The joints of the lower limbs should be in the mid range of movement. The weight of the upper body should be supported evenly by both ischial tuberosities with the pelvis in a slight anterior tilt. The pelvis should rest at 90 degrees flexion, the knees should be flexed to 90 degrees and the feet placed flat on the floor (Collins 1999).

Interface pressure
This is calculated by dividing patient weight by the surface area supported (Burman and O'Dea 1994).

Mattresses

A standard hospital mattress will not be a suitable surface for Mr Jones, Tracey or Marion, and may not be appropriate for Mr Barnes either. The minimum provision for people assessed as vulnerable to pressure ulcers should be a high-specification foam mattress with pressure-relieving properties; this should be instigated in the theatre setting too (Cullum *et al.* 2003; NICE 2003). The National Institute of Clinical Excellence (2003) acknowledges that there is much debate in the literature about the terminology used for pressure-relieving devices and in their guidance they choose to use the term 'pressure-relieving' to cover all devices.

There are two main categories of mattress systems:

■ Systems that increase the area of the body in contact with the support surface. They use materials that mould or contour to the body shape, distributing the load more widely and reducing pressure at bony prominences.
■ Systems that relieve the source of pressure from the surface of the body (Cowan and Woollons 1998). This is usually achieved by alternately inflating cells in a cyclical manner so that the body is supported on one set of cells while the remaining cells deflate away from the body (Fletcher 1997).

There is very little good-quality data to support the selection of any one particular piece of equipment, and more research is needed (NICE 2003). However high-tech devices (e.g. air-fluidised and low-air loss mattresses) are recommended for people who are at high risk of pressure ulcers or where low-tech devices (e.g. foam mattresses, gel/fluid/fibre/air-filled mattresses/overlays) have not been successful, on the basis of professional consensus (NICE 2003). Studies suggest that air-fluidised and low air-loss beds are better than standard beds in promoting pressure ulcer healing (Brown 2001). When choosing a surface, other criteria need to be taken into account too. Patient acceptability is the most important. If the equipment is uncomfortable, increases pain or disturbs sleep then its use must be reconsidered. The other vital consideration is the effects on mobility. The goal of care for all our patients and clients is to increase mobility and therefore using a support system that reduces mobility is not an option.

Reduced mobility may occur for a number of reasons:

■ Lack of a firm edge to the bed so that there is not enough support for people transferring in and out of bed.
■ Increased height of the bed or chair may reduce access, particularly for wheelchair users.
■ Loss of balance with alternating pressure systems.

Other criteria when choosing a support system includes the person's level of risk, the size and weight of the equipment, cost implications and ease of usage (Fletcher 1997).

The National Institute for Clinical Excellence (NICE 2003) has produced evidence-based clinical guidelines for pressure ulcer prevention which are downloadable from their website. However many organisations have developed their own local guidelines, based on available evidence. Their development and implementation is likely to be led by a multidisciplinary team.

Activity

Find out about your local guidelines for pressure ulcer prevention and also find out whether there are locally based tissue viability specialist nurses and how they can be contacted for advice. Also find out how pressure-relieving equipment is ordered locally.

Summary

- Pressure ulcers can have serious consequences so when a patient/client has been identified as at risk of pressure ulcers, it is essential that effective measures are taken to prevent pressure ulcer formation.
- Appropriate preventive measures for people at risk of pressure ulcers need to be planned. These should include providing a suitable support surface which does not impair mobility, using correct moving and handling techniques, promoting adequate nutrition, carer/patient education, pain management, and appropriate skin care.

PREVENTION OF OTHER COMPLICATIONS OF IMMOBILITY

Pressure ulcers are a significant potential problem for people with impaired mobility but there are a number of other possible complications.

LEARNING OUTCOMES

By the end of this section you will be able to:

1. Identify physical and psycho-social problems of immobility.
2. Identify ways in which nurses can minimise the problems of immobility.

Learning outcome 1: Identify physical and psycho-social problems of immobility

Activity

Think of patients/clients you have cared for whose mobility was reduced for some reason. They may have been confined to bed or wheelchair dependent, or physical or psychological problems may have made walking difficult. What physical and psycho-social problems did this limited mobility cause them?

- Circulatory: deep vein thrombosis, pulmonary embolus, orthostatic hypotension
- Respiratory: chest infection
- Gastrointestinal: loss of appetite, constipation
- Urinary: renal calculi, urinary tract infection, incontinence
- Musculo-skeletal: osteoporosis, muscle wasting, contractures
- Psycho-social: loss of self-esteem, frustration, boredom, isolation.

Box 5.3 Physical and psycho-social problems caused by reduced mobility

Compare your answers with the list of problems in Box 5.3. The observation that immobility affects so many bodily functions as well as having psycho-social effects highlights its multidimensional nature. These problems are discussed below.

Circulatory and respiratory problems

Formation of a deep vein thrombosis (DVT) can occur due to one or more predisposing factors: trauma (for example from surgical procedures), blood coagulation factors (dehydration can cause this) and stasis of venous circulation due to bed rest or immobility (Wallis and Autar 2001). Movement of the legs normally contracts the muscles, which press upon the veins and cause them to empty. Legs that are not mobile are unable to maintain the pumping action and the venous blood pools, causing a DVT. There may be no indication that there is a problem until the clot becomes detached and enters the pulmonary circulation into the lungs, causing a fatal pulmonary embolus (Breen 2000). Tracey is at risk as she has no voluntary movement in her legs. The risk of DVT in patients who have had a stroke (e.g. Mr Jones) is high due to the underlying vascular disorder (Gibbon 2002). The Autar DVT scale is available to identify people at risk of DVT (Autar 1996).

Orthostatic hypotension (a fall in blood pressure when moving to an upright position) can quickly develop in chair- and bed-bound patients. Tracey and Marion may feel faint and dizzy when they are transferred from bed to wheelchair. The possibility of orthostatic hypotension should also be considered when Mr Jones starts mobilising.

Decreased cardiac output and reduced tissue perfusion related to immobility can cause venous leg ulcers, particularly if there is associated poor calf muscle function or venous obstruction (Tyrrell 2002).

Impaired mobility can cause reduced ventilation of the lungs. The decreased movement and ventilation causes reduced stimulation for coughing. This leads to a build up of secretions in the bronchi and bronchioles, which can become infected and cause a chest infection. Mr Jones, Tracey and Marion could all be at risk of chest infections. Tracey has paralysis of her abdominal and intercostal muscles, which will reduce lung ventilation and affect her ability to cough, putting her at further risk of a chest infection.

Gastrointestinal problems

Impaired mobility can predispose to constipation and can also affect diet and fluid intake, further increasing the risk. Immobility can impair appetite and people with reduced mobility may find it difficult to pour out their own drinks or feed themselves. For example Marion is unable to feed herself and Mr Jones may not be able to reach his drinks on his locker independently. Constipation not only causes discomfort but also increases the risk of urinary tract infection and urge incontinence (Nazarko 1997).

Urinary problems

Urinary stasis may be caused by reduced mobility, which can cause urinary tract infection or renal calculi (stones). The latter occur when crystalline substances such as uric acid, calcium phosphate and oxalate, which are normally excreted in the urine, crystallise out of solution (Fillingham and Douglas 1997).

People who are immobile rely on staff to take them to the toilet or provide bedpans, urinals or commodes. Impaired mobility may also cause difficulties removing or adjusting clothing. This would be an issue for all the patients/clients in the scenarios and having to be dependent on staff to assist with elimination can threaten their dignity. Older people (such as Mr Jones) do not become aware of the need to empty their bladder (voiding) until the bladder is 90 per cent full (Wilson 2003). This may lead to incontinence when the person is unable to get to the toilet quickly because of impaired mobility.

Musculo-skeletal problems

In immobile parts of the body, muscle wasting commences and this muscle degeneration will deplete the capacity for movement, leading to further impairment. It is estimated that 10–15 per cent of muscle strength can be lost each week (Markey and Brown 2002). The lack of muscle activity will cause degenerative changes involving the release of calcium from the bones (osteoporosis), with loss of bone density.

If joints are allowed to stay in one position too long, the muscle fibres around the joint shorten and the collagen within the joint becomes tightly packed. This combined process causes a contracture (Nussbaum 2000). For Mr Jones a range of positions should be adopted which will discourage the development of abnormal tone and contractures (Gibbon 2002) but Marion already has some joint deformities. Joints particularly at risk are the shoulders, elbows, wrists, neck, fingers, hips, knees, ankles and toes. Contractures are associated with reduced mobility, pain, decreased function, pressure ulcers and institutionalisation (Fox and Wilson 1999). Contractures reduce stability and increase the risk of falls and this can restrict mobility further.

Psycho-social problems

Loss of mobility can cause people to experience loss of self-esteem, and they may feel frustration at being dependent on others.

Children in hospital can have difficulty playing in their usual ways, particularly when they are confined to bed, and can experience boredom. Tracey may find it difficult being bound by hospital rules and regulations and not being able to see her friends when she wants. It can be assumed that Tracey, having fallen from her horse, was an active child prior to her accident; it will take some time to adapt to her current situation where she uses a wheelchair for her mobility.

Older people like Mr Jones, who are admitted to hospital for an acute medical episode, may become functionally impaired, not only because of the disease process but also from the hospitalisation process – some becoming confused and disorientated. They may become depressed and apathetic and it is suggested that up to 75 per cent of functionally independent older people admitted into an acute hospital are no longer independent on discharge (Markey and Brown 2002).

For people like Marion with profound learning and multiple disabilities there may be frustration at having to rely on carers to move her around, and having to make her needs and wishes known with limited communication ability. Mr Jones may also experience feelings of frustration for similar reasons.

Impaired mobility can also affect the ability and opportunity to socialise and communicate with others, leading to isolation, boredom and sensory deprivation. Mr Barnes has had impaired mobility resulting from his accident for some time and this could have contributed to his depression. People can experience despair, loneliness and isolation as family and friends withdraw (Moore and McLaughlin 2003).

Learning outcome 2: Identify ways in which nurses can minimise the problems of immobility

Roper *et al.* (2000) suggest that when planning care, the objective of the plan is:

■ to prevent identified potential problems from becoming actual ones
■ to solve actual problems
■ where possible to alleviate those that cannot be solved
■ to prevent reoccurrence of problems that have been resolved
■ to help the person to cope positively with those problems that cannot be alleviated or solved.

■ **Activity**

We have identified a number of potential and actual problems related to impaired mobility in our four patients/clients. Consider the nursing interventions that could be implemented to prevent or solve these problems.

A few points, which you may have considered, are discussed below.

Deep vein thrombosis/pulmonary embolus

The signs and symptoms of DVT – painful, swollen calf, and of pulmonary embolus – chest pain and cough, are all part of nursing observations. Nurses, in liaison with physiotherapists, can help people with active, passive and isometric exercises of the legs. Passive exercises are where another person puts the limb through a range of movement, while active exercises are when people carry out exercises themselves. Isometric exercises involve muscle contraction with minimal muscle shortening so that there is no movement (Bronte and Gray 1995). Graduated compression stockings are another possible preventive measure. These enhance venous return and blood flow, but there are contraindications to their use, for example leg deformities, severe arteriosclerosis and local skin disorders (Mills 1997). When applying these stockings it is essential to measure the leg carefully so that the correct size is chosen, to achieve optimum prophylaxis and patient acceptability (Wallis and Autar 2001) and to follow the manufacturer's instructions for application. Anticoagulants may also be prescribed for those at high risk. A reduced incidence of DVT has been found in studies in which patients have been prescribed aspirin, as aspirin reduces the 'stickiness' of platelets in the blood, so that aggregation is less likely to occur (Gibbon 2002).

Orthostatic hypotension

In our scenarios, this can be alleviated by gradually sitting Tracey and Marion up in bed before they are transferred into their chairs. Marion's carers will need to be aware of the signs and symptoms of orthostatic hypotension as she may not be able to verbally communicate if she feels dizzy. It is also important to explain to Marion and Tracey what is happening to reduce any anxiety relating to these symptoms.

Chest infection

Frequent repositioning and encouragement to do deep breathing exercises can help to prevent chest infection. The optimal position for breathing can be seen in Fig. 11.1. The person can also be encouraged to cough to clear secretions and prevent them pooling in the lungs. Chapter 11 has a section on observation of sputum which includes tips on how expectoration of sputum can be encouraged.

Loss of appetite and constipation

An adequate fluid and diet intake should be provided, taking individual preferences into account and ensuring that there is sufficient fibre included. Mr Jones should have his food and drinks positioned so that he can reach them. As he has a right-sided hemiplegia he needs to be provided with a non-slip mat to prevent his plate moving, a plate guard to help keep the food on the plate and an appropriate cup for drinking from. Mr Barnes has his dominant arm in plaster, making it difficult to cut up his food. People with profound learning and multiple physical disabilities, like Marion, may have difficulty with eating and drinking and nurses should aim to enhance the quality of their mealtime experience. Chapter 9 'Assessing and meeting nutritional needs' includes more detail about these issues.

Urinary problems: urinary tract infection, incontinence

People who are at risk of urinary tract infection should be observed for signs such as cloudy, foul-smelling urine. In Chapter 9 the section on urinalysis explains how urinary tract infection might be suspected and when a specimen of urine should be sent for microscopy, culture and sensitivity. Marion would require continence aids but consideration must be given to body image, comfort and skin care, and as to how continence can be promoted, rather than only contained. Mr Jones's hemiplegia will make it difficult for him to walk; he may need to be positioned within a short walking distance from the toilet when he starts to mobilise. People who are confused may need guidance to get to the toilet. Making toilets easy to identify by using colour, signs and pictures can help (Nazarko 1997). Tracey will need to be taught how to manage her supra-pubic catheter as blockage, leakage and infection can be a problem (Bardsley 2000). Chapter 8 'Meeting elimination needs' covers all these issues in detail and will help you to develop your practical skills in relation to those who need help with elimination.

Muscle wasting and contractures

This is an issue for Marion because as muscle contraction increases, this further limits joint movement. People with profound learning disabilities who are immobile are particularly at risk of developing deformities. Prevention and management requires a multiprofessional approach with physiotherapy as part of everyday activities, occupational therapy input and devices such as splints and body braces (Wake 1997). Tracey and Mr Jones should be positioned carefully with their limbs kept in symmetry. Splints may be prescribed and physiotherapy and occupational therapy will play an important role in preventing contractures. Botulinum toxin can be used to reduce muscle tone and increase the range of movements in a joint. It can be targeted to individual muscles (Gibbon 2002).

Loss of self-esteem, frustration, boredom and isolation

As discussed in Chapter 1, how nurses carry out care may affect how people feel about themselves. A caring and empathetic approach from nurses can assist in reducing the psycho-social effects of impaired mobility. Chapter 2 looks at the approach of nurses when carrying out practical skills, and emphasises self-awareness. Family and friends have an important role in providing support too. Parental participation is viewed in terms of partnership by Casey (1993), with the emphasis on the family providing care, complemented by nurses. Family-centred care is explored by Lawrence et al. (2003). Most children's units have play therapists and they have an important role with children whose mobility is restricted. The presence of Tracey's parents, her siblings and friends are essential to her psychological well-being, and will relieve potential boredom and isolation. There should also be provision to ensure that Tracey's education is continued, which might reduce some of the psychological effects of her impaired mobility.

Summary

■ People who have reduced mobility are at risk of a number of physical and psycho-social complications.

■ Nurses have an important role in identifying potential complications and implementing preventive care.

ASSISTING WITH MOBILISATION AND PREVENTING FALLS

This is an important role of nurses in many settings, and involves nurses enabling barriers to be overcome and working closely with other members of the multi-disciplinary team, particularly physiotherapists and occupational therapists.

LEARNING OUTCOMES

By the end of this section you will be able to:

1. Identify barriers to mobilisation.
2. Examine ways of preventing falls.
3. Discuss how people can be assisted with mobilisation.

Learning outcome 1: Identify barriers to mobilisation

Activity

What barriers can you identify that could prevent a patient or client from mobilising? How might these apply to the people in the scenarios?

A few possibilities are listed below but you may well have thought of others.

■ Pain or fear of pain may prevent a person from maintaining or regaining their mobility, and this is an important issue for Mr Barnes. Therefore pain must be assessed and strategies implemented to control it. Pain management is focused on in Chapter 12.

■ Lack of motivation, perhaps where people have depression or dementia, may lead to reluctance to move around. Mr Barnes's depression could therefore present a further barrier to mobilisation.

■ Foot problems such as untrimmed toenails, callus and corns can impede mobility by causing pain and discomfort (Love 1995, Tyrrell 2002). These factors could be relevant to Mr Jones and Mr Barnes. Bunions and arthritic feet make it difficult to wear normal shoes.

■ Unsuitable footwear makes mobilising difficult and dangerous; when Mr Jones starts mobilising this is an important consideration. Slip-on shoes or slippers will increase the tendency to shuffle; shiny or plastic soles will cause a frightened, small-step gait. Narrow shoes inhibit normal foot movement, reducing normal toe function and preventing normal toe 'push off', which affects gait pattern and weight transference (Finlay and Fullerton 1996). Ill-fitting shoes can cause blisters, corns, callus and bursae, which are painful and can lead to ulceration (Tyrrell 2002).

■ Arthritic knees can cause instability and falls, which in turn can lead to loss of confidence.

■ Shortening of one leg may occur after the surgical correction of a fractured neck of femur, making it difficult for the person to put both feet on the ground together.

■ Fear of falling is a common problem and this can cause a fear of going outside, and even lead to agoraphobia. When a person, like Mr Barnes, has already had one fall resulting in a significant injury, fear of another fall and a lack of confidence in mobilising is understandable.

Learning outcome 2: Examine ways of preventing falls

The prevention of falls is the focus of one of the sections in *The National Service Framework for Older People* (Department of Health 2001c) and falls in older people is a problem that is being addressed nationally and internationally (Swift 2002). However, people in other age groups can, like Mr Barnes, be at risk of falling too. The effects of falls extend beyond physical injury and cost to the health services. Fear of subsequent falls can lead to restricted mobility and independence. This contributes to functional decline, which in turn contributes to an increased risk of falls. Another potential result of a fall is social isolation due to self-restriction of social activities (Rawsky 1998).

■ **Activity**	Consider people you have cared for in practice who were in hospital as the result of a fall, or perhaps fell while in hospital. List the reasons for their falls.

People you have cared for may have fallen for the following reasons:

■ Poor vision due to age-related deterioration or other visual problems. People may trip over objects in the dark, trip on carpets or uneven floors or miss stairs and fall.

■ Poor mobility with age-related changes in gait, posture and balance. Changes in the inner ear affect a person's sense of balance.

■ Loss of muscle strength and flexibility may make it difficult to hold handrails or get out of chairs.

■ Medications and alcohol can cause dizziness, blurred vision, weakness, poor balance and drowsiness. Mr Barnes's medication for his depression could have these effects. Diuretics and laxatives increase the number of trips to the toilet, often in a hurry. Polypharmacy (taking more than four different medicines) is a recognised predisposing factor in falls (Department of Health 2001d).

- Chronic diseases increase the tendency to fall. For example, Parkinson's disease causes people to stoop, lean forward and develop a short-stepped, shuffling gait; diabetes may cause decreased sensation in legs and feet; stroke affects mobility and balance.
- Fear of falling is contributed to by both physiological and psycho-social factors. People may experience a morbid fear of falling (Walker 1998).

The National Service Framework for Older People recommends that older people who have fallen should be referred to a specialist falls service, which can carry out a comprehensive assessment (Department of Health 2001c). All nurses should be aware of risk factors for falls and be aware of the falls service and how referrals are made.

 Activity | Now think of some ideas as to how falls can be prevented for people who are considered to be at risk.

The following interventions can be effective in preventing falls:

- Muscle strengthening and balance retraining
- Home hazard assessment and modifications to a person's home
- Withdrawal of psychotopic drugs and sedatives
- Regular eye examinations and provision of the correct prescription lenses, walking sticks or walking frames
- Regular exercise to improve gait, posture and flexibility (Gatti 2002; Walker 1998).

The Department of Trade and Industry's website contains useful information on preventing falls (www.dti.gov.uk/homesafetynetwork).

Learning outcome 3: Discuss how people can be assisted with mobilisation

Activity | Focus on the practice scenarios and identify strategies and equipment, which might assist with mobilisation.

You probably considered involvement of the multidisciplinary team, and will have encountered mobility aids. Helping a person to mobilise certainly requires a multidisciplinary approach. For example the orthotist will be able to supply callipers, shoes or knee braces to overcome some of the barriers to mobility. Physiotherapists will assess people for mobility aids such as crutches, or walking frames – standard, or wheeled ones for those who cannot lift a standard frame. Gutter frames can help people with arthritis. Those unable to walk, like Marion and Tracey, will be supplied with wheelchairs. Special chairs with cushions that rise slowly can be helpful for people who have difficulty getting up from a chair. For Mr Jones the physiotherapist will develop a plan, for example the Bobath technique prescribes how a patient is to be handled and moved (Gibbon 2002).

- Specific verbal strategies, involving thoughtful wording, e.g. encouraging and reinforcing, using simple terms: 'Keep going', 'You're doing well'.
- Non-verbal strategies, making use of cues, e.g. holding out your hand towards the person and using touch.
- Strategies to minimise the fear of falling, such as filling the empty space in front of the person with a solid object such as a chair, or ensuring that there is a rail to hold onto by the side.
- Movement strategies, where the carer interprets the environment for the person with dementia. This might entail getting the person to follow you, and copy how you are walking.

Box 5.4 Restoring or minimising loss of mobility in people with dementia (Oddy 1996)

Restoring or minimising loss of mobility in people with dementia is challenging but Oddy (1996) has suggested an approach that uses both communication and movement strategies (see Box 5.4). These strategies are used to bridge the gap that keeps people with dementia disconnected from their environment and from those around them.

Dressing and undressing Marion, who has severe contractures, can be very difficult and the occupational therapist can advise about suitable clothing. Splints and braces can help to maintain body and limb posture. Arm gaiters help to minimise involuntary muscle action so that she might be able to use an adapted motorised wheelchair, thus increasing her independence in mobilising (Wake 1997).

When helping a person to mobilise the safety of both the individual and the nurse must be a major consideration. As we have already discussed, some people may be unsteady on their feet or have lost confidence. Therefore a risk assessment must be carried out before any attempt is made to assist with mobilising. You have probably looked at risk assessment within moving and handling training sessions, and will be aware of the importance of documentation.

Moving and handling risk assessment

You will probably have seen moving and handling assessment tools being used in practice for carrying out and documenting a systematic assessment. They are likely to include sections relating to task, individual capability, load and environment. For example:

- **Task**: What exactly is the manoeuvre to be carried out? For example the task might be to move Tracey out of bed and into her wheelchair.
- **Individual capability**: Here nurses need to assess their own ability and what they are capable of.
- **Load**: How much can the person do for themselves? Tracey is fit, has no communication problems and with support and training will eventually be

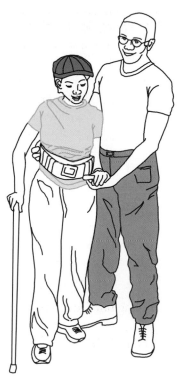

Figure 5.3 Helping a person to walk.

able to transfer from bed to wheelchair using a lateral transfer board. Marion, although not particularly heavy, is unable to move and therefore needs a hoist to move her out of bed.

■ **Environment**: Is there enough room for you and the person to work in? Slippery floors are a danger for people like Mr Jones who are learning to walk or who are unsteady on their feet.

If people cannot move themselves then equipment must be used. You will be able to practise using different equipment in your moving and handling sessions.

Assisting a person to walk

When assisting a person to walk, you stand beside them, facing forward so you both move the same way. The use of a transfer belt around the person's waist gives you something to hold. For example, Mr Jones has a slight weakness on the right side, so you stand at his right side in a walk stance, with your left hand holding the belt around his waist, and his right hand in your right hand, using a palm to palm grip (see Fig. 5.3). On the command 'Ready, brace, stand', you both move forward as you transfer your weight from the back leg to the front. You can now use this hold to give the person confidence to walk. You will have the opportunity to practise these techniques under supervision in the classroom. A very important aspect is not to hurry the person, maintaining a slow steady pace.

Summary

- Building people's confidence and self-esteem is an important aspect of mobilisation and nurses are part of a multidisciplinary approach to the care and management of people with problems of mobility.
- Nurses should be aware of barriers to mobilisation, in order that these can be addressed.
- It is important to identify people who are at risk of falling and implement interventions to prevent falls.
- When assisting with mobilising, risk assessment is essential and must be documented.
- Appropriate mobility aids should be provided for each individual and nurses can give encouragement and support to people who are regaining mobility.

CHAPTER SUMMARY

The underlying reasons for impaired mobility are wide ranging, and may be temporary or permanent. However, the possible complications of impaired mobility can lead to much discomfort and further health problems, so nurses must take a proactive role to prevent these ill-effects. Pressure ulcers were focused on in some depth within this chapter, as their incidence remains widespread even though it is well recognised that they are largely preventable. This chapter has emphasised the importance of identifying potential problems, so that effective preventive strategies for each individual can be implemented. The promotion of mobility wherever possible is the key to preventing many of these problems, and a multidisciplinary approach to this should be taken. Finally, it is essential when caring for people with impaired mobility, that correct moving and handling techniques are used to protect both clients and nurses. It was beyond the scope of the chapter to address this topic in depth. These techniques need to be learnt under supervision and attendance at moving and handling sessions is essential.

REFERENCES

Arblaster, G. 1998. Reducing pressure sores after hip fractures. *Professional Nurse* **13**, 749–52.

Armstrong, D. and Bortz, P. 2001. An integrative review of pressure relief in surgical patients. *AORN Journal* **73**, 645, 647–8.

Autar, R. 1996. Nursing assessment of clients at risk of deep vein thrombosis (DVT): the Autar DVT scale. *Journal of Advanced Nursing* **23**, 763–70.

Bardsley, A. 2000. The neurogenic bladder. *Nursing Standard* **14**(22), 39–41.

Bergstrom, N., Braden, B.J., Laguzza, A. and Holman, V. 1987. The Braden scale for predicting pressure sore risk. *Nursing Research* **36**, 205–10.

Breen, P. 2000. DVT what every nurse should know. *RN* **63**(4), 58–61.

Bronte, M. and Gray, A. 1995. Care implications of disorders of the cardiovascular system. In Peattie, P. and Walker, S. (eds) *Understanding Nursing Care,* fourth edition. Edinburgh: Churchill Livingstone, 385–439.

Brown, S. 2001. Bed surfaces and pressure sore prevention: an abridged report. *Orthopaedic Nursing* **20**(4), 38–40.

Burman, P.M.S. and O'Dea, K. 1994. Measuring pressure. *Journal of Wound Care* **3**, 283–6.

Butcher, M. 1999. Identifying and combating the risk of pressure. *Nursing Standard* **14**(3), 58, 60, 62–3.

Casey, A. 1993. Development and use of the partnership model of care. In Glasper, A. and Tucker, A. (eds) *Recent Advances in Child Health Care*. London: Scutari, 183–93.

Clark, M. 2002. Pressure ulcers and quality of life. *Nursing Standard* **16**(22), 74–8, 80.

Collins F. 1999. Preventing pressure sores in the seated patient. *Nursing Standard* **13**(42), 50–4.

Collins, F. 2001. Sitting: pressure ulcer development. *Nursing Standard* **15**(22), 54–8.

Cook, G., and Nendick, C. 1999. Manual handling: what factors do nurses assess? *Journal of Clinical Nursing* **8**, 422–30.

Cowan, T. and Woollons, S. 1998. Dynamic systems for pressure sore prevention. *Professional Nurse* **13**, 387–94.

Culley, F. 1998. Nursing aspects of pressure sore prevention and therapy. *British Journal of Nursing* **7**(15), 879–80, 882, 884.

Cullum, N., Deeks, J., Song, F. and Fletcher, A.W. 2003. Beds, mattresses and cushions for pressure sore prevention and treatment (Cochrane review). In *The Cochrane Library*, issue 3. Oxford: Update Software.

Dealey, C. 1997. *Managing Pressure Sore Prevention*. Salisbury: Quay Books, Mark Allen Publishing.

Department of Health 1993. *Pressure Ulcers: A key quality indicator*. London: DH.

Department of Health 2001a. *Valuing People: A new strategy for learning disability for the 21st century*. London: DH.

Department of Health 2001b. *The Essence of Care. Patient-focused benchmarking for health care practitioners*. London: DH.

Department of Health 2001c. *The National Service Framework for Older People*. London: DH.

Department of Health 2001d. *Medicines and Older People: Implementing medicines-related aspects of the NSF for older people*. London: DH.

Dunford, C. 1998. Managing pressure sores. *Nursing Standard* **12**(24), 38–42.

EPUAP (European Pressure Ulcer Advisory Panel) 2003. *Pressure Ulcer Classification*. http://www.epuap.org/puclas/theory. Accessed 18 December 2003.

Ferguson M., Cook A., Rimmasch H. *et al.* 2000. Pressure ulcer management: the importance of nutrition. *MEDSURG Nursing* **9**(4), 163–80.

Fillingham, S. and Douglas, J. 1997. *Urological Nursing*, second edition. London: Baillière Tindall.

Finlay, O. and Fullerton, C. 1996. Feet and footwear in older people. In Squires, A.J. (ed.) *Rehabilitation of Older People*, second edition. London: Chapman and Hall, 167–93.

Fletcher, J. 1996. The principles of pressure sore prevention. *Nursing Standard* **10**(39), 47–55.

Fletcher, J. 1997. Pressure-relieving equipment: criteria and selection. *British Journal of Nursing* **6**, 323–8.

Fox, D. and Wilson, D. 1999. Parents' experiences of general hospital admission for adults with learning disabilities. *Journal of Clinical Nursing* **8**, 610–14.

Gatti, J. 2002. Cochrane for clinicians: putting evidence into practice. Which interventions help to prevent falls in the elderly? *American Family Physician* **65**, 225–8.

Gibbon, B. 2002. Rehabilitation following stroke. *Nursing Standard* **16**(29), 47–52, 54–5.

Gould, D., James, T., Tarpey, A. *et al.* 2000. Intervention studies to reduce the prevalence of pressure sores: a literature review. *Journal of Clinical Nursing* **9**, 163–78.

Hampton S.1998. Can electric beds aid pressure sore prevention in hospitals? *British Journal of Nursing* 7, 1010–17.

Harris, M. 2000. The patient in need of rehabilitation. In Alexander, M., Fawcett, J. and Runciman, P. (eds) *Nursing Practice, Hospital and Home. The Adult*, second edition. Edinburgh: Churchill Livingstone, 983–7.

Hawkins, S., Stone, K. and Plummer, L. 1999. An holistic approach to turning patients. *Nursing Standard* **14**(3), 51–2, 54–6.

James, H. 1998. Classification and grading of pressure sores. *Professional Nurse* **13**(10), 6–10.

Lewis, B. 1998. Nutrient intake and the risk of pressure sore development in older patients. *Journal of Wound Care* **7**, 31–5.

Lawrence, C., Gibson, F. and Zur, J. 2003. Care delivery: the needs of children. In Hinchliff, S., Norman, S. and Schober, J. (eds) *Nursing Practice and Health Care*, fourth edition. London: Arnold, 177–202.

Love, C. 1995. Nursing or chiropody? Nurses' attitudes to toe nail trimming. *Professional Nurse* **10**, 241–4.

Lowthian, P. 1987. The practical assessment of pressure sore risk. *Care – Science and Practice* **5**(4), 3–7.

Lowthian, P. 1997. Notes on the pathogenesis of serious pressure sores. *British Journal of Nursing* **6**, 907–12.

Markey, D. and Brown, R. 2002. An interdisciplinary approach to addressing patient activity and mobility in the medical-surgical patient. *Journal of Nursing Care Quality* **16**(4), 1–12.

Mills, C. 1997. Pulmonary embolus. *Nursing Times* **93**(51), 50–3.

Moore, K. and McLaughlin, D. 2003. Depression: the challenge for health care professionals. *Nursing Standard* **17**(26), 45–52, 54–5.

Nazarko, L. 1997. Continence. The whole story. *Nursing Times* **93**(43), 63–4, 66, 68.

NICE (National Institute for Clinical Excellence) 2003. *Pressure Ulcer Prevention: Pressure ulcer risk assessment and prevention, including the use of pressure-relieving devices (beds, mattresses and overlays) for the prevention of pressure ulcers in primary and secondary care. Clinical guideline 7.* London: NICE. Available from http://www.nice.org.uk.

Norton, D., Exton-Smith, A. and McLaren, R. 1962. *An Investigation of Geriatric Nursing Problems in Hospital.* London: National Corporation for the Care of Old People.

Nussbaum S. 2000. Contracture management. In Nesathurai, S. (ed.) *The Rehabilitation of People with Spinal Cord Injury*, second edition. Massachusetts: Blackwell, 67–74.

Oddy, R. 1996. Strategies to help people keep moving. *Journal of Dementia Care* **4**(4), 22–4.

Olding, L. and Patterson, J. 1998. Growing concern. *Nursing Times* **94**(38), 76–9.

Pang, S. and Wong, T. 1998. Predicting pressure sore risk with the Norton, Braden and Waterlow scales in a Hong Kong rehabilitation hospital. *Nursing Research* **47**, 147–53.

Penzer, R. and Finch, M. 2001. Promoting healthy skin in older people. *Nursing Standard* **15**(34), 46–52, 54–5.

Pickersgill, J. 1997. Taking the pressure off. *Paediatric Nursing* **7**(8), 25–7.

Rawsky, E. 1998. Review of the literature on falls among the elderly. *Image Journal of Nursing Scholarship* **30**(1), 47–52.

Roper, N., Logan, W. and Tierney, A.J. 2000. *The Roper-Logan-Tierney Model of Nursing.* Edinburgh: Churchill Livingstone.

Rush, K., and Ouellet, L. 1993. Mobility: a concept analysis. *Journal of Advanced Nursing* **18**, 486–92.

Russell, L. 1998. Physiology of the skin and prevention of pressure sores. *British Journal of Nursing* **7**, 1088–100.

Schoonhoven, L., Defloor, T. and Grypdonck, M. 2002. Incidence of pressure ulcers due to surgery. *Journal of Clinical Nursing* **11**, 479–87.

Simpson, A., Bowers, K. and Weir-Hughes, D. 1996. *Pressure Sore Prevention.* Gateshead: Athenaeum.

Smith, L., Booth, N., Douglas, D. *et al.* 1995. A critique of 'at risk' pressure sore assessment tools. *Journal of Clinical Nursing* **4**, 153–9.

Stephens, F. and Bick, D. 2002. Organisational perspective: a pressure ulcer risk assessment and prevention audit: a pilot. *Nursing Management* **9**(3), 24–9.

Strachan-Bennett, S. 2003. Tool aims to standardise nurses' nutritional care. *Nursing Times* **99**(46), 7.

Swift, C. 2002. The NHS English National Service Framework for Older People: opportunities and risks. *Clinical Medicine* **2**, 139–43.

Tingle J. 1997. Pressure sores: counting the cost of nursing neglect. *British Journal of Nursing* **6**, 757–8.

Tyrrell, W. 2002. The causes and management of foot ulceration. *Nursing Standard* **16**(30), 53, 54, 56, 58, 60, 62.

Young T. 1997. Pressure sores: incidence, risk assessment and prevention. *British Journal of Nursing* **6**, 319–21.

Wake, E. 1997. Profound and multiple disabilities. In Gates, B. (ed.) *Learning Disabilities*, third edition. Churchill Livingstone, Edinburgh.

Walker, B. 1998. Preventing falls (as America ages). *RN* **61**(5), 40–3.

Wallis, M. and Autar, R. 2001. Deep vein thrombosis: clinical nursing management. *Nursing Standard* **15**(18), 47–57.

Waterlow, J. 1985. Pressure sores: a risk assessment card. *Nursing Times* **81**(48), 49, 51, 55.

Waterlow, J. 1988. The Waterlow card for the prevention and management of pressure sores: toward a pocket policy. *Care – Science and Practice* **6**(1), 8–12.

Wiechula R. 1997. Pressure sores – Part 1: Prevention of pressure related damage. *Australian Nursing Journal* **5**(5) Best Practice 1–7.

Wilson, L. 2003. Focus on older people. In Getliffe, K. and Dolman, M. (eds) *Promoting Continence: A clinical research resource*, second edition. London: Baillière Tindall, 135–84.

Principles of wound care

Deirdre Thompson and Janine Jones

The maintenance of skin integrity and management of acute and chronic wounds is a major component of nursing care, relevant to all care settings (Bryant 2000), and has even been referred to as the 'bread-and-butter' of nursing (Williams and Young 1998). Waldrop and Doughty (2000) note that an ageing population and an increasing incidence of chronic disease necessitates a sound foundation in the principles relating to wound care. The aim of this chapter is to assist you to develop a knowledge and understanding of the breadth of issues involved with wound healing, and to apply this to your practice.

Wound management is a vast topic with an ever-expanding and developing knowledge base, to which whole books and journals are dedicated. You are therefore advised that, while this chapter provides a foundation, further reading will be necessary, and you need to continually update your knowledge base; the Cochrane Library and the National Institute for Clinical Excellence (NICE) (discussed in Chapter 1) are good sources. There are a number of other chapters in this book that are directly relevant to wound care: Chapter 3 'Preventing cross-infection', Chapter 5 'Caring for people with impaired mobility', Chapter 7 'Meeting hygiene needs' and Chapter 9 'Assessing and meeting nutritional needs'. These chapters will increase your awareness of some elements of care that help to maintain skin integrity and promote healing. You should also take every opportunity when in the practice setting to increase your knowledge in this field, and there are specialist nurses (e.g. tissue viability and dermatology nurses) and other members of the multidisciplinary team (e.g. podiatrists) who will be valuable resources.

This chapter includes:
- The phases of wound healing
- Classification of wounds and their management
- Factors affecting wound healing
- Wound assessment
- Wound management.

Although you can study this chapter at any stage of your programme, it is particularly recommended that you work through the sections when based in a setting where you have patients/clients with different wounds. There is no substitute for looking at real wounds, and applying theory to practice. Note that Chapter 3 'Preventing cross-infection', is essential prior reading, as when managing wounds an understanding of how microorganisms are transmitted, and adherence to handwashing and non-touch technique, is paramount.

Recommended biology reading:

The following questions will help you to focus on the biology underpinning this chapter's skills. Use your recommended text book to find out:

- What characteristics must skin possess?
- What are the major layers of the skin?
- Which layer is avascular?
- What are the major functions of the skin? What role does skin play in homeostasis?
- How does the skin protect itself against damage and infection?
- What factors can lead to a breakdown in skin integrity? What would the consequences be?
- What is the goal of wound healing? What factors influence the degree of scarring?
- How does age alter the skin's characteristics? Consider the skin at birth, adolescence, young adulthood and old age.
- How does the appearance of skin change, during illness, injury or stress?
- What factors are necessary to maintain normal healthy skin?

An understanding of the physiology of wound healing is essential when assessing and managing wounds, and is therefore included in this chapter.

PRACTICE SCENARIOS

The following practice scenarios illustrate different situations where wound care is required, and are referred to throughout this chapter.

Adult

Mrs Warner is 78 years old, and has a history of type 2 diabetes, which is managed with oral hypoglycaemic medication. Since her husband died 2 years ago she has lived alone with her two cats and has been treated for depression. After falling in her kitchen she was unable to get off the floor, and was found by a neighbour some hours later. After assessment in Accident and Emergency (A&E) she was diagnosed with a stable fracture of her pelvis. She was also found to have an ulcer (open sore) on one of her toes, which had an offensive discharge. Her blood glucose was high. She was transferred to a ward for rehabilitation and pain management. A few days later a large area of black necrotic (dead) tissue developed on her sacrum, and discoloured areas on both her elbows. These appeared to have been caused by the period of prolonged pressure on the kitchen floor. Mrs Warner is keen to get home as soon as possible as she is worried about her cats. She normally smokes ten cigarettes a day and is overweight. Her diet is high in fat and carbohydrates and she rarely eats fruit or vegetables.

Child

Thomas is 4 years old and was brought to A&E after being bitten on his face by the family dog. He and his mother were very upset. He had a number of varied wounds and these were irrigated thoroughly before being closed with sutures, tissue adhesive and steristrips. He was prescribed antibiotics but now, four days later, he has returned to A&E with pain and swelling around the wounds and they have an offensive discharge.

Learning disability

Susan is 32 years old and has a moderate learning disability. She lives in a small group home and was recently in hospital having her acutely inflamed appendix removed. She has been discharged home and has a small abdominal wound, which seems to be healing well. However Susan is concerned about the wound and is worried about getting it wet when she showers, and drying and dressing afterwards in case she harms the wound. She is due to have her sutures removed by the practice nurse. The community nurse for learning disability, who is Susan's **health facilitator**, is visiting regularly to give some support in this situation.

Mental health

Colin is 28 years old, and is being treated as an in-patient in the acute mental health unit, after deterioration in his mental health, which has affected his self-care ability. He has a diagnosis of substance abuse and schizophrenia, which is currently being treated by **clozapine**. Colin requires careful blood monitoring, as clozapine can affect white blood cell levels. While on the unit he complained of pain in his left upper buttock. A large, hot, swollen area was found, which was diagnosed as being an **abscess**. Colin says that he has had several of these before. Incision and drainage took place in theatre and he has now returned to the unit, with a pack *in situ* in the wound. Antibiotics have been prescribed.

THE PHASES OF WOUND HEALING

A wound can be defined as 'a disruption of normal anatomical structure and function which results from pathological processes beginning internally or

Health facilitator
A member of the community learning disabilities team (often a nurse) who supports a person with learning disabilities to access the health care they need. See *Valuing People* (Department of Health 2001).

Clozapine
An atypical antipsychotic drug which has been proved to have efficacy in treatment-resistant schizophrenia and ameliorating negative schizophrenic symptoms (King 1998).

Abscess
A localized collection of pus. Pus is a thick fluid containing leucocytes, bacteria and cellular debris, and indicates infection.

externally to the involved organ' (Lazarus *et al.* 1994). Injury to tissue initiates a complex and orchestrated range of cellular and extracellular events to occur within the wounded area (Schultz 2000). Different wounds do not necessarily follow the same pattern in the healing process. Waldrop and Doughty (2000) explain that:

- Wounds confined to the epidermis and partial-thickness dermis can heal by regeneration.
- Wounds extending through the whole dermis heal by scar formation.

In order to understand the phases of wound healing, it is necessary to examine the cell biological processes involved in normal healing.

LEARNING OUTCOMES

By the end of this section you will be able to:

1. Distinguish the phases of healing and recognise tissue appearance at each stage.
2. Show awareness that healing does not in reality occur in a simple linear fashion.
3. Recognise problems with wound healing and the appearance of scar tissue.

Learning outcome 1: Distinguish the phases of healing and recognise tissue appearance at each stage

The process of wound healing is usually described in three distinct phases. Williams and Young (1998) state that this is a false division, which is done in an attempt to simplify this very complex process. Some authors describe four or more phases/stages but these variations are simply an expansion on the three phases described. Similarly you may find that different terminology is used to describe the phases within the texts which you refer to. This chapter employs the approach that there are three interdependent phases during the process of wound healing.

The inflammatory phase

This phase prepares the tissue for repair. After wounding, blood loss is controlled by a complex series of events, known as haemostasis. This protective mechanism aims to minimise injury and initiate the healing response (Williams and Young 1998). The cellular aspect of this phase occurs within hours of wounding (Krizek *et al.* 1997). The primary function is to attract phagocytes to the inflamed area to kill bacteria and remove debris from dead and dying cells within the tissue spaces (Kloth and McCulloch 1995). This process is known as phagocytosis. The five cardinal signs of inflammation are: heat, redness, pain, swelling and loss of function.

The proliferative phase

This phase rebuilds the tissue through three separate processes:

- **Granulation** leads to the formation of new blood vessels (angiogenesis) in a collagen-rich matrix. Fibroblasts and endothelial cells are the primary cells in this phase. Fibroblasts from the surrounding tissue need to become activated in order to be able to replicate (Witte and Barbul 1997). Granulation tissue is characterised by a reddish velvety carpet in the base of the wound.
- **Contraction** is the approximation of the wound edges believed to be caused by the 'push' and 'pull' effect of the myofibroblasts (Witte and Barbul 1997).
- **Epithelialisation** resurfaces the wound by regeneration of epithelial cells.

In full-thickness wounds regeneration occurs from wound margins, while in partial-thickness wounds remnants of partially ablated hair follicles also contribute to re-epithelialisation (Waldrop and Doughty 2000). Contraction and epithelialisation can be identified by a marginal zone of smooth tissue.

The maturation phase

This phase involves remodelling the tissue to form a scar. This can take a year or more as cellular activity reduces and the number of blood vessels in the wound decreases (Krizek *et al.* 1997).

Activity

Prior to observing and assessing wounds, you need some underpinning theoretical knowledge. Prepare notes on the phases of healing, which are outlined briefly above, from your recommended biology textbook. Clancy and McVicar's (1997) paper explains the homeostatic responses of wound healing, so this is also a useful source. Try to focus in your reading on the requirements for each phase of the healing process.

Your reading should have helped you to understand that the wound healing process is a complex interplay of events leading to complete healing.

Activity

Aim to observe an uncomplicated surgical wound, or a minor traumatic wound – this could even be a laceration on your own skin. Compare the appearance of the wound to the described criteria for different phases of healing. Discuss with a practitioner which phase of healing is predominant at present.

At different phases of wound healing, the tissue has a different appearance.

- When observed in the **inflammatory** phase, the wound appears swollen and red, and the surrounding tissue feels warm and can be painful. Recognising these signs (which occur due to local vasodilation) can be difficult at first. Note that in the inflammatory phase, the wound is usually kept covered to prevent contamination.

- In the **proliferative** phase, signs of wound contraction commence. The appearance of tiny red buds is the first sign of primitive blood vessels emerging, acting as a transport system for nutrients, oxygen, cells and growth factors essential for the development of connective tissue (Witte and Barbul 1997). This friable tissue which fills the deficit at the wound bed is also referred to as granulation tissue. New epithelial cells divide and using a leapfrog action migrate from wound edges and any remaining islands of epidermal cells that may encompass sebaceous glands and hair follicles.

- A wound in the **maturation** phase may remain in this phase for up to 2 years. It will appear smaller, and may be white and hard (scar tissue), and fixed to surrounding tissue, or similar in appearance to surrounding tissue, indicating a healed mature wound. The maximum tensile strength post injury is 70–85 per cent (Levenson *et al.* 1965).

Casey (1999) summarises the implications of the different colours of wounds as:

- **Black**: Necrotic (dead) tissue and therefore no healing has begun (Plate 1)
- **Yellow**: Slough (made up of dead cells). Occurs near the end of the inflammatory stage (Plate 2)
- **Red**: Granulation tissue (Plate 3)
- **Pink**: Epithelialisation (Plate 4).

■ *Activity*	Now that you have some understanding of the phases of healing and the possible appearance of wounds at different phases, consider how the community nurse for learning disabilities might reduce Susan's anxiety about her wound, and prepare her for suture removal.

Points that you might have considered are:

- The community nurse will need to have assessed Susan's cognitive and physical ability to care for her wound and would then be able to approach helping Susan to understand the wound's healing, and the care it requires, from this informed basis.
- The nurse can use effective communication skills to ascertain Susan's understanding of the healing process, and her anxieties about this. Use of diagrams might be helpful. The nurse could encourage Susan to look at the wound and point out the signs of healing, explaining about the sutures being removed when the wound is healed.
- Once Susan understands how the wound is healing, the nurse can build on this to explain why she need not be afraid of showering, and give her practical advice about drying herself without rubbing the wound itself and about wearing clothing that will not rub the wound.

- The nurse must similarly ensure that Susan's carers understand these issues so they can reinforce the information and be consistent in their reassurance and explanation.
- The nurse can prepare Susan for her suture removal and will be able to ensure that the practice nurse removing Susan's sutures knows how Susan communicates and how she has been prepared.
- If there is anyone who has a healed surgical wound, perhaps Susan could, with the person's permission, talk to them. Actually seeing a healed wound might help to allay her anxiety, if this is possible to arrange.

All the above aspects should be incorporated in Susan's **Health Action Plan**.

Health Action Plan
A personal action plan developed for each individual with a learning disability, containing details of their health interventions, medication taken, screening tests, etc. See *Valuing People* (Department of Health 2001).

Learning outcome 2: Show awareness that healing does not in reality occur in a simple linear fashion

Due to a number of factors, wound healing is not always a straightforward process. A review of wounds caused by trauma, pressure or ulceration illustrates these issues. These wounds are considered in further detail in the later section 'Classification of wounds and their management'.

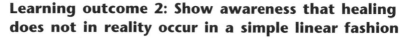

Activity

If possible, select a patient with a wound caused by trauma, pressure or ulceration, in discussion with your practice mentor. Try to find out about the history of the wound, and its healing process to date.

Compare your investigations with the discussion below.

Trauma

Traumatic wounds vary greatly in nature. While minor wounds may heal in a straightforward manner, others involve extensive skin loss and contamination, which can affect the healing process and may require surgical intervention. As you have read, Thomas's wound healing is not progressing well due to the infection caused by its contamination.

Pressure ulcers

Wounds such as pressure ulcers follow a progressive path. The impairment of the circulation to the skin for even short periods is problematic in susceptible individuals, such as people who are frail, older or malnourished. Mrs Warner, as an older person who also has diabetes and had a period of immobility on a hard surface (the kitchen floor), was obviously a high risk individual (see section in Chapter 5 on 'Pressure ulcer risk assessment'). The discoloured areas on Mrs Warner's elbows could potentially develop into necrotic ulcers similar to her sacral pressure ulcer.

Leg and foot ulceration

There are many causes of leg/foot ulceration, each having different distinguishing features, underlying pathology and treatment, but the majority are associated with circulatory problems (Nelson and Bradley 2003). For example:

- Diffusion – problems arise when the distance between the capillary and tissue cells is increased, for example oedema.
- Perfusion – occurs when there is arterial or venous insufficiency.

Ulcers are an increasingly common chronic wound, and are often an extensive and longstanding problem (Dealey 1999). Plate 5 shows a large venous leg ulcer, which the patient concerned has had for many years. It is estimated that 400 000 people in the UK have leg ulcers; of these 25 per cent need treatment at any one time (Audit Commission 1999). Seventy per cent are venous in origin and 25 per cent are arterial (Nelson and Bradley 2003). Goldstein *et al.* (1998) explain that a non-healing ulcer of the lower extremity can be multifactorial in origin, and discuss how diagnosis can thus be made. A useful overview of lower leg ulceration can be found in Doughty *et al.* (2000). There are also a number of books devoted entirely to leg ulcers and their management (see Cullum and Roe 1995; Morison and Moffat 1994; Negus 1995). Diabetic ulcers can occur on the feet of people with diabetes; these are complex wounds by nature and cause unacceptably high levels of morbidity and mortality (Foster 1999). Plate 1 shows how severe these ulcers can potentially be. A systematic review indicated that education of people with diabetes can reduce foot ulceration in high-risk patients (Valk *et al.* 2003). However Mrs Warner's depression could affect her ability to carry out this self-care (see Chapter 7, Box 7.3 'Foot care').

You should now be aware that some wounds progress in a complicated fashion due to underlying health problems. These complex wounds often necessitate a multidisciplinary team approach in diagnosis and management, with investigations performed to ensure an accurate identification of the problem.

Learning outcome 3: Recognise problems with wound healing and the appearance of scar tissue

A scar is the end result of healing, but the formation of a mature scar can be a slow process. Understanding how Susan's scar is likely to develop over the coming months will mean that people caring for her can be supportive and reassuring.

To gain understanding of scar tissue, you need to observe what appears to be a healed wound, with no scab, open wound or discharge. Select a client who does not have an obvious wound-healing problem in the inflammatory or proliferative phase of healing. Your practice mentor may be able to guide you towards a suitable individual, and remember to be sensitive and tactful. If the person is happy to show you the wound scar, carry out the activity below to examine its appearance and explore its stage of maturity (eventual appearance). Provided the wound is not too personal most people will provide a very good history of events, and be happy to show the scar to you. This can provide useful information relating to assessing potential problems with any surgery to be undergone, or if new wounds appear. If it is difficult to access a person with a scar in the practice setting, you yourself may have a scar, which you could examine, or perhaps a friend/relative would help you with this exercise.

Remember that you need warm hands, as some wounds are extremely sensitive to the cold. Do not touch unhealed wounds with bare hands – potential risk of contamination to the client and/or you! You need paper and pen to record your findings.

Activity

Examine the healed wound as discussed above and observe:

- The appearance: Is the scar white or pink? Is it surrounded by normally coloured or discoloured tissue? Are stretch marks visible?
- The size: How big is the scar? Draw a diagram especially if large.
- The location: Where is it located? Scars located on joints and pressure points such as the sacrum or elbows can create potential problems in the future.
- Features of the scar: Is it intact, or has it signs of breakdown and repair? This will often relate to the location, as scars on joints undergo continuous stretching and contraction, and are likely to be damaged.
- The texture of the scar: Is it hard or soft, does it feel mobile or attached to surrounding tissue?

A scar is the product of many cells. However specialist myofibroblast cells have a key role in healing, by shrinking the wound by contraction. Note that 75 per cent of normal wound healing is by contraction, which results in a smaller, less visible scar. A scar initially consists of raised vascularised tissue – hence the red colour. Gradually, the redness disappears, as the number of blood vessels reduces, and the colour changes to white. As noted earlier, the new tissue will not be as strong as previously and may predispose an individual such as Mrs Warner to increased risk of pressure ulcer damage.

Some individuals have problems with hypertrophic scars and keloids. A **hypertrophic scar** is a raised, healed red scar that is uncomfortable and tight. This is the result of an increased deposition of collagen within the area of the original wound (Weiss 1995). A **keloid** is a firm mass of scar caused by excessive collagen deposition, but it extends outside the wound boundaries (Weiss 1995). While hypertrophic scars can regress, keloid scars do not. Management of both of these problems requires a specialist and multidisciplinary team approach, for both the physical and psychological problems that may accompany them.

Summary

- Wound healing is a complex process involving phases of healing through which the wound must pass in order to heal adequately.
- The process is theoretically sequential, but in reality parts of different phases occur concurrently.
- The end result is a scar of uncertain appearance and weakened structure in comparison to surrounding undamaged tissue.

CLASSIFICATION OF WOUNDS AND THEIR MANAGEMENT

In the exploration of healing in the previous section, it was noted that surgical wounds and minor traumatic wounds heal relatively quickly if no complications occur. These are acute wounds and are called acute because of their sudden occurrence, short duration and minimal need for external interventions. Waldrop and Doughty (2000) suggest that as an acute wound begins with an injury that initiates haemostasis, this triggers the wound healing cascade, thus promoting rapid healing, especially in a healthy individual.

Chronic wounds are usually caused by underlying health problems so haemostasis is absent from the process, and the individual's ability to heal is often impaired. As Waldrop and Doughty (2000) emphasise, wound healing is a 'systemic process and is therefore significantly affected by systemic conditions' (p. 34). Features of chronic wounds include their problematic and slow nature of healing and the accompaniment of other health, social and psychological problems. In chronic wounds, the inflammatory response is continually stimulated by the underlying disease process, resulting in a prolonged and excessive inflammatory phase of wound healing (Williams and Young 1998).

Learning to classify wounds will enable you to appreciate issues affecting their management, and so plan more effective care. When exploring the classification of wounds, be aware that there are a variety of ways of performing this but this chapter uses a simple classification based on the cause.

LEARNING OUTCOMES

By the end of this section you will be able to:

1. Distinguish between acute and chronic wounds.
2. Discuss the principles of wound closure for different types of acute and chronic wounds.

Learning outcome 1: Distinguish between acute and chronic wounds

Activity

Table 6.1 shows a classification of wounds and Table 6.2 shows a classification of surgical wounds. Working from these tables, how would you classify the wounds of Mrs Warner, Susan, Colin and Thomas?

You should have identified that Mrs Warner's sacral wound is a chronic pressure ulcer and her toe wound is probably a chronic diabetic foot ulcer. Thomas's wounds are acute bites. Susan and Colin both have acute surgical wounds. However while Susan's would be considered a clean contaminated wound,

Table 6.1 Wound classification

Classification	Types of wound	Causes and features
Acute	Penetrating wounds	Wounds penetrating the skin provide the opportunity for infection to gain access. Causative objects could include missiles (e.g. bullets, explosion debris) or hand-held objects (knives, billiard cues etc.)
Acute	Lacerations	Healing of lacerations is affected by the cause, i.e. whether it is a clean wound or is contaminated by dirt/debris, age of the wound and the individual. Wounds involving the eyes and joints are priorities
Acute	Abrasions	Abrasions tend to be caused by a part of the body being dragged against an abrasive surface, thus removing surface epithelium. They can be very painful and sensitive as nerve endings are exposed, and if they are not meticulously cleaned, 'tattooing' results from the dirt trapped in the dermis and epidermis, which is almost impossible to remove (Evans and Jones 1996)
Acute	Bites	These are a common cause of wounds, most of which are caused by dogs, but human bites account for a substantial proportion too (Higgins *et al.* 1997). Infection is a particular concern due to the large number of microorganisms to be found in mouths
Acute	Surgical	As these wounds are planned, risks (e.g. of infection) can be reduced to a minimum (Dealey 1999). Infection rates vary according to the type of surgery (see Table 6.2). Mishriki *et al.* (1990) found an overall infection rate of 7.3% but this was affected by a number of variables, e.g. age, surgeon. Bremmelgaard *et al.* (1989) found infection rates ranging from 2.3% (clean wounds) to 27.1% (dirty wounds)
Acute	Burns	Burns can be thermal (caused by flame, hot fluid or radiation), chemical (acid or alkali), or electrical. Burns can damage the epidermis only (superficial), the epidermis and the dermis (partial thickness) or extend into deeper tissue (full thickness). The extent of the burn is very important to assess, as fluid resuscitation may be needed

(*continued*)

Table 6.1 (*continued*)

Classification	Types of wound	Causes and features
Chronic	Venous leg ulcers	Caused by damage to the venous system in the leg, especially the valves, resulting in pooling and distending of vessels. By-products of this process cause tissue death and ulcer formation. Risk factors include varicose veins and rheumatoid arthritis. Ulcers usually shallow and situated in the gaiter area, with irregular edges, and cause pain that may be severe or described as dull or aching (Doughty *et al.* 2000)
Chronic	Arterial leg ulcers	Occur when impairment of the blood supply by a variety of causes leads to areas of skin death, as the blood vessel supplying the area becomes occluded. Located on tips of toes or pressure points of feet and have well defined borders and cause cramping or a constant deep ache (Doughty *et al.* 2000)
Chronic	Diabetic neuropathic or neuro-ischaemic foot ulcers	Chronic hyperglycaemia can cause impairment of the nerve supply to the foot and lower limb. The resulting loss of sensation can lead to pressure damage, repeated trauma and/or penetration by foreign bodies. These ulcers are neuropathic in origin. In neuro-ischaemic ulcers, the combination of neuropathy and arterial disease produces a very complex wound with a poor prognosis
Chronic	Pressure ulcers	Prolonged pressure on the skin produces obstruction of small vessels, resulting in death of skin, and sometimes deeper tissues, due to lack of blood supply. Shearing and friction can also contribute to their development
Chronic	Infection-induced	Opportunistic organisms gain access through the skin via a small wound, and produce an ulcer. Tropical ulcers are one of the most common forms of these
Chronic	Ulcers caused by cancer	Referred to as fungating wounds, these can complicate cancers in a number of different areas of the body and present as a rapidly growing fungus or with a cauliflower-like appearance which may ulcerate (Goldberg and McGynn-Byer 2000)

Table 6.2 Classification of surgical wounds (Cruse and Foord 1980)

Type	Features	Infection rate
Clean	Surgery without infection present and no entry into hollow muscular organs. Appendicectomy, cholecystectomy and hysterectomy are also included in this category if there is no acute inflammation	1.5%
Clean contaminated	Hollow muscular organ penetrated, but minimal spillage of contents occurred	7.7%
Contaminated	Hollow muscular organ opened with gross spillage of contents,or acute inflammation but no pus found. Traumatic wounds less than 4 hours since occurrence	15.2%
Dirty	Traumatic wound over 4 hours old. Surgery where there is presence of pus or a perforated viscus	40%

Colin's is a dirty wound as it contained pus. Plate 6 shows the wound of a man who had a hip replacement 10 days previously and has now had his skin closures removed. This wound would be categorized as a clean surgical wound. Now try using the table to classify wounds of patients/clients in the practice setting, in the following activity.

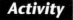 **Activity** | Tables 6.1 and 6.2 provide you with information to distinguish the majority of wounds that are met in the care environment. Now explore the nature and cause of wounds that you have identified recently within your practice setting. Do all the wounds clearly fit into a category type? Are there any wounds that started as acute, and have ended up as chronic? If so why?

You may have identified that wounds are not always easy to place in a category; acute surgical wounds can break down and sometimes appear similar to pressure ulcers, i.e. these wounds started as acute and ended as chronic. The reasons for this are not always clearly understood, but often relate to the physical health of the individual. It is estimated that about 21 000 surgical wounds per year in England and Wales become difficult to heal, i.e. they do not heal in the normal way (NICE 2001). Plate 7 shows an abdominal wound, 5 days after surgery. The distal part has broken down due to infection and the clips have had to be removed early.

Learning outcome 2: Discuss the principles of wound closure for different types of acute and chronic wounds

If possible you should relate this next section's content to the practice setting which you are working in. In a useful overview of wound closure techniques, Gottrup (1999) identifies that wounds may be closed through:

- Primary closure
- Early (delayed primary) closure, that is 4–6 days (performed before there is visible granulation tissue)
- Late (secondary) closure, that is 10–14 days
- Grafting using skin or artificial skin products
- No closure (leaving the wound to heal by granulation).

When wounds are closed (i.e. the skin edges are brought together), the wound is said to be healing by **primary** intention. Plate 6 shows a good example of a surgical wound which has healed by primary intention. When wounds are left open, this is termed healing by **secondary** intention. Although the wound in Plate 7 was planned to heal by primary intention, the lower part may have to heal by secondary intention unless the wound is reclosed after the infection has cleared. **Tertiary** intention consists of wound closure via surgical reconstruction techniques.

Activity

Try to find out how and when wounds are closed by observing in practice and asking practitioners. Consider:

- A surgical wound (such as Susan's abdominal wound)
- A traumatic wound (like Thomas's bites)
- A chronic wound (such as Mrs Warner's pressure ulcer)

Also find out:

- How long are closure materials (clips, staples or sutures), if present, left in the wound before removal and does the site of the wound have any effect on this?

Surgical wounds

Clean or clean-contaminated wounds are managed by primary closure, using sutures, staples or clips, at the end of surgery, with the aim of protecting the wound from the bacteria circulating in a hospital environment (see Chapter 3 'Preventing cross-infection') and promoting the best cosmetic result. Thus Susan's wound will have been managed by primary closure at the end of her operation, as were the wounds shown in Plates 6 and 7.

With contaminated or dirty surgical wounds, delayed primary closure may be preferable, and in some cases the wound may be left open, to heal by secondary intention. A dirty, infected wound, such as Colin's, will be left open to enable continuing drainage; closing the wound would allow build up of pus and a further abscess.

Traumatic wounds

Management of traumatic wounds depends on the degree of contamination (taking into account where and how the wound occurred), the extent of skin damage/skin loss, the site of the wound, and how long ago the injury occurred. Gottrup (1999) advises that a clean incisional wound, with little tissue damage, that occurred less than 6 hours previously (caused by a knife for example) can be irrigated, debrided and managed by primary closure. However he suggests that if the injury is more than 6 hours old, or is heavily contaminated, for example by soil, then primary closure should be delayed.

There may be differing priorities though. As Higgins *et al.* (1997) explain, while bites should usually be left to heal by secondary intention due to their infection risk, exceptions are made where cosmetic effects are paramount, or restoring function takes priority. Although Thomas's wounds were heavily contaminated, being facial wounds, after thorough cleansing and irrigation, primary closure was applied to the lacerations. Facial wounds do have an excellent blood supply and rarely become infected (Higgins *et al.* 1997). However, as stated in the scenario, Thomas was unlucky and developed an infection. It would be difficult to irrigate the wounds really thoroughly in such a young child without a general anaesthetic.

Incised wounds and lacerations can be closed with tapes, sutures or tissue adhesive, the choice depending on factors such as size, depth and site. For example, tissue adhesive could be very suitable for a small scalp wound, but should not be used for lacerations of the mouth or eye (Young 1997). A systematic review confirmed the acceptability of tissue adhesive for simple traumatic lacerations, with the benefits of decreased procedure time and less pain (Farion *et al.* 2003). Where extreme accuracy of alignment is essential for cosmetic reasons, e.g. a lacerated nostril, lip or eyebrow, suturing is preferable (Young 1997). As you read, a variety of skin closures were used for Thomas as his wounds were varied in size and depth.

If a person with a traumatic wound has delayed seeking attention, then prolonged bacterial access will have occurred. Usually the wound will be cleansed with the aim of free drainage and/or detection of infection, followed by delayed primary closure by suturing at 4–6 days. Gottrup (1999) explains that secondary closure (at 10–14 days) is used when a wound is heavily contaminated, and that although this leaves a broader scar than after primary (early or delayed) closure, it is still cosmetically preferable to that achieved through the healing of an open granulating wound.

Chronic wounds

Chronic wounds are usually allowed to heal by secondary intention. Granulation tissue fills the defect, and new epidermis covers the surface. While satisfactory, this is slow and time-consuming, and provides poor protection against risks such as repeated pressure. It can, nevertheless, provide a successful outcome.

Mrs Warner's pressure ulcer will need to heal by secondary intention. When surgical excision of necrotic tissue as in a pressure ulcer is performed, the aim is also for healing to occur by secondary intention. Attempts to directly close large defects by bringing the edges of the wound together have often been unsuccessful, since the tension on the suture line pulls the wound apart. An alternative is to use surgical techniques such as skin grafting and skin flaps, examples of tertiary intention; Gottrup (1999) gives a brief overview of these techniques.

When to remove skin closures

The decision on when to remove skin closures depends on a number of factors including:

- Site: The face heals faster – sutures are often removed in 5 days. The feet heal more slowly so sutures may remain *in situ* for 7–10 days.
- Factors such as ageing and diabetes can affect the rate of healing (see section on 'Factors affecting wound healing').

It is important to ensure that patients being discharged from hospital with skin closures *in situ* are informed of exactly when and where the skin closures will be removed. Susan's sutures would probably be ready for removal at 7 days, and she can attend her local health centre for their removal by the practice nurse. Sometimes it is necessary to arrange for the district nurse to visit a patient's home for skin closure removal, for example, if it is difficult for the person to leave the house due to poor general condition or lack of mobility. Adhesive glue has the advantage of not needing removal. Thomas's facial sutures and paper strips would normally be removed at 5 days but due to the infection may be removed early to allow drainage of pus.

Summary

- Acute wounds usually heal more uneventfully and quickly, but can in certain situations become chronic.
- Different types of wounds are managed in different ways: in general, clean surgical wounds by primary direct closure, contaminated traumatic wounds by delayed primary closure, and chronic wounds by secondary intention healing.

FACTORS AFFECTING WOUND HEALING

Factors influencing wound healing are many and complex; the range of biological, psychological and sociological elements that influence wound healing in individuals cannot yet be explained. Nevertheless there are some common elements that can be identified and addressed in order to achieve a successful outcome. It is important to identify factors that may influence wound healing for individuals, as a perpetuating wound will result if underlying causes are not addressed (Waldrop and Doughty 2000). A multidisciplinary approach may be needed to address these factors. Patients with acute wounds that are healing by primary intention usually require less input, but each individual should be assessed.

LEARNING OUTCOMES

On completion of this section you will be able to:

1. Explore the range of factors that can affect wound healing.
2. Identify how a multidisciplinary approach can address factors affecting wound healing.

Learning outcome 1: Explore the range of factors that can affect wound healing

Miller (1995) suggests that when assessing an individual with a wound, the following two questions are necessary.

- What factors are interfering with wound healing?
- Which of these can be changed in order to move the wound healing process forward?

The following exercise is based on this framework.

 Activity

With the guidance of your practice mentor, identify a patient/client (like Mrs Warner) who has a problematic wound and carry out the activity below.

1. Look at the patient's assessment documentation. Identify factors that have been recorded that could influence wound healing (several have already been referred to in this chapter), and try to provide a rationale for your selection of these factors. Remember to consider the person (biologically and psychologically) as a whole, as well as the wound itself.
2. Then ask yourself, can these factors be altered/changed? Try to think of what action could be required.

Table 6.3 includes factors that might have been identified for Mrs Warner. Compare the list you prepared for your patient with this. You may well have identified a much wider range of issues, depending on your individual patient (see also Miller 1999a, Mulder *et al.*1995, Partridge 1998).

You probably considered general health, age and nutrition. Chronic conditions that affect wound healing include respiratory and cardiovascular disease, due to their effect on tissue oxygenation (Williams and Young 1998). Plate 8 shows how a lack of blood supply affects skin and deeper tissues. This patient had heart failure and a lack of circulation to her feet causing necrosis. This highlights that an adequate blood supply to the skin and underlying tissues is essential, both to prevent wounds and promote wound healing. Are you aware of the

Table 6.3 Factors influencing Mrs Warner's wound healing

Factor	Rationale for identification	Can be influenced?	Action required
Smoking	Effects of smoking on tissue function are outlined by Siana and Gottrup (1992). Smoking causes a compromised blood supply to the wound, and impairs the cardiovascular system, delaying healing. It leads to inhibition of epithelialisation and a reduction in wound contraction (Williams and Young 1998)	Potentially	Reduction in smoking balanced against quality of life issues
Diabetes mellitus and elevated blood glucose level	People with diabetes have impaired wound healing (Davidson et al. 1984; Silhi 1998). A wide range of underlying pathologies are responsible	Yes	Blood glucose monitoring, medication and dietary consideration
Depression	Depression affects ability to self-care, for example to manage her diabetes, relieve pressure, and care for her feet	Yes	Pharmacology and therapeutic approach
Poor nutritional intake	Adequate nutrients required for wound healing (see Table 6.4)	Yes	Promote nutritious and balanced diet
Ageing	The skin's ability to repair reduces with ageing (Desai 1997). The disease processes that often accompany ageing may impair healing (Partridge 1998)	Indirectly by improving overall health	General health promotion
Stress and anxiety about being in hospital	Stress delays healing (Boore 1978; Kiecolt-Glaser et al. 1995)	Potentially	Develop nurse–patient relationship, identify and address sources of anxiety
Infection in toe wound	Infection compromises healing, places stress on body, and impairs diabetes stabilisation	Yes	Investigations (e.g. X-ray to identify whether there is bone infection). Wound management and antibiotics
Necrotic tissue in sacral ulcer	Necrotic tissue prevents wound healing	Yes	Debride necrotic tissue using suitable method

effect of steroids on wound healing? The anti-inflammatory response of steroids reduces the inflammatory response, and affects the function of the macrophages, thus slowing healing (Williams and Young 1998). Did you also identify stress and anxiety as a factor? This too can have a major influence on wound healing (Partridge 1998); provision of information can contribute to healing (Boore 1978). Colin has a longstanding mental health problem, and the discomfort associated with his wound may be a further source of stress. Susan, too, has been through a stressful experience. Now that she is back in her own environment with familiar staff members, it will be important to be supportive and reassuring. Thomas and his mother will be upset about the initial incident and now anxious that healing is not progressing smoothly. Thus nurses should aim to relieve their stress and anxieties and help them to relax (see Chapter 2). Casey (1999) notes that even minor wounds can have a significant psychological impact on both the child and the parents, and that there is often associated parental guilt. Box 6.1 summarises common fears and anxieties that parents of children with wounds can experience.

Chapter 9 'Assessing and meeting nutritional needs' highlights the need for an adequate and increased nutritional intake for wound healing. However, there is evidence that many people with chronic wounds, such as pressure ulcers, have poor nutritional intake and risk factors for malnutrition, as do other community patients (Green *et al.* 1999). Williams and Young (1998) suggest that every patient with a wound should be assessed nutritionally. Table 6.4 outlines the key nutrients required for wound healing and their role in the process. Stotts (2000) extensively reviews the literature linking nutrition and wound healing.

Finally, you may also have identified factors to do with the condition of the wound and how it is being managed. Miller (1999a), acknowledging the systemic nature of wound healing, states that the wound itself is the last place practitioners should look at when questioning why a wound is not healing. Relevant factors include aspects to do with the wound itself, for example the presence of necrotic (dead) tissue or infection – both factors relevant to Mrs Warner. How the wound is being managed is also relevant, for example frequent and excessive exposure of the wound causes a drop in temperature at the wound bed and inappropriate use of antiseptics or certain wound products, which could damage fragile new tissue. All these factors could delay healing and are considered later in this chapter in the section 'Wound management'.

- Dealing with their child's anxiety
- Their child's pain, particularly during dressing removal
- How to manage dressings and keep them in place
- How to keep the child amused
- Subsequent scarring.

Box 6.1 Sources of parental anxiety in relation to wound care (based on Casey 1999)

Table 6.4 Nutrients required for wound healing and their function (adapted from Williams and Young 1998, pp. 26–7)

Nutrient	Function
Carbohydrate	Energy source for increased cellular activity during wound healing
Fat	An alternative energy source. Fat-soluble vitamins are essential for the building of new cell membranes in wound repair
Protein	Essential for building the new wound bed, i.e. collagen formation. Patients already protein depleted before wounding are worse effected
Vitamin A	Supports epithelial proliferation and consequent migration across granulation tissue. More efficient when given prior to wounding
Vitamin B	Assists formation of collagen mesh which supports new blood vessels as they move into granulating tissue
Vitamin C	Assists formation of collagen mesh
Vitamin E	With vitamin C, attacks damaging oxygen free radicals that are present in infected wounds and during the inflammatory phase of wound healing
Minerals: zinc, copper and iron	Required for collagen formation. Zinc also has an antibacterial effect, mainly against gram-positive bacteria

Learning outcome 2: Identify how a multidisciplinary approach can address factors affecting wound healing

Addressing factors affecting healing requires multidisciplinary team working, including relatives and the client; involvement of patients and/or carers is essential in the process of wound healing (Williams and Young 1998).

 Activity

> Look back at Table 6.3 and list members of the multidisciplinary team who might be involved in addressing the factors affecting Mrs Warner's wound healing. Make a note of what their specific roles might be.

Mrs Warner, who has chronic wounds, would require considerable multidisciplinary teamwork in order to address the factors affecting her wound healing. Compare your list with Table 6.5, which gives some ideas; you may have thought of others.

If psychological adjustment relating to a wound is problematic, input from a psychologist is sometimes necessary. Voluntary organisations can also play a part in supporting individuals, Diabetes UK in Mrs Warner's case. For children, there would be involvement of the Hospital Play Therapist to provide preparation for procedures, and support and distraction during procedures. When the

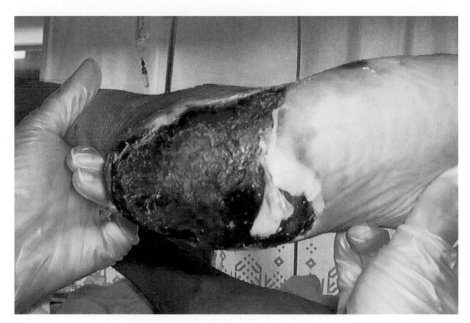

Plate 1 A diabetic ulcer which developed on this patient's heel. The tissue bed is covered in hard black necrotic tissue. The wound will not heal until this is removed. Unfortunately this ulcer eventually led to amputation of the patient's lower leg and foot.

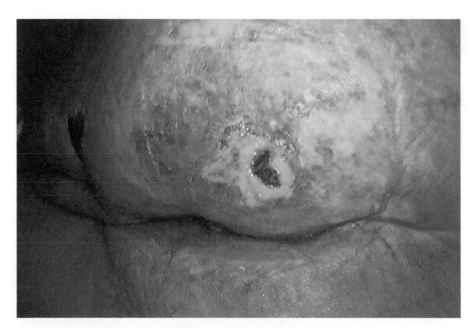

Plate 2 This pressure ulcer (Stirling scale 3.4) developed on the sacrum of a patient with multiple sclerosis. The wound bed is covered with yellow slough, except for a central necrotic area. Slough is soft necrotic tissue containing dead phagocytes, and the wound will not heal until it is removed. Surrounding this ulcer are other areas of pressure damage, evidenced by discolouration and superficial ulceration (Stirling scale 1.2–2.2).

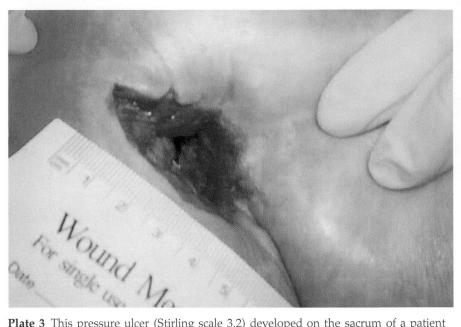

Plate 3 This pressure ulcer (Stirling scale 3.2) developed on the sacrum of a patient with a spinal injury. The ulcer was covered with 60 per cent slough prior to debridement by maggots. The wound is now almost filled with red granulation tissue. This photo also shows how a ruler placed by the side of a wound before the photo can provide a more accurate record of its dimensions.

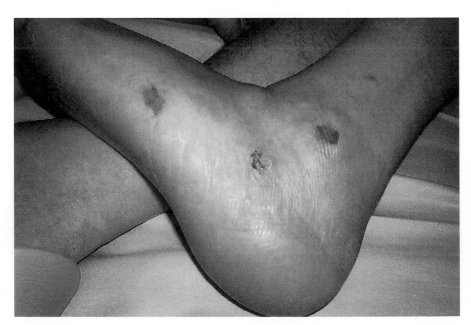

Plate 4 These are pressure ulcers (Stirling scale 2.2) on the side of the foot/ankle of a patient who has multiple sclerosis. They are now almost healed with tissue beds showing mainly pink epithelialising tissue.

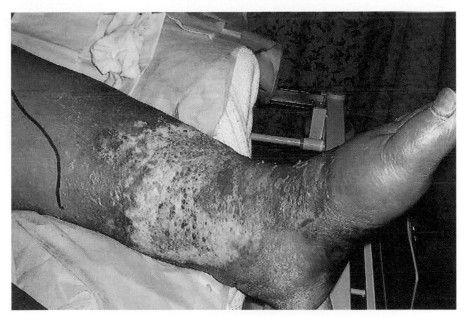

Plate 5 This is a venous leg ulcer which has been a long-standing problem for the patient concerned. There are large areas of yellow slough and areas of red granulation tissue covering the wound. The lower foot looks oedematous and there is hard scaly skin (hyperkeratosis) present. The surrounding skin also looks red suggesting cellulitus.

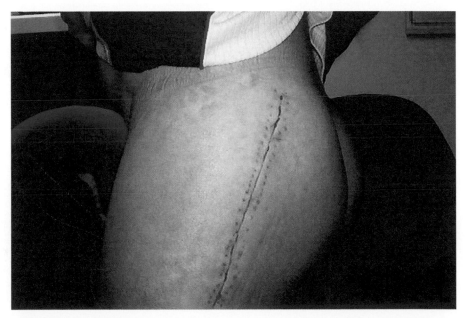

Plate 6 This is the hip wound of a man who had a total hip replacement, ten days previously, and just had his skin closures (clips) removed. This is a good example of a clean surgical wound which has healed as planned by primary intention.

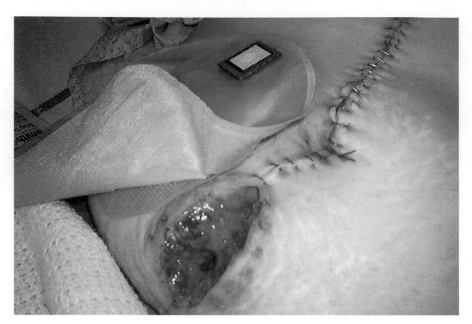

Plate 7 This is an abdominal wound of a woman who has had an abdominoperineal resection, with colostomy formation, for ulcerative colitis. The colostomy has been sited very close to the wound. The photo was taken on the fifth post-operative day. The wound had started to ooze pus from the distal part of the wound, and had dehisced. The clips from this area have been removed. Towards the top of the wound and the central area there is slight inflammation. In the dehisced area, some small patches of red granulating tissue can be seen but other areas look unhealthy. There is a dark centre to this area, which was found to be a sinus.

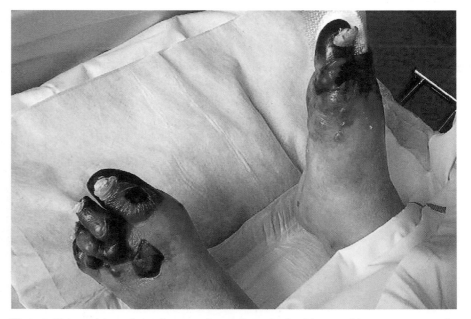

Plate 8 This patient, whose feet are shown here, had a history of heart surgery and heart failure and over two weeks developed black necrotic toes which spread to the distal area of her feet due to the lack of arterial circulation.

Table 6.5 Addressing factors affecting wound healing: suggested multidisciplinary involvement for Mrs Warner

MDT member	Role
Ward nurse	Blood glucose monitoring, improving nutritional status, relieving stress/anxiety, etc., mobilisation, pressure-relieving strategies, wound assessment and appropriate wound care, education of patient/carer and health promotion, support and information giving, liaison with other nurses, relatives and MDT
Specialist nurses: infection control, diabetes, nutritional support, tissue viability, dermatology, discharge liaison	Specialist advice, education and support for patient and family, and ward team, to address the factors affecting wound healing and advise on appropriate strategies. Equipment provision and resources
Physiotherapist	Promote mobility and correct positioning: education and advice
Occupational therapist	Positioning, mobility and dressing aids, seating, adaptations/equipment for home
Social worker	Discharge arrangements and support at home, e.g. home care, arranging meals on wheels, day centre, financing of home adaptations/equipment
Podiatrist	Foot care
Doctor	Blood glucose control, prescribing medication, surgical debridement of wounds (if needed), identifying and treating other health problems which may delay healing, liaison with GP
Pharmacist	Advice on wound care products
Dietician	Assessment and advice re dietary supplements
Primary Health Care Team: district nurse, health visitor, GP, practice nurse	Medical and nursing care in the community after discharge. Assessment of health needs in the community
Chaplain	Spiritual needs and support

child is discharged, the community children's nurse can provide support and follow-up in the community.

Summary

■ A range of factors can potentially interfere with the healing process of a wound. These factors relate to the individual's general health status, the condition of the wound, and the care being received.

■ Nurses should identify factors affecting wound healing in individuals and plan strategies to address them where possible, involving the multidisciplinary team appropriately.

WOUND ASSESSMENT

As discussed in the previous section, when assessing a wound you need to consider the whole person, so factors that could interfere with healing can be addressed wherever possible. This section now prepares you to assess the wound itself, based on your accumulated knowledge of the phases of wound healing, the ability to classify wounds, and finally an awareness of the range of wider issues that affect wound healing. All these aspects underpin the assessment process. Useful articles relating to wound assessment include Miller (1996, 1999b).

LEARNING OUTCOMES

By the end of this section you will be able to:

1. Discuss the features of a wound assessment and how wound assessment tools/charts can be used.
2. Record key information in a useful format that can be used to plan appropriate interventions.

Learning outcome 1: Discuss the features of a wound assessment and how wound assessment tools/charts can be used

When considering wound assessment tools/charts, ensure that you distinguish these from pressure ulcer risk assessment tools for example the Waterlow Scale (Waterlow 1985, 1988), and the Braden Scale (Bergstrom *et al.* 1987). The function of these is to assess the risk of an individual developing a pressure ulcer (see Chapter 5). Grading tools on the other hand, aim to provide information on the wound itself. Some, for example the Stirling Scale (Reid and Morison 1994) are used to grade the type of pressure ulcer, and when used on a chart may include a diagram of the body for marking the location of the wound(s). The Stirling Scale was shown in Chapter 5 as it is included on the second side of the Waterlow card (Fig. 5.2), and is referred to in Plates 2–4, which are all photos of pressure ulcers. The Red-Yellow-Black system (RYB) (Cuzzell 1988) is based on assessing the condition of the wound bed, but has had little uptake in the UK. Cooper (2000) warns that although this tool is useful, it oversimplifies wound assessment, as it considers only a single variable. However Rolstad *et al.* (2000) present how it can be used as a basis for dressing selection. If you look at Plates 1–5, you can see how the colours in the RYB system could be applied (e.g. Plate 1 – black).

Assessment and on-going Record of Wound Care
(Each wound should be assessed on a separate form)

Name... Wound Site..

Date of Birth.................................... Date wound present.................................

Named Nurse.................................... Previous treatments (if any).......................

Wound Type..................,,,,,,,,,,........... Allergies/Systemic medication................................

Date of assessment				
Photo (Tick)				
Dimensions (mm)				
Max length × max breadth				
Max depth				
Wound Base (%)				
Epitheliasing				
Granulating				
Sloughy				
Necrotic				
Exudate				
Amount (+, ++, +++)				
Odour				
None/mild/offensive				
Infection				
Date swab/specimen sent				
Result				
Wound Edges (Tick)				
Healthy/normal				
Rolled				
Punched out				
Hard/fibrous				
Condition of surrounding skin (Tick)				
Healthy				
Erythema				
Eczema				
Cellulitis				
Moist/macerated				
Pain				
Location				
Frequency				
Intensity				
Duration				
Woundcare				
Cleansing Agent				
Dressing				
Dressing Frequency				
Signature				
Date of re-assessment				

Figure 6.1 An example of a wound assessment chart.

Figure 6.1 gives an example of a wound assessment chart, and its features are discussed below in relation to Mrs Warner's sacral pressure ulcer. Note: she would require a chart like this for each of her wounds as each must be assessed separately.

- **Wound type**: This relates to the wound classification discussed earlier so for Mrs Warner will be recorded as a pressure ulcer.
- **Wound site**: As stated earlier, a body map can be used to indicate this as well as writing 'sacrum' at the top of the chart.
- **Date wound present**: Here the date that the ulcer on Mrs Warner's sacrum was first noticed should be recorded.
- **Previous treatments**: For Mrs Warner's sacral ulcer this is not applicable but would be useful to note for other patients, and might be appropriate to note for her toe ulcer (if previously dressed by community staff).
- **Allergies/systemic medication**: Mrs Warner could have a known allergy to a dressing product, which should be noted, and could be taking medication that will affect wound healing.
- **Photo**: Increasingly photos are used in wound assessment and carry a number of advantages but consent from the patient must be given, preferably in writing (Flanagan 1997). Often a ruler is placed by the side of the wound when taking the photograph, showing the wound's size as well as its appearance (see Plate 3). Clearly the sacral area would be a sensitive area to photograph and the reasons for doing so need careful explanation. However the photos can be shown to Mrs Warner to help her to appreciate the nature of the wound, and how its healing is progressing.
- **Dimensions**: Recorded in millimetres as width by length. Depth is difficult to measure but a wound probe or sterile wound swab can be used and then measured against a ruler. Sometimes a tracing is made, which creates a record of shape as well as size, and this can be attached.
- **Wound base**: The wound base may have several different types of tissue present. For example Plate 5 shows a wound base that has both sloughy areas and granulation tissue. Nurses assessing this wound would need to estimate the percentage of the wound bed covered with slough, and the percentage covered with granulation tissue, and record this on the chart. For Mrs Warner the recording will be 100 per cent necrotic, but in due course there will be sloughy areas, and then hopefully some granulation tissue, and then areas that are epithelialising. Necrotic tissue (as in Mrs Warner's sacral pressure ulcer and Plate 1) prevents or delays the healing process (Kiernan 1999), and therefore needs removing to enable healing to progress.
- **Exudate**: This is fluid arising from the wound due to increased permeability of capillaries. Estimating the amount of exudate ($+$, $++$ or $+++$) is not easy. However the presence and extent of exudate will influence your dressing choice. The production of large or increased amounts of exudate or pus could indicate infection, but other signs and symptoms (as discussed below) should be taken into account too.
- **Odour**: A slight odour can occur due to wound occlusion and is associated with some types of dressings. However an offensive odour is often a sign

of infection. Necrotic wounds, like Mrs Warner's sacral pressure ulcer, and also fungating wounds, are often malodourous. Assessing odour can help to identify infection, as one of a range of criteria, but also helps with dressing choice as some dressings are deodorising.

- **Infection**: Several signs discussed so far will help to identify whether infection is present, and this should be assessed at each dressing change as the presence of infection will delay wound healing. Wound swabs taken should be recorded but they have limitations. How and when to take wound swabs is discussed in Chapter 3 'Preventing cross-infection'. A detailed examination of the criteria for identifying a wound infection can be found in Cutting and Harding (1994).

- **Wound edges**: In large and/or deep wounds, the edge of the wound when in the inflammatory phase is oedematous and very red. As this progresses towards the proliferative phase, a white border will appear which is new epidermal tissue, fragile and easily removed. Edges that are rolled in can delay healing time. In chronic wounds, the edges can have a punched out appearance and small satellite wounds can be present. Wound edges that are hard and fibrous indicate a chronic wound.

<hr>

Macerated skin

Macerated skin is soft and breaking down due to prolonged contact with excessive amounts of fluid, e.g. wound exudates (see Cutting 1999).

- **Condition of surrounding skin**: This is important in considering the type of dressing to be used. For example if the skin is moist/**macerated** a more absorbent dressing is needed. If eczema is present great care will need to be taken in choice of dressing and how it is secured. Cellulitis would need to be reported if a new feature as it indicates infection is present and systemic antibiotics are needed.

- **Pain**: Assessment of pain relating to the wound indicates whether the current pain management strategy is effective. If the pain only occurs during dressing removal, a different product may be required. If the pain has increased and is associated with other signs and symptoms such as malodour, inflammation, increased exudate, and delayed wound healing, a wound infection may be present (Miller 1998).

As you can see in Fig. 6.1, the wound chart includes spaces for recording wound care, which is planned on the basis of the assessment.

Assessing a wound might also include considering any of the following:

- Is the wound open or closed? Remember from earlier in this chapter: an open wound is one healing by secondary intention, a closed wound is predominantly healing by first intention. Thus Susan's wound is healing by first intention but Mrs Warner's sacral wound is healing by secondary intention. A dehisced wound is one where tissue has become separated from deeper tissue owing to the presence of infection, and this complicates some surgical wounds.

- Extent of tissue involvement: does the wound involve epidermis, dermis, fat, fascia, muscle and/or bone?

- Presence of foreign bodies: These delay the healing process. Foreign bodies like dirt or grit can also increase infection risk, and lead to permanent marking (Fletcher 1997).

- Presence of a fistula (an abnormal connection between two spaces such as skin surface and bowel) or a sinus. A sinus is a tract that ends in a blind cavity; these are frequently found in deep pressure ulcers. A sinus should heal from its base, as if it heals at the surface, fluid will accumulate within, promoting an abscess, which will subsequently break through to the surface. In Plate 7, the darkened central area of the dehisced part of the wound was found to be a sinus.

- Wound drain and drain site. Wound drains are inserted into some surgical wounds to promote the removal of fluid that would otherwise accumulate and form a potential growing medium for infection, or interfere with healing.

■ Activity

Find out whether there is a wound assessment tool/chart used in your local practice setting, and try to access this. Otherwise use one from the literature or the one in Fig. 6.1. You also need a measuring instrument, e.g. ruler (disposable ones are available from wound product manufacturers), and good light. Under supervision of a practitioner assess a client's wound and document your assessment. After carrying out this exercise, consider: should a wound assessment tool/chart be used for all wounds?

Minor straightforward wounds do not require a formal recorded assessment. If the wound is judged to be healing uneventfully, a record of this in the patient's notes will suffice. This would have been adequate for Susan's surgical wound when she was in hospital, and also for the wound shown in Plate 6, which is a straightforward clean surgical wound which healed without complication. Judging when to use a tool/chart involves issues such as a wound that is not healing as expected, possibly reverting to a previous stage, wounds with problems or where required as a legal record, for example after an assault. The assessment of the patient's wound in Plate 7 should be documented on a wound assessment chart as it is complicated by infection causing dehiscence. Mrs Warner's pressure ulcer and ulcerated toe (which could, as a diabetic ulcer, deteriorate) are both chronic and problematic wounds and so the use of assessment tools/charts would be advantageous.

Leg ulcer assessment

All patients presenting with a leg ulcer should be screened for arterial disease by Doppler ultrasound measurement of ankle brachial pressure index (ABPI) by staff trained to carry out this investigation (Royal College of Nursing 1998), alongside a thorough clinical investigation. Often a specific leg ulcer assessment chart is used to record this assessment, which will include documenting assessment of factors affecting wound healing (e.g. smoking, nutritional status) as discussed earlier. The ABPI is calculated by dividing the brachial systolic blood pressure by the ankle systolic blood pressure. A normal ABPI reading is about 1 and if the reading is 0.8 or above compression therapy can usually be applied (Royal College of Nursing 1998). Compression therapy aims to provide graduated compression, with the highest pressure at the ankle and the lowest at the knee, thus returning blood from the lower limb and preventing pooling in distended lower leg veins. An arterial ulcer is caused by an inadequate arterial blood supply to the area and a patient suspected of having an arterial ulcer may require vascular surgery. **Note: Applying compression to a limb with an arterial ulcer will have catastrophic results for the ulcer and the patient, potentially leading to loss of the limb affected. Thus accurate assessment is essential.**

Learning outcome 2: Record key information in a useful format that can be used to plan appropriate interventions

Activity

Review the material that you recorded by using the wound assessment tool/chart earlier, and consider: is it specific and comprehensive enough to help you to plan the wound's management, and to promote continuity of care?

Consider the following points in relation to your assessment:

- The tools employed are generally very wound specific. They have to be simple to use, yet all-encompassing, but not so inclusive as to waste valuable time and so deter usage.
- These are legal documents. Have you accurately described the wound environment? Have you avoided the use of colloquialisms, such as 'wound bed appears fine': what does 'fine' mean? Ensure that you use descriptive language that can be interpreted by anyone, not just yourself. This helps to promote continuity of care. As referred to in learning outcome 1, a photograph of the wound can be particularly useful for recording wound assessment, and may provide a more objective record of the wound's status, alleviating potential variation in the use of descriptive terms and their interpretation.
- Can the assessment help you to plan the management of the wound? Has it identified, for example, any problems with the existing approach to the dressing, for example is the dressing allowing the wound to dry out, or the surrounding skin to become macerated? Was the dressing painful to remove?

Summary

- Wound assessment requires a holistic approach involving assessment of the whole person and the wound together.
- Documentation is becoming increasingly important, for management as well as litigation reasons.
- Accuracy in recording assessment is an important skill to develop and does much to promote continuity of care, as well as a firm basis for planning interventions.

WOUND MANAGEMENT

You have already considered factors affecting wound healing and a multidisciplinary approach. In this section you focus on care of the wound itself. When carrying out any wound management it is important to be aware of the psychosocial effects of wounds, so that you can be supportive; this is relevant to both acute and chronic wounds. The effects on body image of acute wounds can result in a range of psychological reactions including a grief response, anxiety and depression (Magan 1996). Neil and Barrell (1998) point out that the skin is 'a major factor in a person's body image', with denial, anxiety, pain, immobility and altered body image experienced by people with chronic wounds. Being aware of this can help health professionals to be understanding, and effective assessment can promote helpful interventions, referrals and information provision (Neil and Barrell 1998). Wounds can also impact on a child's body image; see Price (1993) for further discussion on this aspect.

LEARNING OUTCOMES

By the end of this section you will be able to:

1. Discuss how wound dressings are conducted.
2. Explain methods of debridement and cleansing.
3. Identify a range of wound dressings showing awareness of how they are selected for individuals.
4. Outline ways of reducing pain and discomfort associated with wounds.

Learning outcome 1: Discuss how wound dressings are conducted

Non-touch technique to maintain asepsis is outlined in Chapter 3 'Preventing cross infection', and how this can be carried out for a wound dressing is discussed. A sterile technique has traditionally been used for wound care but there is some argument that it holds no advantage over a clean technique in some situations. Hollinworth and Kingston (1998) clarify that in both instances, prevention of transmission of microorganisms is intended. Clean technique should not, therefore, be a sloppy version of sterile technique leading to risks of cross-infection. In essence, when using sterile technique, equipment, fluids and dressings are sterile, while with a clean technique, clean but non-sterile single-use gloves can be used, with tap water (that is safe to drink) used for cleansing.

Activity	How do you think you might identify when a sterile technique would be essential and when a clean technique might be sufficient?

Williams and Young (1998) suggest that risk to the individual patient should be assessed. You might have identified that some patients are particularly vulnerable to infection; this was discussed in Chapter 3. A sterile technique must be used if the patient is immuno-compromised or has undergone surgery, which carries a high infection risk. However, chronic wounds are likely to be colonised with bacteria and therefore a clean rather than sterile procedure may be sufficient. Young (1997) suggests that maintaining asepsis when caring for a traumatic wound, prior to removing the contaminating debris, is probably pointless. Hollinworth and Kingston (1998) outline how a clean technique has been used for wound dressings with no detrimental effects for a number of years in one specified hospital. However the dressings were carried out in a central treatment suite, with positive pressure controlled air changes and a team of expert nurses; these conditions are not available within all hospitals currently, and may hold disadvantages in that ward nurses could become de-skilled.

Effective handwashing and gloving techniques are essential, whether a sterile or clean technique is used for wound care, and nurses also need to protect themselves from patient's body fluids when carrying out dressings (see Chapter 3 for detailed discussion of these issues). Some dressings are very difficult to apply using gloves – hand hygiene is then essential to prevent contamination of the dressing (Williams and Young 1998). As discussed, gloves can perforate, and their use should not compromise hand hygiene. Wound dressings, whether applied using a sterile or a clean technique, must be sterile. Use of dressings from an opened pack, even if for the same patient, could introduce contamination and thus delay healing (Williams and Young 1998).

Learning outcome 2: Explain methods of debridement and cleansing

Debridement

Debridement is 'the removal of devitalised or infected tissue, fibrin, or foreign material from a wound' (NICE 2001, p. 2). The body can naturally carry out debridement but if large quantities of such debris are present it delays healing and predisposes to infection (NICE 2001). It was identified earlier in this chapter that Mrs Warner's sacral wound requires debridement due to the presence of necrotic tissue. Debridement can be carried out in a number of ways (Box 6.2).

Autolysis

This involves applying the body's own mechanisms, by using a dressing that creates a moist environment. This liquefies the necrotic tissue, enabling it to separate from the wound bed. Both hydrogels (used in conjunction with occlusive and semi-occlusive dressings) and hydrocolloids can be used for this purpose. They should usually be left *in situ* for 1–3 days, and then renewed.

Larvae therapy

The use of larvae (maggots) for debridement is gaining interest and has been found to be effective. The larvae are applied directly to the wound, held in place with a dressing and left undisturbed for 3 days.

Surgical debridement

This involves removal of the dead tissue with scalpel or scissors, which can be performed by a doctor or an experienced nurse. Sometimes a softening dressing is needed first so that the tissue is easier to remove. Analgesics may be required.

Enzymatic agents

Enzymatic solutions will digest slough and necrotic tissue without damaging healthy tissue.

Box 6.2 Methods of debridement (based on Kiernan 1999)

The National Institute for Clinical Excellence (NICE 2001) reviewed the evidence on debridement for difficult to heal surgical wounds. It was concluded that no particular method could be supported so choice of debriding agent should be according to the individual and issues around comfort and odour control.

Dressings promoting autolysis and bio-surgical methods (sterile maggots) may be more acceptable to patients and less painful (NICE 2001). Maggots liquefy and ingest necrotic tissue (Thomas *et al.* 1996, 1998). A study by Sherman *et al.* (2001), which used maggots to debride non-healing wounds in outpatients, found maggot therapy to be safe, effective and acceptable to most people. Plate 3 shows a deep sacral pressure ulcer the day after maggots had been removed after 3 days *in situ*. The ulcer, which was 60 per cent covered with slough, is now about 85 per cent granulation tissue. Vacuum-assisted closure uses negative pressure to remove slough and loosen necrotic tissue from the wound bed (Hampton 1999). The use of honey in wound care is also gaining interest. It has been found to have a debriding action as well as many other beneficial effects, for example antibacterial activity (Molan 1999, Cooper *et al.* 2002). However Fox (2002) found the current evidence base for honey to be weak.

As regards wound cleansing this has sometimes been carried out ritualistically without sound rationale for practice.

You have probably seen wound cleansing carried out in practice. Think about the following: Why are wounds cleansed? How are wounds cleansed? What are wounds cleansed with?

Now compare your thoughts to the points below.

Purpose of wound cleansing

The aim of wound cleansing is to remove contaminated/foreign material from the wound bed, i.e. slough, necrotic tissue, exudate and dressing debris. Nurses must decide whether this can be achieved by cleansing or whether debridement, as discussed earlier, is needed. Williams and Young (1998) emphasise that cleansing should not be done unless it is clearly indicated. For example if the wound is granulating, cleansing is not necessary and may even damage the new tissue; dressing renewal is all that is required. Surface exudate is beneficial to wound healing, but excessive exudate macerates surrounding skin (Fletcher 1997, Cutting 1999), and can provide a good culture medium for bacteria (Casey 1999).

Further reasons for wound cleansing are so that the wound can be assessed, and to maintain hygiene and enhance well-being, particularly when there is excessive exudate and malodour (Fletcher 1997). When there is excessive production of exudate, as in infected or large surface area wounds, excess exudate should be removed to prevent maceration of surrounding skin, while leaving sufficient fluid in the wound bed to enhance the wound healing process (Williams and Young 1998).

Methods of cleansing

As Fletcher (1997) identifies, there are a number of documented methods for wound cleansing. We will consider swabbing, irrigation and bathing/showering.

- **Swabbing**: Swabbing of wounds, using gloves or forceps and gauze swabs, is a traditional method of wound cleansing but Thomlinson's (1987) study demonstrated that this merely led to redistribution of microorganisms.
- **Irrigation**: Irrigation of wounds is often considered preferable to swabbing. To irrigate you can use a syringe with a needle or quill, an aerosol spray, a showerhead, or simply pour the fluid over the wound from a sachet or capsule. You will need to collect fluid in a container such as a kidney bowl. The pressure of the irrigation may be difficult to measure or regulate. To dislodge debris from a wound, high-pressure irrigation can be achieved by using a 30 mL syringe with a large gauge needle, and pushing the plunger with maximum force from a distance of 2 cm above the wound (Young 1997).

> - A wound that presents early (within 6 hours of injury), has a clean incision, is uncontaminated and was caused by low energy trauma should be irrigated with tepid water or saline.
> - A wound that presents late (more than 12 hours after injury), has ragged edges, is contaminated, and was caused by high energy trauma requires more extensive cleansing and debridement.

Box 6.3 Cleansing of traumatic wounds: key points (based on Young 1997)

■ **Bathing**: Williams and Young (1998) recommend that bathing a patient with a contaminated sacral pressure ulcer is the most efficient wound cleansing method, and is comforting for the patient. If there is no wound infection present, cleaning of the bath with normal detergent is adequate but if the wound is infected, the bath should be cleaned with hypochlorite solution. This would be necessary therefore if Colin baths, which could well be a soothing method of wound cleansing for him.

How traumatic wounds should be cleansed depends on a number of factors; see Box 6.3. Bites, in particular, need very thorough cleansing (Higgins *et al.* 1997). In Thomas's case this may not have been done sufficiently, resulting in infection.

Solutions for wound cleansing

A review by Leaper (1996) highlights the clinical controversy surrounding use of antiseptics in open wounds, particularly in relation to:

■ whether these solutions are toxic to healing tissue
■ whether they actually promote healing.

Leaper (1996) notes that many of the studies to determine the effects of these solutions have been conducted in laboratories rather than clinical trials, and that this evidence is therefore not necessarily applicable to the practice setting. However, whilst antiseptics are undoubtedly antibacterial, they have been found to be quickly inactivated when in contact with body tissues and fluids, pus and necrotic tissue (Hugo and Russell 1992, cited by Leaper 1996). A detailed review of the qualities of povidine-iodine identified that it can prevent colonisation of wounds with pathogenic bacteria, which could prevent some from becoming infected, which may be particularly important in the prevention of **MRSA** infections (Lawrence 1998). However Young (2000) notes that there is no consensus on the use of antiseptics (e.g. povidine-iodine and chlorhexidine) for wounds containing MRSA. Casey (1999) suggests that as healing tissue is very delicate, a good strategy is never to use an antiseptic that we would not wish used in our eyes.

While a wide selection of solutions have been used to cleanse wounds, normal saline is often considered the solution of choice, as it is isotonic and non-toxic to healing tissue (Fletcher 1997). However, a randomised study conducted with

MRSA

Methicillin-resistant *Staphylococcus aureus* is a highly resistant microorganism and is discussed in Chapter 3 in the section on source isolation.

705 soft tissue wounds that were less than 6 hours old compared the use of sterile saline with tap water for cleansing acute traumatic wounds, and found that tap water appeared to be preferable (Angeras *et al.* 1992). Williams and Young (1998) note that chronic wounds always contain large numbers of bacteria, which do not delay wound healing; only systemic infection does this. They therefore suggest that tap water is a satisfactory cleansing agent, and that for patients with leg ulcers it can be comforting, and psychologically enhancing, to bathe their legs in a bucket lined with a waterproof plastic bag, which can then be disposed of afterwards.

A systematic review of the use of water for wound cleansing advises that, based on limited evidence, tap water (as long as it is of good quality) can be used for wound cleansing (Fernandez *et al.* 2003). Solutions used for cleansing/irrigating should be used at body temperature if possible, thus reducing the cooling of the wound bed which adversely affects healing (Myers 1982).

Learning outcome 3: Identify a range of wound dressings showing awareness of how they are selected for individuals

Before considering which dressing to apply, see Box 6.4 which gives an overview of the requirements of the ideal dressing, based on research findings.

Activity

Read the summaries in Box 6.4 and relate this to the range of products you have access to in the practice setting and/or the skills laboratory. Do any of them meet all the necessary criteria? How might you choose which to use? If possible, discuss with a practitioner how a specific dressing is chosen for an individual. You may find that there are local clinical guidelines and if so, try to locate them.

Before asking which dressing to use, your question might sometimes be: Does the wound require a dressing at all? In an extensive study, involving 3674 wounds Weiss (1983) demonstrated that wound dressings are unnecessary for clean surgical wounds after 24 hours, and suggests that dressings are expensive, time-consuming, can interfere with breathing and cause discomfort. Susan's wound dressing could, therefore, have been removed after 24 hours and the wound left open. However a more recent though small study indicated that a film dressing left *in situ* until skin closure removal promotes pain relief (Briggs 1996). Susan might feel more comfortable and less worried about her wound if it is kept covered with a film dressing.

Your choice of dressing will relate to your wound assessment, while taking into account the attributes of an effective wound care product. Particularly important to consider are of course, stage of wound healing, site of wound, pain relief, and amount of exudate, but many other individual factors too. Key groups of dressings, and their uses, are summarised in Table 6.6. Foster and Moore (1999) note that despite the vast range of dressings that are available, many require more sound evidence for their use than is currently available as trials have often used insufficient numbers of people. A systematic review of wound

Effective wound dressings:

1. **Possess high thermal insulation**. A study by Lock (1979) (cited in Myers 1982) with pigs found 108 per cent increased cell division at the edge of wounds maintained (through use of a film dressing or a polyurethane foam) at a high temperature (30–35°C), when compared with wounds left open (attaining a temperature of 21°C), or covered with a gauze dressing (attaining a temperature of 25–27°C). It has been demonstrated that 40 minutes is required for a wound to return to room temperature after cleaning, and 3 hours for mitotic cell division and leucocyte activity to restart (Myers 1982).

2. **Maintain a high humidity at the wound/dressing contact**. Winter (1962), in a classic piece of research, dispelled the myth of dry wounds being necessary to prevent bacterial infection. Instead he demonstrated that film dressings increased humidity at the wound surface, doubling the rate of epithelialisation. A moist surface enabled the epithelial cells to migrate across the wound more easily than when the wound was dry.

3. **Remove excess exudate from the wound surface**. The aim here is to prevent the wound becoming macerated by the profuse exudate in certain types of wounds such as pressure ulcers, burns, fistulae and drain sites. This remains a difficult task for a dressing to achieve, but there are products aimed specifically at heavily exudating wounds.

4. **Are impervious to microorganisms**. Thus preventing air-borne bacteria from reaching the wound through the dressing and bacteria on the wound surface from entering the environment causing cross-infection (Dealey 1999).

5. **Do not shed any fibres or leak out toxic substances**. Dressings that leave particles in wounds prolong the inflammatory response, thus delaying healing (Wood 1976). Gauze, gamgee and cottonwool should not be in contact with wound beds but can be used to help maintain temperature as a secondary dressing.

6. **Allow easy removal from the wound without causing damage to the newly formed tissue**.

Handling qualities of an effective wound dressing are that it should (Dealey 1999):
- Be easy to apply and remove
- Conform well to the wound surface
- Be comfortable
- Not require frequent dressing changes.

Box 6.4 Criteria for effective wound dressings

Table 6.6 Wound dressings (based on Foster and Moore 1999, Dealey 1999, except where stated otherwise)

Dressing type	Examples	Description	Uses
Simple	Mepore	Simple wound covering which provides protection from contamination and absorbs mild exudate	Wounds healing by primary intention, e.g. a straightforward surgical wound
Adhesive film dressings	Opsite, Tegaderm, Bioclusive	A transparent, vapour-permeable adhesive film dressing which acts as a barrier to bacteria and water, and therefore allows bathing/showering. Allows observation of wound. Can be left in place for several days	Primary wound closure, e.g. a straightforward surgical wound. To protect skin susceptible to damage from shearing. Shallow granulating and epithelialising wounds, with low to moderate exudate. Abrasions. Can be used as secondary dressings with alginates, or with hydrogels if there is hard necrotic tissue present
Tulles: medicated and non-medicated	Jelonet (impregnated with soft paraffin), Bactigras (with chlorhexidine), Inadine (with povidine-iodine)	Open weave cotton or rayon dressing impregnated with soft paraffin, antiseptics or antibiotics. Granulation tissue cells can move through the open weave of the dressing, causing damage and pain on removal, and fibres can be left in the wound. Non-absorbent	Infected wounds healing by secondary intention, with minimal exudate, abrasions, minor burns
Hydrogels	Intrasite gel, Purilon, Aquaform, Granugel	A dressing based on starch polymers, which provides a moist wound environment, and promotes debridement	Dry, necrotic and granulating wounds. Light to moderately exuding wounds. Abrasions. Require a secondary dressing
Foam dressings	Allevyn, Tielle, Biatain, Cavicare, Flexipore, Truform	A highly absorbent dressing made from polyurethane or silicone. Available as a flat dressing and a cavity dressing	Heavily exudating wounds, full thickness cavity wounds healing by secondary intention. Granulating and epithelialising wounds
Hydrocolloids	Granuflex, Comfeel plus, Tegasorb, Combiderm, Hydrocol	A polyurethane foam sheet fixed onto a semi-permeable film. Provides a moist environment, promotes debridement, granulation and epithelialisation. A protective barrier against microorganisms. Can cause maceration of surrounding skin. Also available as a paste or powder for cavity wounds	Has wide application, for both chronic wounds, and acute wounds such as abrasions. Moderately but not heavily exudating wounds. Necrotic, infected, sloughy, granulating or epithelialising wounds. Can be left in place for several days and bathing/showering can take place with the dressing *in situ*

(continued)

221

Table 6.6 (*continued*)

Dressing type	Examples	Description	Uses
Alginates	Kaltostat, Sorbsan	Made from the sodium and calcium salts of alginic acid – a seaweed-derived polymer. Reacts with wound exudate to form a gel which, it is believed, promotes wound healing. This can be irrigated off leading to a less painful dressing change. Highly conforming and encourages clotting. Available as a flat dressing, rope and ribbon	Used for moderately to heavily exudating wounds, including infected wounds. Can be used to pack puncture and cavity wounds. For sloughy and granulating wounds. May require a secondary dressing
Hydrofibre dressings	Aquacel	An absorbent dressing which provides a moist wound healing environment	Infected wounds, and acute surgical wounds healing by secondary intention. Can be left in place for up to 3 days
Hydro-capillary and capillary dressings	Alione, Transorbent, Vacutex, Versiva	Used to absorb and manage large amounts of exudates and are generally composed of two or more layers of material	Moderate to heavily exudating wounds, granulating and epithelialising wounds
Cadexomer iodine dressings (see Collier 2002)	Iodosorb, Iodoflex	Dressings contain hydrophilic beads impregnated with iodine. Following contact with wound fluid the beads absorb excessive moisture and release iodine into the wound bed	Wounds with low to moderate exudates. Infected wounds healing by secondary intention
Silver-impregnated products (see Lansdown *et al.* 2003)	Acticoat, Actisorb Silver 220, Aquagel Ag, Contreet, Advance	Metallic silver and its salts have antibacterial properties and bind to DNA of the bacteria which then impairs cell production. Effective broad-spectrum antimicrobial effect	Infected wounds
Topical negative pressure (see Birchall *et al.* 2002)	VAC	Applies localised subatmospheric negative pressure to a wound bed via a computerised therapy unit	Assists in the removal of excessive exudate, reduces oedema, improves circulation, stimulates granulation tissue formation and wound contraction, and reduces bacterial loading

care management found little evidence as to which dressings or topical agents are the most effective in treating chronic wounds (Bradley *et al.* 1999). However there was evidence to support the use of hydrocolloids for pressure ulcers, and that low adherent dressings are as effective as hydrocolloids beneath compression bandaging for venous leg ulcers. Note that the dressing should keep the wound bed warm (Myers 1982), and that dressing changes can cool the wound and slow down the healing. This should be taken into account when planning dressings and carrying the dressing out. Also, always consult the manufacturer's instructions when applying dressings.

The ideal dressing for a diabetic foot ulcer should:

- Perform well in the enclosed environment of a shoe, and not take up too much space
- Absorb large quantities of exudate but enable drainage
- Withstand the pressures and shear of walking
- Not be associated with side effects
- Not depend for its maximum effect on being left in place for long periods as diabetic ulcers can deteriorate very rapidly
- Be easy to remove/lift for inspection.

Box 6.5 The ideal dressing for a diabetic ulcer (Foster *et al.* 1994)

Dressings for diabetic foot ulcers must be chosen with particular care (Foster 1999), but Gill (1999) identifies that many dressing trials exclude people with diabetes, making it difficult to make evidence-based decisions on product choice. A systematic review found much uncertainty over how to effectively prevent and treat diabetic foot ulcers (O'Meara *et al.* 2000). The use of hydrocolloids for these wounds appears to be particularly controversial but Gill (1999), in a critical review, suggests that this product has often been used in an incorrect manner, i.e. left in place for too long a time, without inspecting the wound. The criteria for an ideal dressing for a diabetic foot ulcer, as suggested by Foster *et al.* (1994), can be found in Box 6.5. A trial by Foster *et al.* (1994), compared the use of alginates with polyurethane dressings for non-infected diabetic ulcers, and found that the ulcers healed with either dressing, but the polyurethane dressing handled better. In addition to dressing the ulcer, general foot care (see Chapter 7, Box 7.3) is also essential.

As noted at the start of this chapter, there are constantly new products being developed. This chapter has incorporated available systematic reviews and clinical guidelines but there are many more in progress; check the Cochrane Library and the National Institute for Clinical Excellence for their latest publications.

All patients/clients need education about their wound care and dressings and this has been discussed a little in relation to Susan and her wound already.

Activity

If you were being discharged home with a dressing *in situ*, or had had a dressing applied by the community nurse, what sort of things would you want to know?

You would probably want to know some of the following:

- Can I get the dressing wet? If not, how can I manage activities such as washing?
- When should the dressing be redone, and by whom?
- What should I do if the dressing becomes loose, uncomfortable, too tight, falls off or soaks through?

■ What should I expect of the wound? For example when will it heal?
■ Will the wound be painful? If so, how can I deal with this?
■ How would I know if the wound was getting infected?
■ Are there any special instructions that I should follow?

Remember that education about all these matters should involve relatives/carers as applicable. For Susan, her carers should have been educated prior to her discharge, and explanations should have been given to Susan using the appropriate methods of communication. You might have thought of other things that you would want to know too, and remember that this information is also important to people receiving in-patient care in order to allay anxiety, build confidence and promote self-care. Parents will wish to know similar things about their child's dressing, but may have special concerns such as how to keep the dressing in place. Certainly, with children there are particular considerations when choosing a wound dressing. For example, Casey (1999) notes that for children in nappies it can be difficult to prevent contamination of the wound by faeces or urine if it is in the nappy area, but that occlusive, waterproof dressings can help. It is also important that wounds are kept free of contamination by dirt etc. while playing. Young children may be inquisitive or resent the addition of a dressing to their bodies when they are still developing a clear picture of their own physical self. Therefore dressings need to be securely applied and 'finger proof'. Written information is useful to back up verbal instructions, because it is difficult for people to retain a lot of new information, particularly when under stress. Written patient information should be readable, understandable and culturally relevant however, if it is to be effective in promoting self-care and relieving anxiety (Wilson and McLemore 1997).

Leg ulcer bandaging

A systematic review by Cullum *et al.* (2003) concluded that compression increases venous ulcer healing rates when compared with no compression, that multilayered systems are more effective than single-layered systems, that high compression is more effective than low compression but that there are no clear differences between different types of high compression. Clinical guidelines for the management of venous leg ulcers, based on a systematic review of available evidence, were developed by the Royal College of Nursing (1998) and endorsed by the National Institute of Clinical Excellence. More recently, in 2002 the European Wound Management Association published an evidence-based pathway for the use of compression therapy in the treatment of venous leg ulcers (Ashton 2003). However compression should only be used in the absence of significant arterial disease, and therefore, as discussed earlier in this chapter, arterial blood supply must first be assessed. Treatment needs to be continued after healing, as without compression, the underlying problem – venous hypertension – will return, and a leg ulcer will form once more (Williams and Young 1998). When the ulcer is healed, continuing to use compression (of the strongest tolerable) is associated with reduced rates of recurrence (Nelson *et al.* 2003). Therefore patient education and involvement are essential.

Before selecting a compression bandage, each patient is assessed individually and lifestyle considered (Williams and Young 1998). Bandaging should extend from the base of the toes to the knee (Scully 1999). Royal College of Nursing guidelines (1998) state that leg ulcer bandaging should be applied by a trained practitioner, have adequate padding and be capable of sustaining compression for at least a week. You should get the opportunity to observe leg ulcer bandaging in practice, possibly at a clinic, or with the district nurse. Try to find out about a local leg ulcer clinic, and arrange a visit.

Learning outcome 4: Outline ways of reducing pain and discomfort associated with wounds

Unfortunately patients often associate their wounds with pain. A study of 694 patients with a variety of chronic wounds found that almost half experienced pain (Lindham *et al.* 1999). Any care in relation to wounds can cause fear and distress, be this removal of a surgical drain, a dressing change or removal of skin closing devices such as staples, clips or sutures. A person with a traumatic wound, such as Thomas, has already experienced pain when the injury occurred, and the thought of having a wound dressing could be very distressing. A summary of factors contributing to pain associated with wounds, and possible solutions, can be found in Table 6.7. Chapter 12 considers assessment and management of pain in detail. A few points, particularly relevant to wound pain, are covered below.

Table 6.7 Factors causing pain associated with wounds, and possible solutions (adapted from Hollinworth 1997)

Factors	*Solution(s)*
Use of cold fluids for cleansing/irrigation	Use fluid at body temperature
High-pressure irrigation	Consider reducing pressure, and use of analgesics and other pain-relieving strategies
Use of forceps on sensitive tissue	Use gloves instead
Use of plastic spray which stings	Consider benefits of use versus discomfort. If used, warn patient, and be supportive
Pain on removal of dressings	1. Careful choice of product 2. Information giving and explanations about the procedure 3. Correct dressing removal technique. Refer to manufacturer's instructions 4. Use of analgesics, and other pain-relieving strategies such as relaxation, distraction

It is important that pain is assessed and that the source of pain is identified, so that measures can be taken to alleviate this. Clear links have been found between anxiety and pain, and providing information can reduce this (Hayward 1975). The administration of analgesics prior to dressing change may be required, particularly with children (MacQueen 2000), opiates being necessary if pain is severe, but otherwise non-steroidal anti-inflammatory drugs or simple analgesics. Sufficient time should be allowed for them to take effect before the dressing change (Emflorgo 1999). Nitrous oxide (entonox) can also help some people, and can be effective even for young children (Casey 1999). Other pain-reduction strategies include use of relaxation and distraction. MacQueen (2000) suggests that children can remove their own dressings while bathing/showering, which makes the experience less frightening. The Hospital Play Therapist can accompany a child during the dressing procedure, providing support and employing distraction strategies to help the child cope with the experience.

Casey (1999) notes the importance of giving children the opportunity to express concerns about dressing changes. An infant or small child can sit on his or her parent's lap while the dressing takes place. However, while parental presence during dressings is beneficial to the child, parents can find observing painful procedures being performed on their children emotionally distressing (Callery 1997). Nurses should, therefore, be sensitive to the parents' needs for support. MacQueen (2000) also suggests the use of play, and that dressing times for children should be kept to a minimum, thus reducing discomfort. Planning carefully and preparing everything in advance is essential, as well as choosing an uncomplicated dressing that takes minimal time to apply. Casey (1999) emphasises that pain management must be effective from the start, as the child would otherwise quickly start to associate wound dressings with pain. This statement could equally apply to adults, particularly where there is a chronic wound that requires ongoing wound dressings.

Adherent dressings, for example gauze or paraffin gauze, cause pain on removal because they dry out, and tissue can grow through the fabric. Therefore never use gauze as a primary dressing, and if using paraffin gauze, redress daily. Some products are much less painful to remove (e.g. hydrocolloids, alginates, foam, hydrogels), so give preference to these, which are also generally more comfortable to wear. Some products, e.g. hydrocolloids and film dressings, lose their adhesion as days go by, so leaving them *in situ* for the maximum time possible promotes easy removal. Irrigation can ease removal with some dressings. To remove film dressings, lift the edge, and stretch the dressing up and away rather than peeling it back which is more painful (Jones and Milton 2000).

■   *Activity*

Drawing on the material in this section, identify possible strategies for wound care for Mrs Warner, Colin, Susan and Thomas. Remember to consider: use of clean or sterile technique, debridement/cleansing, wound dressing and pain management.

Points that you might have identified can be found in Table 6.8.

Table 6.8 Possible wound management strategies for Colin, Mrs Warner, Susan and Thomas

	Colin	Mrs Warner	Susan	Thomas
Wound type	Dirty surgical wound on buttock	1. Necrotic sacral pressure ulcer 2. Infected diabetic neuropathic ulcer on toe	Clean contaminated surgical wound on abdomen	Contaminated and infected bites on face
Use of sterile or clean technique?	Sterile	Clean	Sterile	Clean
Debridement needed?	Was performed surgically	Yes. Identify an appropriate option for this individual	Not required	May need to be performed surgically
Cleansing?	Yes, bathing, showering or irrigation with warm saline	Could bath or shower, or the wounds could be irrigated with warm saline when the dressings are renewed. Consider use of antiseptic for infected toe ulcer (Miller 1998)	Not required. Can bath or shower as she wishes	Irrigation will be necessary but this may be performed under a general anaesthetic
Which dressing?	Pack wound with alginate or hydrofibre, then apply secondary dressing	1. Hydrogel, hydrofibre or hydrocolloid to sacrum 2. Toe could be dressed with an alginate, hydrofibre or foam dressing	Not necessary after first 24 hours (Weiss 1983) but Susan may find it more comfortable if her wound is covered with a film dressing until her sutures are removed	If required film dressings would be appropriate. In practice, facial wounds are rarely dressed
Pain management	Assess client. Information giving and explanations. Regular analgesics, e.g. non-steroidal anti-inflammatory drugs. The alginate or hydrofibre dressing should be comfortable to wear and painless to remove	Assess client. Information giving and explanations. Hydrogel, hydrofibre, hydrocolloid, foam and alginate dressings are all comfortable to wear and their removal should be painless. Regular analgesics if needed. Neuropathic ulcers are usually painless	Assess pain. Information giving and explanations. Regular analgesics may be needed. Removal of film dressing with care. Removal of skin closures will need careful preparation, reassurance and support	Assess pain. Information giving and explanations. If dressings are present, remove with care. Regular analgesics may be needed. Removal of skin closures needs careful preparation, reassurance and support

Summary

- Wound assessment must precede effective wound management, which requires the application of suitable cleansing methods, the most appropriate dressing to cover the wound, and pain-relieving strategies.
- Application of these skills in the care of each individual is the product of knowledge and experience.

CHAPTER SUMMARY

This chapter aimed to introduce an understanding of how wounds heal, with an emphasis on the systemic nature of wound healing, and the range of factors that may impair wound healing. An awareness of how wounds can be assessed and managed, taking into account their underlying causes, has also been promoted. The chapter emphasised an individualistic and holistic approach to wound care, and discussed different options available for managing wounds.

The reader has been encouraged to take the opportunity to apply knowledge to practice and to start to gain experience in observing wounds and identifying their stage of healing. Involving patients/clients and their families, working with the multidisciplinary team, accessing expert knowledge, and being aware of the need to continually update have all been addressed. This chapter did not attempt to include specialist knowledge and it is intended that further in-depth reading in relation to individual topics such as leg ulcers and burns would be undertaken by the reader.

To conclude, an understanding of wound care is important for all nurses; this chapter aimed to introduce key principles to act as a foundation for future learning.

REFERENCES

Angeras, M.H., Brandberg, A., Falk, A. and Seeman, T. 1992. Comparison between sterile saline and tap water for the cleansing of acute traumatic soft tissue wounds. *European Journal of Surgery* **158**, 347–50.

Ashton, J. 2003. A review of a recommended management pathway in the treatment of venous leg ulcers. *Nurse2Nurse Magazine* **3**(3), 46–8.

Audit Commission 1999. *First Assessment: A review of district nursing services in England and Wales*. London: Audit Commission.

Bergstrom, N., Demuth, P.J. and Braden, B.J. 1987. A clinical trial of the Braden Scale for predicting pressure sore risk. *Nursing Clinics of North America* **22**, 417–28.

Birchall, L., Street, L. and Clift, H. 2002. Developing a trust-wide centralised approach to the use of TNP … topical negative pressure. *Journal of Wound Care* **11**, 311–14.

Boore, J. 1978. *Prescription for Recovery*. London: RCN.

Bradley, M., Cullum, N., Nelson, E.A. *et al.* 1999. Systematic reviews of wound management: (2) dressings and topical agents used in the healing of chronic wounds. *Health Technology Assessment* **3**(17 Part 2), 1–135.

Bremmelgaard, A., Raahave, D., Beier-Holgersen *et al.* 1989. Computer aided surveillance of surgical infections and identification of risk factors. *Journal of Hospital Infection* **13**, 1–18.

Briggs, M. 1996. Surgical wound pain: a trial of two treatments. *Journal of Wound Care* **5**, 456–60.

Bryant, R.A. 2000: Preface. In Bryant, R.A. (ed.) *Acute and Chronic Wounds: Nursing Management*, second edition. St Louis: CV Mosby, ix–x.

Callery, P. 1997. Paying to participate: financial, social and personal costs to parents of involvement in their children's care in hospital. *Journal of Advanced Nursing* **25**, 746–52.

Casey, G. 1999. Wound management in children. *Paediatric Nursing* **11**(5), 39–44.

Clancy, J. and McVicar, A. 1997. Wound healing: a series of homeostatic responses. *British Journal of Theatre Nursing* **7**(4), 25–34.

Collier, M. 2002. Wound care.Wound bed preparation. *Nursing Times* **98**(2), 55–7.

Cooper, D.M. 2000. Assessment, measurement and evaluation: their pivotal roles in wound healing: In Bryant, R.A. (ed.) *Acute and Chronic Wounds: Nursing Management*, second edition. St Louis: CV Mosby, 51–83.

Cooper, R., Halas, E. and Molan, P. 2002. The efficacy of honey in inhibiting strains of Pseudomonas aeruginosa from infected burns. *Journal of Burn Care and Rehabilitation* **23**, 366–70.

Cruse, P. and Foord, R. 1980. The epidemiology of wound infection, a ten year prospective study of 62,939 wounds. *Surgical Clinics of North America* **60**, 27–40.

Cullum, N. and Roe, B. 1995. *Leg Ulcers: Nursing management, a research based guide*. Harrow: Scutari Press.

Cullum, N., Nelson, E.A., Fletcher, A.W. and Sheldon, T.A. 2003. Compression for venous leg ulcers (Cochrane review). In *The Cochrane Library*, Issue 2. Oxford: Update Software.

Cutting, K.F. 1999. The causes and prevention of maceration of the skin. *Journal of Wound Care* **8**, 200–1.

Cutting, K.F. and Harding, K.G. 1994. Criteria for identifying a wound infection. *Journal of Wound Care* **3**, 198–201.

Cuzzell, J. 1988. The new RYB color code. *American Journal of Nursing* **88**, 1342–6.

Davidson, N.J., Sowden, J.M. and Fletcher, J. 1984. Defective phagocytosis in insulin controlled diabetics: evidence for a reaction between glucose and opsonising proteins. *Journal of Clinical Pathology* **37**, 783–6.

Dealey, C. 1999. *The Care of Wounds: A Guide for Nurses*, second edition. Oxford: Blackwell Science.

Department of Health 2001. *Valuing People: A new strategy for learning disability for the 21st century*. London: DH.

Desai, H. 1997. Ageing and Wounds: Healing in old age. *Journal of Wound Care* **6**, 237–9.

Doughty, D.B., Waldrop, J. and Ramundo, J. 2000. Lower-extremity ulcers of vascular etiology. In Bryant, R.A. (ed.) *Acute and Chronic Wounds: Nursing management*, second edition. St Louis: CV Mosby, 265–300.

Emflorgo, C.A. 1999. The assessment and treatment of wound pain. *Journal of Wound Care* **8**, 384–5.

Evans, R.C. and Jones, N.L. 1996. The management of abrasions and bruises. *Journal of Wound Care* **5**, 465–8.

Farion, K., Osmond, M.H., Hartling, L. *et al.* 2003. Tissue adhesives for traumatic lacerations in children and adults (Cochrane Review). In *The Cochrane Library*, Issue 4. Chichester: John Wiley and Sons.

Fernandez, R., Griffiths, R. and Ussia, C. 2003. Water for wound cleansing (Cochrane Review). In *The Cochrane Library*, Issue 4. Chichester: John Wiley and Sons.

Flanagan, M. 1997. A practical framework for wound assessment 2: methods. *British Journal of Nursing* **6**(1), 6–11.

Fletcher, J. 1997. Wound cleansing. *Professional Nurse* **12**, 793–96.

Foster, A. 1999. Diabetic ulceration. In Miller, M. and Glover, D. (eds) *Wound Management: Theory and practice*. London: NT Books, 72–83.

Foster, L. and Moore, P. 1999. Acute surgical wound care 3: fitting the dressing to the wound. *British Journal of Nursing* **8**, 200, 202, 204, 206, 208–10.

Foster, A.V.M., Greenhill, M.T. and Edmonds, M.E. 1994. Comparing two dressings in the treatment of diabetic foot ulcers. *Journal of Wound Care* **3**, 224–8.

Fox, C. 2002. Honey as a dressing for chronic wounds in adults. *British Journal of Community Nursing* **7**, 530–4.

Gill, D. 1999. The use of hydrocolloids in the treatment of diabetic foot. *Journal of Wound Care* **8**, 204–6.

Goldberg, M.T. and McGynn-Byer, P. 2000. Oncology-related skin damage. In Bryant, R.A. (ed.) *Acute and Chronic Wounds: Nursing management*, second edition. St Louis: CV Mosby, 367–86.

Goldstein, D.R., Vogel, K.M., Mureebe, L. and Kerstein, M.D. 1998. Differential diagnosis: assessment of the lower extremity ulcer . . . is it arterial, venous or neuropathic? *Wounds: A Compendium of Clinical Research and Practice* **10**(4), 125–31.

Gottrup, F. 1999. Wound closure techniques. *Journal of Wound Care* **8**, 397–400.

Green, S.M., Winterberg, H., Franks, P.J. *et al.* 1999. Nutritional intake in community patients with pressure ulcers. *Journal of Wound Care* **8**, 325–30.

Hampton, S. 1999. Choosing the right dressing. In Miller, M. and Glover, D. (eds) *Wound Management Theory and Practice*. London: NT Books, 116–28.

Hayward, J. 1975. *Information: A prescription against pain*. London: Royal College of Nursing.

Higgins, M.A.G., Evans, R.C. and Evans, R.J. 1997. Managing animal bite wounds. *Journal of Wound Care* **6**, 377–80.

Hollinworth, H. 1997. Less pain, more gain. *Nursing Times* **93**(46), 89, 91.

Hollinworth, H. and Kingston, J.E. 1998. Using a non-sterile technique in wound care. *Professional Nurse* **13**, 226–29.

Jones, V. and Milton, T. 2000. When and how to use adhesive film dressings. *NTPlus* **96**(16), 3–4

Kiernan, M. 1999. Wet, sloughy and necrotic wound management. *Nurse Prescriber/Community Nurse* **5**(3), 51–2.

Kiecolt-Glaser, J.K., Marucha, P.T., Malarkey, W.B. *et al.* 1995. Slowing of wound healing by psychological stress. *Lancet* **346**, 1194–6.

King, D.J. 1998. Atypical antipsychotics and the negative symptoms of schizophrenia. *Advances in Psychiatric Treatment* **4**, 53–61.

Kloth, L.C. and McCulloch, J.M. 1995. The inflammatory response to wound healing. In McCulloch, J.M., Kloth, L.C. and Feedar, J.A. (eds) *Wound Healing Alternatives in Management.* Philadelphia: FA Davis.

Krizek, T.J., Harries, R.H.C. and Robson, M.C. 1997. Biology of tissue injury and repair. In Georgiade, G.S., Riefkohl, R. and Scott-Levin, L. (eds) *Georgiade Plastic Maxillofacial and Reconstructive Surgery,* third edition. London: Williams and Wilkins, 3–9.

Lansdown, A.B.G., Jensen, K. and Jensen, M.Q. 2003. Contreet foam and contreet hydrocolloid: an insight into two new silver-containing dressings. *Journal of Wound Care* **12**, 204–10.

Lawrence, J.C. 1998. The use of povidine iodine as an antiseptic agent. *Journal of Wound Care* **7**, 421–5.

Lazarus, G.S., Cooper, D.M., Knighton, D.R. *et al.* 1994. Definitions and guidelines for assessment of wounds and evaluation of healing. *Archives of Dermatology* **130**, 489–93.

Leaper, D. 1996. Antiseptics in wound healing. *Nursing Times* **92**(39), 63–4, 66.

Levenson, S.M., Geever, E.F. and Crowley, L.V. *et al.* 1965. The healing of rat skin wounds. *Annals of Surgery* **161**, 293.

Lindham, C., Bergsten, A. and Berglund, E.1999. Chronic wounds and nursing care. *Journal of Wound Care* **9**, 5–10.

MacQueen, S. 2000. Wound care. In Huband, S. and Trigg, E. (eds) *Practices in Children's Nursing: Guidelines for hospital and community.* Edinburgh: Churchill Livingstone, 317–18.

Magan, M.A. 1996. Psychological considerations for patients with acute wounds. *Critical Care Nursing Clinics of North America* **8**, 183–93.

Miller, M. 1995. Principles of wound assessment. *Emergency Nurse* **3**(1), 16–18.

Miller, M. 1996. Best practice in wound assessment. *Community Nurse* **2**(3), 41–2, 44, 47.

Miller, M. 1998. How do I diagnose and treat wound infection? *British Journal of Nursing* **7**, 335–8.

Miller, M. 1999a. Wound assessment. In Miller, M. and Glover, D. (eds) *Wound Management Theory and Practice*. London: NT Books, 23–36.

Miller, M. 1999b. Nursing assessment of patients with non-acute wounds. *British Journal of Nursing* **8**(10), 12–14.

Mishriki, S.F., Law, D.J. and Jeffrey, P.J. 1990. Factors affecting the incidence of post-operative infection. *Journal of Hospital Infection* **16**, 223–30.

Molan, P.C. 1999. The role of honey in the management of wounds. *Journal of Wound Care* **8**, 415–18.

Morison, M. and Moffat, C. 1994. *A Colour Guide to the Assessment and Management of Leg Ulcers*, second edition. London: Mosby.

Mulder, G.D., Brazinsky, B.A. and Seeley, J.E. 1995. Factors complicating wound repair. In McCulloch, J.M., Luther, C., Kloth, L.C. and Feedar, J.A. (eds) *Wound Healing Alternatives in Management*, 2nd edition. Philadelphia: FA Davis, 47–59.

Myers, J.A. 1982. Modern plastic surgical dressings. *Health and Social Service Journal* **92**, 336–7.

Negus, D. 1995. *Leg Ulcers: A practical approach to management*, second edition. Oxford: Butterworth-Heinemann.

Neil, J.A. and Barrell, L.M. 1998. Transition theory and its relevance to patients with chronic wounds. *Rehabilitation Nursing* **23**, 295–9.

Nelson, E.A. and Bradley, M.D. 2003. Dressings and topical agents for arterial leg ulcers (Cochrane Review). In *The Cochrane Library*, Issue 4. Chichester: John Wiley and Sons.

Nelson, E.A., Bell-Syer, S.E.M. and Cullum, N.A. 2003. Compression for preventing recurrence of venous ulcers (Cochrane Review). In *The Cochrane Library*, Issue 4. Chichester: John Wiley and Sons.

NICE (National Institute for Clinical Excellence) 2001. *Guidance on the Use of Debriding Agents and Specialist Wound Care Clinics for Difficult to Heal Surgical Wounds*. London: NICE.

O'Meara, S., Cullum, N., Majid, M. and Sheldon, T. 2000. Systematic reviews of wound care management: (3) antimicrobial agents for chronic wounds; (4) diabetic foot ulceration. *Health Technology Assessment* **4**(21).

Partridge, C. 1998. Influential factors in surgical wound healing. *Journal of Wound Care* **7**, 350–3.

Price, B. 1993. Diseases and altered body image in children. *Paediatric Nursing* **5**(6), 18–21.

Reid, J. and Morison, M. 1994. Towards a consensus: classification of pressure sores. *Journal of Wound Care* **3**, 157–60.

Rolstad, B.S., Ovington, L.G. and Harris, A. 2000. Principles of wound management. In Bryant, R.A. (ed.) *Acute and Chronic Wounds: Nursing management*, second edition. St Louis: Mosby, 85–112.

Royal College of Nursing 1998. *The Management of Patients with Venous Leg Ulcers*. London: RCN.

Scully, C. 1999. In on a limb. *Nursing Times* **95**(27), 59–60, 62, 65.

Schultz, G. S. 2000: Molecular regulation of wound healing. In Bryant, R.A. (ed.) *Acute and Chronic Wounds: Nursing management*, second edition. St Louis: Mosby, 413–69.

Sherman, R.A., Sherman, J., Gilead, L. *et al.* 2001. Maggot debridement in outpatients. *Archives of Physical Medicine and Rehabilitation* **82**, 1226–9.

Silhi, N. 1998. Diabetes and wound healing. *Journal of Wound Care* **7**, 47–51.

Stotts, N.A. 2000. Nutritional support and assessment. In Bryant, R.A. (ed.) *Acute and Chronic Wounds: Nursing management*, second edition. St Louis: Mosby, 41–50.

Thomas, S., Jones, M., Shutler, S. and Jones, S. 1996. Using larvae in modern management ... maggot therapy. *Journal of Wound Care* **5**(2), 60–69.

Thomas, S., Andrews, A. and Jones, M. 1998. The use of larvae therapy in wound management. *Journal of Wound Care* **7**, 521–524.

Thomlinson, D. 1987. To clean or not to clean. *Nursing Times* **83**(9), 71, 73, 75.

Valk, G.D., Kriegsman, D.N.W. and Assendelft, W.J.J. 2003. Patient education for preventing diabetic foot ulceration (Cochrane Review). In *The Cochrane Library*, Issue 4. Chichester: John Wiley and Sons.

Waldrop, J. and Doughty, D. 2000: Wound healing physiology. In Bryant, R.A. (ed.) *Acute and Chronic Wounds: Nursing management*, second edition. St Louis: Mosby, 17–39.

Waterlow, J. 1985. A risk assessment card. *Nursing Times* **81**(48), 49, 51, 55.

Waterlow, J. 1988. The Waterlow card for the prevention and management of pressure sores: towards a pocket policy. *Care – Science and Practice* **6**(1), 8–12.

Weiss, E.L. 1995. Connective tissue in wound healing. In McCulloch, J.M., Luther, C., Kloth, L.C. and Feedar, J.A. (eds) *Wound Healing Alternatives in Management*, second edition. Philadelphia: FA Davis, 16–31.

Weiss, Y. 1983. Simplified management of operative wounds by early exposure. *International Surgery* **68**, 237–40.

Williams, C. and Young, T. 1998. *Myth and Reality in Wound Care*. Dinton: Mark Allen Publishing.

Wilson, F.L. and McLemore, R. 1997. Patient literacy levels: a consideration when designing patient education programs. *Rehabilitation Nursing* **22**, 311–17.

Winter, G. 1962. Formation of the scab and the rate of epithelialization of superficial wounds in the skin of the young domestic pig. *Nature* **193**, 293–4.

Witte, M.B. and Barbul, A. 1997. General principles of wound healing. *Surgical Clinics of North America* **77**(3), 509–28.

Wood, R.A.B. 1976. Disintegration of cellulose dressings in open granulating wounds. *British Medical Journal* **1**, 1444–5.

Young, T. 1997. Wound care in the accident and emergency department. *British Journal of Nursing* **6**, 395–6, 398, 400–1.

Young, T. 2000. Managing MRSA wound infection and colonisation. *NTPlus* **96**(14), 14–16.

USEFUL WEBSITES

- The **World Wide Wounds** website covers all aspects of wound management and can be found at www.worldwidewounds.com.
- The E-jottings in **Tissue Viability** website has lots of photos of wounds and clear explanation about different types of wounds and how they can be assessed. It can be found at www.ejtv.co.uk.

Meeting hygiene needs

7

Chrissie Major

Assisting people to meet their hygiene needs is a fundamental and vital part of nursing care. The Department of Health (2001a) reinforced this view by including 'Personal and oral hygienc' as a section in *The Essence of Care*. Meeting hygiene needs greatly contributes to comfort, gives an opportunity for observing physical and psychological needs, and provides a chance to build a trusting relationship, which is at the heart of good nursing. Hygiene is one of those activities which most people learn to perform for themselves. However disability and/or physical and mental health problems may lead to the need for assistance, either on a temporary or on a permanent basis. Henderson's definition of nursing emphasised this point, stating that 'the unique function of the nurse is to assist the individual … in the performance of those activities contributing to health … that he would perform unaided if he had the necessary strength, will or knowledge' (Henderson 1960). As with any procedure, hygiene care must be discussed with the person beforehand, and consent obtained. As this chapter is focusing on the care of the body, last offices – care of the body after death – is also included.

The principles of care (e.g. observation, comfort, communication, safety and prevention of cross-infection) discussed in this chapter are generally relevant to anyone of any age. How they are carried out for each individual varies, and for a child will take developmental stage into account. Young babies' immune systems are not yet fully developed, and therefore prevention of cross-infection (see Chapter 3) is particularly important (Simpson 1998/9). For babies and small children, parents are usually resident and attend to their child's hygiene. However, if parents are unable to be present, the nurse would need to meet the child's hygiene needs.

This chapter includes:
- Rationale for meeting hygiene needs and potential hazards
- Bathing a person in bed
- Washing a person's hair in bed
- Bathing and showering in the bathroom
- Facial shaving
- Oral hygiene
- Last offices.

> ### Recommended biology reading:
>
> You are advised to revise the layers of the skin. In addition, the following questions will help you to focus on the biology underpinning this chapter's skills. Use your recommended text book to find out:
>
> - The skin and oral cavity hosts a range of microorganisms. Which of these are potentially pathogenic?
> - What is saliva composed of? Where is it produced, and what is its role in maintaining a healthy mouth?
> - What protective mechanisms do eyes have which help to prevent them becoming infected?
> - Distinguish between transient and resident bacteria found on the skin. Which of these cannot be removed with handwashing? (Chapter 3 'Preventing cross-infection' and the section 'Hand hygiene', will help you).
> - How does the skin maintain its waterproof properties?
> - Why does the skin on the palms of the hands and soles of the feet wrinkle when soaked in water?
> - How does ageing affect the skin?
> - Why do we sweat and what does sweat contain?
> - Why does stale sweat smell?
> - What is the 'acid mantle' and how can it be destroyed?

PRACTICE SCENARIOS

The following practice scenarios are referred to throughout this chapter in relation to meeting hygiene needs.

Adult

Metastases

Secondary deposits of cancer which have spread from the primary site, either directly or via blood or lymph.

William Newton, who likes to be called 'Bill', is a retired accountant, aged 73 years. He is terminally ill with a history of oesophageal cancer and **metastases** in his lungs. He is cared for by his wife at home with the support of community nurses and the Macmillan nurse. He is taking regular oral morphine for pain control. He has a very low haemoglobin and has been admitted for a blood transfusion. He is weak, breathless and his general condition is poor. He has a **Body Mass Index** (BMI) of 16. He can swallow only very small amounts of liquidised food and drink. He has some of his own teeth but also a partial denture which he likes to wear although it is now ill-fitting. His tongue appears coated and his mouth is dry.

Body Mass Index

BMI is explained in Chapter 9 in the section 'Assessing nutritional status and developing a plan of action'. A BMI of 16 indicates a person is underweight.

Child

Chickenpox

An infectious disease caused by a virus (varicella-zoster virus, a member of the herpesvirus family). It results in skin lesions that are intensely itchy and that can result in permanent scarring if scratched, with resulting bacterial infection.

Laura Cox is 4 years old and is in hospital with a chest infection but has developed **chickenpox**. She is being nursed in the isolation area of the children's ward and has to remain in the cubicle at all times. Laura has many skin lesions all over her body, some of which are beginning to crust over. Lesions on her vulval area sting when she passes urine, making her reluctant to go to the toilet. Consequently, she sometimes wets the bed when she is asleep. She is pyrexial, lethargic, and reluctant to eat or drink anything. The family decided that Laura's father would remain with her in hospital while her mother would care for Molly, Laura's 8-month-old sister, at home. Both Laura's parents have had chickenpox but her sister has not.

Learning disability

Ellen Grey is a 47-year-old woman with a learning disability. She lives in sheltered accommodation in her own flat. There is a communal lounge. She has always managed her own personal hygiene adequately. However, recently she has developed an unpleasant smell and other residents have begun to avoid her because of this. The community nurse for learning disabilities has been asked to assess the situation and she finds out that the reason Ellen's personal hygiene has become compromised is because of the recent development of nocturnal incontinence. As well as her bed linen being wet, this situation has disrupted Ellen's usual hygiene routine.

Mental health

Miss Smith, aged 83 years, was admitted to an in-patient assessment unit for older people following concerns from her social worker and GP about her ability to cope at home. She lives on her own with only her pet dog for company. As she can no longer climb her stairs she has been sleeping in an armchair downstairs. Her poor mobility also prevented her from reaching the bathroom. Although Miss Smith is in reasonable physical health her clothing has obviously not been changed for many months and is encrusted with dirt and excrement. Her hair is badly knotted and matted and her skin is in poor condition. She also has poor oral hygiene which she has obviously neglected for some time. Miss Smith was initially distrusting of staff and resisted all attempts to help her have a bath and clean clothes. Eventually she agreed to do this but remained hostile towards staff, accusing them of stealing her dog and her house. However nurses explained that her dog had been taken to the local RSPCA kennels and was in good health. Gradually Miss Smith became more accepting of her new surroundings and began to engage nurses in conversation without her previous hostility or suspicion.

RATIONALE FOR MEETING HYGIENE NEEDS AND POTENTIAL HAZARDS

LEARNING OUTCOMES

By the end of this section you will be able to:

1. Identify why facilitating patients/clients to meet their hygiene needs is a beneficial nursing action.
2. Discuss possible hazards and problems associated with meeting hygiene needs.

Learning outcome 1: Identify why facilitating patients/clients to meet their hygiene needs is a beneficial nursing action

 Activity

Many benefits have been associated with bathing patients (Whiting 1999). Why might it be important for nurses to assist with hygiene needs? Consider how you might feel if you were incapacitated, mentally or physically, and unable to attend to your hygiene.

You may have included the following points.

■ Feeling clean and comfortable is an important social need for most people; to feel well groomed and not offensive to others can help to maintain self-esteem (Rader 1994). Thus for Ellen to be aware that she has an unpleasant odour which others are discussing could cause her some distress. Miss Smith's poor mobility has prevented her maintaining her hygiene and this is probably upsetting for her.

■ Cleanliness is also important within culture and religion. For example, for Muslims, cleanliness has both a spiritual and physical dimension and a very high standard of hygiene is required (Rassool 2000). Muslims must wash before they pray (Holland and Hogg 2001). A study of older South Asian patients' experiences of culturally sensitive care highlighted that maintaining their hygiene was essential for dignity (Clegg 2003).

■ The act of assisting people with personal hygiene needs allows nurses to build up a trusting relationship (Winkworth 2003). It is a private time where communication may be facilitated. Brawley (2002) points out that for people living in care homes bathtime may be one of the only opportunities for individual attention.

■ A number of valuable observations can be made, for example the condition of the skin. This will be important for all the people in this chapter's scenarios.

■ Cleansing the skin removes potentially harmful microorganisms and also sweat, dead skin cells and the bacteria which produce body odour.

■ Washing stimulates the circulation; the movement associated with this and the effect of warm water on the skin is beneficial, both physiologically and psychologically (Sloane *et al.* 1995).

■ Bathing has been described as one of the 'great pleasures in life' (Brawley 2002, p. 38).

As identified above, observant nurses can learn a great deal about people when assisting with their hygiene needs.

Activity

Make a list of the things you can observe while assisting a person with hygiene. Looking at the scenarios might give you some clues.

You may have thought about the following:

■ **Condition of the skin**: Is there any redness, any breaks in the skin, skin infections or bruising? This will be important for Bill because of advancing disease, but is also highly relevant to Laura, Ellen and Miss Smith.

■ **Hydration and nutrition**: Does the skin feel dry and loose, or oedematous? Any of the people in this chapter's scenarios could potentially become dehydrated due to poor fluid intake, and their skin could become dry. Chapter 9 emphasises that visually observing skin is important in nutritional assessment.

■ **The person's mental state**: Is the person anxious, calm, depressed, demotivated, cheerful, lethargic or confused? This would be an important observation with all the people in this chapter's scenarios.

■ **Physical ability**: To what extent can the person do things for him/herself? Does activity cause breathlessness or fatigue? This will be a factor in Bill's ability to self-care. Is there any apparent limb weakness or difficulty/discomfort on movement? Nurses assisting Miss Smith will be able to observe what aspects of hygiene she can manage and what aspects she needs help with or for which aids might be needed.

■ **Condition of any wound, drain or IV sites**: This could apply to Laura and Bill in particular. You could note oozing, scabbing of Laura's lesions or inflammation of surrounding skin, for example, as well as Bill's IV site.

Learning outcome 2: Discuss possible hazards and problems associated with meeting hygiene needs

As discussed above, meeting hygiene needs should be a therapeutic activity, and yet there are a number of potential difficulties.

| ■ *Activity* | What could be possible hazards or problems associated with hygiene care? |

You might have identified the following:

■ Bathing may cause disturbance to a very ill patient (such as Bill) who has limited reserves of energy may be breathless. Laura is lethargic and uncomfortable, and therefore may not want to have a wash.

■ People can become chilled if large areas of the body are exposed. Bill is underweight, and thus is even more likely to become cold if care is not taken. Small babies are also susceptible to the cold (Kay 2000). Specific care relating to the hygiene needs of babies, for example baby bathing, top and tailing, are not discussed in this chapter, but are covered in detail by Kay (2000).

■ Rather than removing harmful microorganisms, the procedure may actively contaminate the skin by redistributing microorganisms from heavily colonised areas such as the perineum, to other areas (Gould 1994). Cross-infection from other patients may be facilitated if nurses are careless about infection control procedures, such as handwashing between patients.

- Excessive washing and the use of harsh soaps may remove essential oils and the protective natural flora of the skin (Skewes 1997; Thaipisuttikul 1998).
- Having to allow other people, strangers, to perform intimate personal tasks can be a source of shame or embarrassment. In Chapter 1 (Box 1.3) there is an example of the fear of being seen naked when being assisted with a shower. Miss Smith may never before in her adult life have been assisted with bathing and dressing and could find this very demeaning. There may be cultural differences in the gender and relationships of who is permitted to perform these procedures, so you will need to be aware of this and be sensitive to each individual. For example, modesty is a requirement of Islam and therefore exposure of the body for both men and women can be very upsetting (Holland and Hogg 2001). Age can also be a factor. An Australian study found that for intimate procedures like washing younger women in particular preferred care to be given by female nurses, while men did not appear to mind if the nurse who washed them was a man or a woman (Chur-Hansen 2002). Consider how each of the patients/clients described in the scenarios may feel under these circumstances. How would you feel?

Many of the above difficulties can be minimised by careful assessment of individuals. *The Essence of Care* (Department of Health 2001a) emphasises the role of assessment in meeting hygiene needs, with its benchmark of best practice: 'All patients/clients are assessed to identify the advice and/or care required to maintain and promote their individual personal hygiene' (p. 52). This assessment will identify the level of help needed which could range from total assistance to verbal support and encouragement in other instances. Unfortunately there have been reports of people not receiving the help with hygiene they need: 'A friend gave me a full bath after three days … I had one bath during an eleven day stay' (Health Advisory Service 2000 1998, p. 19). *The Essence of Care* (2001a) emphasises that the level of support people need to maintain their hygiene may vary so evaluation and reassessment must be carried out as needed.

Summary

- Assisting people to meet their hygiene needs can greatly increase comfort and provide an excellent opportunity for observation.
- People may not find being assisted with their hygiene a pleasant experience and there are associated hazards. Assessment of each individual and a caring approach are key principles necessary to carry out this care in a therapeutic manner.

BATHING A PERSON IN BED

Bathing a person in bed is necessary to meet hygiene needs when people are unable to get out of bed for medical reasons (e.g. after certain surgery or injuries), or when people are too unwell or weak to be able to get out of bed. Bill may need this option at present, and Laura, being isolated in her cubicle and feeling very unwell, may also be washed in bed. The procedure described in this section – bedbathing – involves washing a patient's body while they are in bed using a bowl of water and cloths. An alternative technique involves covering the face and body with warm towels which have been soaked in emollient/water solution in a plastic bag, referred to as a 'bag bath' (Lentz 2003) or 'soft towel' method (Hancock *et al.* 2000). Hancock *et al.* (2000) found this method to be preferred by patients and nurses; in particular the method kept patients warmer.

While this section focuses on bathing in bed, some patients who are unable to wash in the bathroom are able to sit out in a chair to wash, using a bowl. Nurses need to give assistance according to individual needs, based on assessment, and the principles discussed in this section can be adapted to each situation.

LEARNING OUTCOMES

By the end of this section you will be able to:

1. Discuss ways of maintaining patients' dignity and enhancing comfort when bathing a person in bed.
2. Describe the procedure for carrying out bedbathing.

Learning outcome 1: Discuss ways of maintaining patients' dignity and enhancing comfort when bathing a person in bed

As mentioned earlier, there is a risk that assisting people with hygiene needs can threaten dignity and cause discomfort.

Activity

> How might you maintain dignity and comfort for people while bathing them in bed?

Points which you might have identified include:

■ Ensuring privacy by drawing cubicle curtains.
■ Encouraging people to do as much as possible for themselves and allowing sufficient time to do so.
■ Not exposing any more of the patient's body than is necessary for the task being carried out.
■ Being aware that clothing may have special significance within some religions. For example some Hindus wear a white cotton thread (*janeu*) over the right shoulder and round the body. This is sacred and should not be removed unless absolutely essential (Holland and Hogg 2001).
■ Appropriate communication. Your approach to people will do much to promote dignity (see Chapter 2 'The nurse's approach'). Walsh and Kowanko's (2002) study found that patients appreciated nurses using

small talk to reduce embarrassment, with one patient saying that the nurse discussed current affairs while she was bathing him: 'mainly about the morning topics, like the news or something like that. Just to keep your mind off the fact that there is a woman standing in front of you bathing you' (p. 149).

The *National Service Framework for Older People* (Department of Health 2001b) states that service users and carers should be able to expect that personal hygiene needs are carried out sensitively and in privacy. The importance of providing an appropriate environment for hygiene needs to be met is emphasised in *The Essence of Care* (Department of Health 2001a) with the following benchmark of best practice: 'Patients/clients have access to an environment that is safe and acceptable to the individual' (p. 52).

Learning outcome 2: Describe the procedure for carrying out bedbathing

Before commencing the bathing of a person in bed, you need to make an assessment of the individual.

Assessment

Activity

What items should you include in your assessment? Consider Laura and Bill, for example.

You may have thought of the following:

- The person's usual hygiene routine – some people bath in the morning, others in the evening. Not everyone baths every day. If possible, try to maintain the person's usual routine. For a child in hospital, this provides comfort and reassurance (Kay 2000). Consider: can you fit the routine to the patient, rather than the patient to the routine?
- How does the person feel today? For example, is Bill anxious to be clean and groomed, or feeling so ill and fragile that the bare minimum will suffice until he feels more comfortable? Is Laura feeling too unwell to be bothered with a wash at present? A sick child is better left undisturbed unless there is a good indication otherwise (Kay 2000). Particularly when a person is unwell or fatigued, try to combine other care with hygiene needs, so that they can then be left to rest. For example if the person needs repositioning for pressure relief, bathing can be timed to coincide with turning. Ensure that pain is controlled as bathing inevitably involves movement, which would cause further pain.
- How much assistance is needed? Can you promote independence in any way, or is some time and care needed to re-establish self-care? A recent survey of patients who had been assessed as self-caring found that many of them felt that they would have liked to have been offered some degree of assistance with washing at some time (Hartley 2003).

■ Does the person want a nurse to help, or is there a relative coming in whose help they would prefer instead? For example Bill's wife may have been assisting him to wash at home and might prefer to continue to do this while he is in hospital. Laura's father is resident, and with children nurses should negotiate with parents the extent to which they would like to be involved in their child's care (Coyne 1995a; Kawik 1996). A small study conducted by Coyne (1995b) suggested that parents all expected to carry out everyday care such as bathing. However, they may need assistance or guidance, particular when their child has dressings in place, and movement is impaired. In Laura's case her father might need guidance about care of her skin with the many lesions, and also prevention of cross-infection, for example handwashing (see Chapter 3). For some parents of chronically sick children, it may be a relief if nurses carry out their child's hygiene care (Kay 2000). This can also be the case with informal carers of adults. Bill's wife may be exhausted and benefit from a break.

■ Does the person need to empty their bladder or bowels before commencing the bath? Offer this facility. Chapter 8 discusses assisting with elimination in detail.

■ What toiletries do they usually use? Use of toiletries is quite individual; it might be interesting to make a list of your own requirements, and compare it to a friend's. If people have been admitted as emergencies they may not have been able to bring their own, in which case single-use toiletries should be available for them (Department of Health 2001a).

■ What time is available – do you have the time now, or will you have more time later? Will you need another nurse to help you? Other health care professionals for example, physiotherapists or dieticians, may need access to the patient too.

Equipment

Having made this assessment, you will be ready to gather the equipment needed. Always try to think ahead and collect all that you will need at the start, thus avoiding having to leave the person during the procedure. Box 7.1 lists

---

- Patient's own washing bowl
- Soap or liquid skin cleanser
- Disposable flannels
- Towels
- Comb and/or brush
- Toiletries as required
- Clean bedlinen and nightclothes
- Linen skip
- Plastic apron and disposable gloves.

Box 7.1 Preparing to bath a patient in bed: equipment required

likely equipment you will need but there may be additional items, depending on the individual person's needs, for example a clean incontinence pad, a slide sheet for moving the person.

Procedure

Listed below is a suggested procedure for bathing a person in bed, which is likely to maintain comfort and prevent the person from becoming cold. Remember that a sensitive and empathetic approach should be maintained throughout. Ensure that you have introduced yourself to the patient, and that you use the bedbath as an opportunity to build further rapport. Patients you are bathing may be pleased to engage in conversation but they may feel too weak and wish for a minimum of interaction, so be sensitive to non-verbal cues. For a child use play, and try to make this a fun activity.

- Wash your hands and put on the plastic apron (and gloves if needed – see Chapter 3).
- Fill the bowl with comfortably warm water.
- Remove the top bedclothes, leaving the patient covered by a blanket, sheet or towel.
- Remove the pyjama jacket or nightdress. If the patient has a weak arm or has an intravenous infusion attached (as has Bill) remove this arm from the clothing last.

Activity

Practise with a friend or colleague, removing a jacket or cardigan from each other, while pretending that one arm's mobility is impaired. Now try replacing it, inserting the affected arm first.

- Can the patient wash his or her own face? Even quite unwell people may like to do this for themselves. Otherwise, wash the patient's face, using soap if wanted. Never poke inside ears. Rinse off soap, if used, and dry carefully. With eyes, take care to wash from the inner to outer corner of the eye (thus reducing risk of contamination). Always approach any care relating to eyes with gentleness and cleanliness to avoid risk of trauma or cross-infection.

Activity

With a friend or colleague, practise washing and drying each other's face. How did it feel?

Note that people who are unconscious or semi-conscious are at risk of corneal damage and eye infections, as the normal protective mechanisms of the eyes (e.g. adequate lid closure, blink reflex) are impaired. Such people therefore require eye care in order to maintain healthy eyes and prevent future problems. A systematic review of eye care for intensive care patients recommended that ointments and drops are more effective than no eye instillations for reducing corneal abrasions but further research into eye care is urgently needed (JBIEBNM 2002). A flowchart to assess the type and frequency of eye care

- Assessment should include checking whether the eyelids are clean, whether the corneas are dry (i.e. dull, no sparkle from reflected light), whether there is any sign of infection (e.g. redness, discharge), and whether the eyes are closed.
- If eyelids are not clean, wash your hands, and cleanse the eyelids with gauze, moistened with sterile water.
- Instillation of hypromellose eyedrops will prevent the corneas drying out. Lucri-Lube can be prescribed for persistently dry corneas and for open eyes.
- Assessment of eyes and instillation of hypromellose eyedrops should occur at least every 6 hours, but more frequently if corneas are dry.

Box 7.2 Eye care for unconscious or semi-conscious patients, key points (based on Laight 1995, 1996, and further personal communication)

required by unconscious or semi-conscious patients can be found in Laight (1995). Key points relating to eye care can be found in Box 7.2.

- Place a towel under the arm furthest away from you, and wash from the hand to the axilla. Rinse off the soap and dry thoroughly, taking care not to dislodge any cannulae or dressings. Repeat with the other arm.
- Uncover the chest and abdomen and wash and dry this area in the same way, again taking care not to dislodge dressings or attachments. Work gently but quickly to prevent the patient from becoming chilled. Pay special attention to skin folds and under the breasts, as these areas may be moist through sweat and therefore heavily colonised with micro-organisms. A little talcum powder may be applied if liked; shake it into your hand rather than directly onto the patient, as the fine powder can be irritating if inhaled. Cover the chest and abdomen once this is completed. Other toiletries such as antiperspirant or body spray can be applied as wished by the patient.
- Change the water at this point, or at any time if it feels cool or becomes excessively soiled. If water is not changed and the same wash cloth is used for the whole body the water can become full of bacteria and be a potential hazard to patients with breaks in their skin (Ayliffe *et al.* 2001).
- Now remove any lower body clothing (including thrombo-embolic deterrent (TED) stockings), cover the leg nearest you, and place the towel under the opposite leg. Wash the leg from toes to groin, rinse and dry. Apply moisturising lotion if the skin appears dry over the shins or feet. Repeat with the other leg.

Activity | What observations should you be making while washing arms, body and legs?

Your observations should include condition of the skin, checking for dryness, colour, bruises, abrasions, rashes, swelling or oedema. Christmas (2002) advises that people of African-Caribbean origin are particularly prone to skin dryness and skin needs moisturising once or twice a day. Nurses should apply skin moisturisers for any patients as needed. You should also note any tenderness in the limbs, particularly in the calves, which might indicate a deep vein thrombosis (see Chapter 5 'Caring for people with impaired mobility').

■ Note that for some people attention to foot care is particularly important. Those at risk of foot problems include older people and people with diabetes, peripheral vascular disease or peripheral neuropathy (Thompson 1999). Foot problems in people with diabetes are discussed in detail by a number of authors (e.g. Edwards 1998; Foster 1999; Renwick *et al.* 1998; Young 1997), and are also referred to in Chapter 6 'Principles of wound care'. A systematic review indicated that patient education about foot care may reduce foot ulceration and amputations especially in high-risk patients (Valk *et al.* 2003). When people are unable to self-care, nurses must carry out the foot care and observation required, and report any concerns immediately. In some circumstances, nurses can use this opportunity to educate people about foot care. Box 7.3 outlines the key principles.

■ Using a disposable washcloth, wash the genitals and perineal area, working from front to back to prevent contamination of the urethra and/or vagina with faecal matter. Catheter care may be required at this point (see Chapter 8, section on 'Caring for people who have urinary catheters'). Change the water now, and remember the rationale for this (see previous section, Learning outcome 2).

Activity

Recall your thoughts on Learning outcome 1, and how you could maintain dignity during this intimate care. What might be the specific needs of Bill and Laura in the scenarios?

You might have considered that most people, if at all able, would probably prefer to attend to this care themselves, but some people are too physically or mentally impaired to do so. Although Bill is weak, he might be able to do this for himself with facilitation. Laura would need sensitive and gentle assistance because of the painful lesions in this area.

■ At this point, you need to assess how you can wash the patient's back. There are two possibilities: either sitting the person forward or lying them on their side. Sitting Bill forward to wash his back would be best as he might become breathless if lying on his side for long, You can ask/assist him to lean forward, wash, rinse and dry his back, using a clean washcloth. The pillowcases can be changed, and he can be assisted into a clean pyjama jacket. For a woman, a clean nightdress can be put on at this point.

- Wash feet daily, drying them carefully and thoroughly, particularly between the toes.
- Examine feet daily for problems (colour change, swelling, breaks in skin, pain or numbness), and if they occur, report them to a health care professional. People with a foot care emergency (new ulceration, swelling, discoloration) should be seen by a multidisciplinary foot care team within 24 hours). Check the top of the foot, the sole of the foot (patients can be taught to use a mirror to do this), between the toes, and pressure areas, i.e. tips of toes and heels.
- Nail care: check for signs of redness around nail areas and ensure nails do not cut into adjacent toes. Cut immediately after bathing when nails are soft, following the shape of the toe and not down into tissue. If nails are thick and brittle, do not attempt to cut. Refer to podiatrist.
- Make sure that shoes and hosiery fit well.
- Ensure that feet are assessed at least annually by trained personnel.

In addition, people at increased or high risk of foot ulcers (neuropathy, and/or absent pulses or other risk factor) should:

- Have feet reviewed by a foot protection team 3–6 monthly.
- Never walk barefoot.
- Realise that any break in the skin is potentially serious.
- Check bath temperatures carefully (numb feet cannot assess temperature).
- Avoid hot water bottles, electric blankets, foot spas and sitting with feet too close to fires.
- Get help to deal with calluses and corns (avoid over-the-counter remedies).
- Regularly inspect footwear for rough areas, ripped linings, etc.

Box 7.3 Advice about foot care for people with diabetes (adapted from NICE 2004)

■ To wash a person's back if they cannot sit forward, and to wash people's buttocks, you need to turn them on their side and you may require assistance to do this. The bottom sheet can be changed at this time. A slide sheet could be inserted to assist with turning and then moving the patient up the bed on completion of the wash. If you feel assistance is not required, you need to raise a bed side on the opposite side to provide security for the patient when rolling onto their side. Assist the patient to roll over, using the log roll method. Roll up the soiled bottom sheet lengthways, close to the patient. Place a towel along the patient's back, wash, rinse and dry the back and buttocks, noting any skin problems as previously outlined.

■ Activity — Which areas of skin do you think you should pay most attention to while the patient is on their side?

It is important to pay particular attention to the areas most at risk from pressure damage. These include the sacrum, trochanters, elbows and shoulder tips, base of the skull and heels. See Chapter 5 section on 'Pressure ulcer risk assessment' for more details; Box 5.1 outlines how to inspect skin for signs of early pressure damage.

- Now assist with putting on pyjama trousers or adjusting a nightdress. Some people prefer to wear underwear in bed so ensure you help them with putting this on if required. Replace the TED stockings if worn and change the bottom sheet. To do this, roll or concertina fold a clean sheet close to the patient, taking care not to contaminate the clean sheet with the soiled one. Assist the patient to roll back towards you, and support them while your assistant removes the soiled sheet, pulls though the clean one and secures it.

Activity | What might be the infection control issues when disposing of the soiled sheet?

Look back to the principles outlined in Chapter 3 'Preventing cross-infection'. Note that Health Service Guidelines have established a national colour-coding standard for disposal of linen (NHS Management Executive 1995). Used linen (soiled and foul) should be disposed of in white or off-white bags. Infected linen should be placed into a water-soluble bag and then into a red bag.

Activity | You will need two friends/colleagues for this exercise, and access to a bed in the skills laboratory. Practise changing the bottom sheet, taking it in turns to be the 'patient'. Consider whether you felt vulnerable during this. What reassured you?

Finally:

- Using safe moving and handling methods assist the patient into an appropriate and comfortable position, as determined by their condition and care plan.
- Brush or comb the patient's hair into their preferred style. Any other hair care needed at this stage should also be carried out – check with patients their personal requirements and what assistance they need. For example, Christmas (2002) advises that the special hair type of people of African-Caribbean origin needs moisturising every other day or more often if needed.
- Assist with make-up if required by the patient, and with oral hygiene (see later section).
- Place the locker and call bell within reach.
- Wash and dry the bowl, and dispose of soiled equipment appropriately (see Chapter 3 section on 'Waste disposal'). Note that wash bowls should be stored upside down to reduce colonisation by microorganisms, which prefer horizontal surfaces. Also, if wash bowls are not dried properly and

are stacked together bacteria multiply in the moisture trapped between the bowls; contaminated wash bowls have been implicated in infection outbreaks, Gram-negative bacteria being most likely to be found (Ayliffe *et al.* 2001).

■ Document any observations made, and the care given, in the care plan or nursing notes.

Summary

■ It is important to assess the suitability of a bed bath for the individual patient, and negotiate involvement by the patient and family, as desired.

■ Respect for the individual's privacy and dignity, and maintenance of comfort, should be promoted.

■ Adherence to infection control procedures and safe moving and handling techniques is vital.

WASHING A PERSON'S HAIR IN BED

LEARNING OUTCOMES

By the end of this section you will be able to:

1. State the circumstances under which hair washing in bed may be carried out.
2. Describe the procedure for hair washing, considering infection control, and patient comfort and safety needs.

Learning outcome 1: State the circumstances under which hair washing in bed may be carried out

Many people will not be confined to bed for long enough for hair washing to become a problem, and will be able to visit the bathroom where hair washing will be more easily accomplished. In the short term, a dry shampoo can be brushed through the hair, to absorb grease, sebum and remove dead skin cells. However, if patients remain in bed for long periods of time, their hair will become in need of washing. This could be necessary for Bill who, as his disease becomes more advanced, might need to have his hair washed in bed. Some hospitals have a hairdresser who will visit the ward and wash patients' hair in bed. Find out if this facility is available in your area.

Activity   You may have been introduced to the Roper–Logan–Tierney model of nursing (Roper *et al.* 2000). Which activity of living is hair washing associated with?

Hair washing is associated with the 'Personal cleansing and dressing' and 'Expressing sexuality' activities of living. In many cultures, hair and hairstyles play a large part in defining and advertising sexual identity. Hair can be an important part of a person's body image, and its condition may improve or lower self-esteem. These issues are considered in Chapter 2.

Learning outcome 2: Describe the procedure for hair washing, considering infection control, and patient comfort and safety needs

As with bathing in bed, try to think ahead about what you will need. Box 7.4 suggests suitable equipment.

Positioning

First remove the head of the bed, and assist the patient to lie flat.

Activity

Consider patient safety and comfort. Which patients might not be able to lie in this way?

This might not be possible for a number of people, including Bill who is breathless. Other people include those with arthritis of the neck, or patients on skull traction. It is therefore very important before commencing hair washing to assess the individual. If the patient cannot lie down, hair can be washed over a bowl on a bed table.

Procedure

- Place the empty bowl on a chair or bed table at the head of the bed, at a lower level. Consider your own comfort at this point; is the bed at a comfortable height for you to work without stooping?
- Arrange the plastic sheet to protect the mattress, and a towel to protect the patient's shoulders.
- Move the patient, using a slide sheet, so that their head is over the bowl. An assistant may be required to support the patient's head.

- Plastic bowl, shampoo guard
- Plastic sheeting
- Large jug or bowl of hand hot water
- Empty bowl
- Small jug
- Shampoo and conditioner, as requested by the patient
- Towels
- Flannel
- Brush/comb and hairdryer
- Plastic apron.

Box 7.4 Preparing to wash hair in bed: equipment required

- Having checked the temperature of the water, wet the hair using the small jug. The patient may like to protect their eyes with a clean flannel.
- Apply shampoo, massage gently into the scalp, and rinse off. Repeat this if desired. Apply conditioner, if used, comb through, leave for a minute or two, and rinse off until the hair feels clean. You may have to empty the bowl at intervals, before it gets too full.
- Be aware of health and safety issues – mop up any spills immediately.
- Wrap the patient's hair in a clean towel and empty the bowl.
- Slide the patient back onto the bed, and remove the plastic sheet. Make sure the bottom sheet is not damp; replace if necessary.
- Replace the head of the bed, and assist the patient to sit up if able, using a safe moving and handling technique.
- Towel the hair dry, and style the hair as desired, using a hairdryer if necessary.

Activity What health and safety issues should be considered when using hairdryers?

It is important to make sure that:

- The hairdryer is not too hot
- There are no trailing flexes
- The equipment is checked regularly by electricians
- The electric hairdryer and water are not in contact.

Finally, you will need to wash and dry the bowls and jug, and dispose of all equipment in accordance with hospital policy. Leave the patient comfortable, with bed table, locker and call bell within reach. Document the care given in the care plan or nursing notes.

Summary

- If hair washing in bed is required, carefully assess the patient's suitability first.
- Be aware of individual preferences in hair care.
- Maintain health and safety for both yourself and patients.

BATHING AND SHOWERING IN THE BATHROOM

If people are able to visit the bathroom to meet their personal hygiene needs, this is usually preferable for a number of reasons. For some people, actually going in the bath or shower may not be possible or desirable, but they may be able to at least sit and wash at the sink, which is usually preferable to washing in, or by, the bed.

LEARNING OUTCOMES

On completion of this section you will be able to:

1. State the particular benefits and possible problems of meeting hygiene needs in the bathroom rather than at the bedside.
2. Describe the procedure for assisting with bathing/showering in the bathroom, discussing health and safety issues.

Learning outcome 1: State the particular benefits and possible problems of meeting hygiene needs in the bathroom rather than at the bedside

Activity

Which of the people in this chapter's scenarios may be able to visit the bathroom to meet their hygiene needs?

All should be able to at some stage, but as previously mentioned, Bill may be too weak, tired or in pain to do so at present, and Laura will be unable to leave her cubicle while she is infectious. Miss Smith will be able to visit the bathroom but will require mobility aids in order to do so. Ellen will carry out her hygiene care in her own bathroom but it will be necessary to revisit her knowledge and skills and reinforce the importance of good hygiene and a bathing routine. Underlying causes of her incontinence must be investigated (see Chapter 8) and the nurse can support Ellen in accessing the necessary services (e.g. continence advisor). The aim should be for Ellen to regain continence and her ability to maintain her hygiene, and her **Health Action Plan** will need to be amended to address these issues. The nurse will need to be sensitive in broaching the subject with Ellen but it is important to address this so that this short-term problem does not impact on her social integration and relationships in the longer term. It may be necessary for a carer to visit in the mornings and evenings, to help Ellen structure her day and ensure that her hygiene needs are being met.

Ellen will probably not require physical assistance in the bathroom, but prompting, encouragement and praise for success in meeting the assessed and agreed plan for meeting her hygiene needs. As she re-establishes her skills the caring input can reduce until Ellen is self-caring once more.

The presence of a wound is not a contraindication to a shower or bath, as long as the skin edges of the wound are sealed (Briggs 1997). However a shower is preferable to a bath for a person with a wound as there is less risk of cross-infection from a previous user (Gilchrist 1990). Children in particular might prefer to slowly and gently soak off dressings in warm water in the bath or shower, reducing distress and causing less damage to the epithelium (Bale 1996).

Health Action Plan
A personal action plan developed for each individual with a learning disability, containing details of their health interventions, medication taken, screening tests etc. See *Valuing People* (Department of Health 2001c).

Activity

Why might it be preferable for hygiene needs to be met in the bathroom, rather than at the bedside, if at all possible?

You might have considered these points:

- Familiarity: The bathroom is a more familiar environment in which to attend to hygiene, and this is important for someone who is confused, or who is preparing for discharge home. Ellen's teaching programme to meet her hygiene needs will certainly be more effective if carried out in the familiar surroundings of her own bathroom. The bathroom is the most appropriate environment for Miss Smith for whom nurses will be trying to re-establish a routine of carrying out hygiene care.
- Privacy can be more easily maintained in a bathroom than behind curtains at the bedside.
- There is a continuous supply of water and this may be desirable for cultural reasons. Within some religions, for example Hinduism, washing in running water, as in a shower or by pouring water from a jug, is very important (Holland and Hogg 2001). This is easier to achieve in the bathroom.
- For older people, going into a bath is a familiar activity, and some people, for example those with muscle spasm, find a bath relaxing and therapeutic, particularly when used with bath water additives (Tarling 1997).
- For small children, bathtime is usually enjoyable and fun.

As discussed above, there are good reasons why people may be better able to meet their hygiene needs in the bathroom. However, you may be able to think of some possible problems.

| ■ *Activity* | List possible problems with bathing in the bathroom. |

- Patients can become chilled if a suitable temperature cannot be maintained and it can be exhausting for people with few reserves of strength, like Bill. There are also a number of health and safety issues which could cause problems and these are discussed later.
- Bathrooms may cause problems for people whose conditions are unstable – physically and mentally – as unless a nurse stays with them observation is more difficult in bathrooms than when they are behind curtains in the ward.
- Brawley (2002) points out that for a person with dementia who has possible visual and hearing impairment a bathroom can be a noisy and disorientating place, causing fear and confusion.

People with impaired mobility, like Miss Smith, have special moving and handling requirements and need suitable equipment to enable them to access baths or showers. Sound moving and handling practices must be maintained by nurses within the bathroom to prevent injury to patients and nurses. These are discussed in detail by Tarling (1997), and occupational therapists can advise.

There are shower trolleys available, which can be useful for some individuals, for example those with spinal injuries, and other neurological conditions such as cerebral palsy. There is a wide range of other equipment available to assist with bathing and showering; an overview is given by Collins (2001).

Learning outcome 2: Describe the procedure for assisting with bathing/showering in the bathroom, discussing health and safety issues

As with washing a person in bed, it is important to introduce yourself, and build a rapport prior to assisting with personal care. As you read, Miss Smith was initially very resistant to going to the bathroom to be assisted with hygiene but as a relationship with the staff was established, she became more accepting of their help. Nurses need to be patient and understanding in such situations. Assisting with hygiene in the bathroom provides a good opportunity to further the nurse–patient/client relationship, as it involves one-to-one interaction in a private environment.

As discussed previously, parents will usually wish to carry on with bathing their child but may need assistance and support if the child has a physical impairment. The carers of some adults might also wish to continue to be involved in bathing. A person with dementia, for example, may be more comfortable if their usual carer assists. This involvement in care should be negotiated by nurses and not taken for granted, as some informal carers may be exhausted and, as noted previously, might appreciate a break. Involving relatives in bathing can sometimes be important in preparation for discharge, particularly where a person has a new disability. Nurses can take the opportunity to teach relatives about use of equipment and skin observation and care for example.

Equipment

As always, it is important to plan ahead, and gather all equipment likely to be needed. Having to leave the bathroom to fetch items when the person is undressed could lead to chilling and exposure. If a person is unsafe to leave the nurse would have to ring the call bell and wait for help to arrive in such circumstances. As with bathing a person in bed, the toiletries required vary between individuals, so always ask about preferences. With some people this may be indicated through non-verbal rather than verbal communication. You are likely to need towels, soap/shower gel or other cleansing agent, shampoo/conditioner (if hair washing is to be carried out), clean clothing (of the person's choice), brush/comb, toothbrush and toothpaste, and flannel/disposable washcloths.

Some people are prescribed specific skin care agents for use in the bath or afterwards. For children, a selection of bath toys should be available, and for babies, a baby bath should be used.

Preparing the bathroom

After assembling the equipment, check that the bathroom is free, and has been cleaned after any previous user.

Activity | Why is it necessary to check the bathroom prior to taking your patients/clients there?

Apart from any physical soiling, you need to consider potential risk of cross-infection. Always adhere to the relevant infection control policy for your practice setting regarding cleaning of baths/showers between people. You should also check that the floor is not wet or slippery, and that any extra equipment, such as a hoist or shower stool, is in place and in safe working order. Also check the temperature of the bathroom, as some people, particularly if underweight like Bill, are susceptible to the cold, as are very young children and older people like Miss Smith. Warm the bathroom first if necessary.

Bathing or showering procedure

The following steps provide a suggested procedure that will maintain comfort and safety. As with bedbathing, assisting with hygiene in the bathroom requires nurses to be sensitive and respectful.

- If bathing, fill the bath with warm water, using your elbow or a bath thermometer to check the temperature.
- Assist the person to the bathroom, offering them the opportunity to use the toilet first if necessary.
- Consideration should be given to people who have sensory impairment. People with visual impairment can find bathrooms particularly difficult due to the often white walls and white bathroom suite, making it difficult to locate the sink or bath. Therefore always take time to orientate them to the environment, showing them where everything is.
- Assist with undressing, maintaining dignity and comfort and avoiding unnecessary exposure by using towels.
- If the person has a urinary catheter *in situ*, a shower is preferable. However, if a bath is used, then the catheter should be clamped if the catheter has to be lifted above bladder level (e.g. when assisting the person in and out of the bath), to prevent reflux of urine back into the bladder (Getliffe 2003).
- If bathing, check the bath water temperature again, and allow the patient to check for themselves if they are able. Remember that some people have impaired sensation in their feet and will not be able to feel the temperature accurately.
- Using suitable equipment, if necessary, help the person into the bath, or onto the shower chair. If the shower is being used, check the temperature before use.

■ You should aim to promote independence by supporting/enabling people to wash themselves as far as possible. Every encouragement should be given to Miss Smith with the aim of rebuilding her confidence in meeting her hygiene needs. Ellen will need gentle prompting without being patronising.

■ As with bathing in bed, particular attention should be given to skin creases, and areas susceptible to becoming sore for example under breasts, palms of hands which are fixed in tonic flexion. Note also, as in the earlier section 'Bathing a person in bed', the importance of foot care for some people, in particular those with diabetes. Check Box 7.3, to remind yourself of the essential observations and care. Miss Smith's feet could be in very poor condition as with her poor mobility she might not have been able to reach them for some time. She may well need to be referred to a podiatrist.

■ You should only leave a person alone in the bath or shower if you have assessed that it is safe to do so. For example, people who have epilepsy should not be left alone and neither should children, or people who are confused. Always check with the registered nurse, if unsure. If it has been assessed as safe to leave a person, ensure that the call bell is within reach, and working, before leaving.

■ Remember, as discussed earlier, skin condition can be specifically observed, as well as psychological and physical condition, for example any pain or breathlessness on movement, level of motivation to assist. These will all be important observations when assisting Miss Smith.

■ If hair washing is required, as for Miss Smith, use clean water in a washbasin or bowl, and a jug, or shower attachment. Wet the hair, allowing the person to protect their eyes with a flannel. Apply shampoo, and massage gently into the scalp. Rinse and repeat, if necessary, and apply conditioner, as needed. Rinse again, and dry with a clean towel.

■ Before assisting the person out of the bath, it may be easier to let some water out, and dry the upper body. This minimises the time for the person to become chilled. Assist the person out of the bath or shower, using equipment as necessary, and give what assistance is needed to dry, again thinking about maintaining comfort and dignity by avoiding unnecessary exposure. Talcum powder and other toiletries can be applied if liked at this point. Can you recall the safety points about applying talcum powder which were discussed in the section on bathing in bed?

■ Assist the person to dress in clean clothes, to clean teeth (see oral hygiene section), and to brush/style hair as desired. Once again, assess the person's ability to participate in these activities. Both Miss Smith and Ellen may need verbal encouragement and reinforcement.

■ Dispose of used equipment in accordance with waste disposal policy, and leave the bathroom clean and ready for the next user.

■ Document the care given in the care plan or nursing notes.

Summary

- Meeting hygiene needs in the bathroom is preferable for many reasons, for example privacy, availability of running water.
- When assisting with hygiene in the bathroom, always assemble all equipment beforehand, to avoid leaving people alone.
- The bathroom is potentially hazardous; it is important to take active steps to avoid accidents, such as falls or scalding, and only leave people alone if you have assessed that it is safe to do so.
- Maintain privacy and dignity throughout, and promote independence.

FACIAL SHAVING

LEARNING OUTCOMES

On completion of this section you will be able to:

1. Discuss the rationale for shaving male patients/clients who are unable to do this for themselves.
2. List the equipment needed and describe the procedure for shaving.

Learning outcome 1: Discuss the rationale for shaving male patients/clients who are unable to do this for themselves

Facial hair has important social and cultural meanings. In some religions, for example Sikhs, neither facial or hair on the head may be cut. In many Western European cultures, a wide variety of facial hair is socially acceptable, and plays a part in maintaining self-esteem. While facial shaving is usually associated with men, some females (particularly older women) have unwanted facial hair which they prefer to remove. This is important to their body image. If a female patient requests assistance with shaving, always approach this sensitively and matter-of-factly.

Activity

Talk to a male relative or friend who is usually clean shaven. Ask him how he would feel if unable to shave himself.

For many men being clean shaven is important, and being unable to self-care in this way would be distressing. In addition people visiting relatives can be upset to find them unshaven if they are usually clean shaven, and would view such a lack of care as neglectful, leading to a loss of confidence in staff. There are some people for whom shaving may be hazardous. For example, individuals receiving anti-coagulant medication can be at risk of bleeding from minor cuts which could occur. Using an electric razor rather than carrying out a wet shave is safer in such circumstances.

Learning outcome 2: List the equipment needed and describe the procedure for shaving

Equipment

You will need:

- Either a razor, with shaving soap/foam and shaving brush, or the person's own electric razor (communal razors pose a high risk of cross-infection).
- Towel and flannel/disposable washcloth.
- Bowl of hand hot water.
- Aftershave as desired by the client.

The procedure

Assemble the equipment, and assist the person to sit up if possible. Protect the person's chest with a towel. Assess to what extent the person can assist. For some men, careful positioning, provision of a shaving mirror and having all equipment to hand may enable them to be independent with shaving. Note that shaving does require very fine motor control. It is important to always assess the person's capability; consulting the individual's care plan should clarify this, and any particular precautions that need to be taken.

Wet shaving

- Wet the brush and apply the soap to the face, or use the foam, working up a good lather.
- Work in the direction of the hair growth, starting with the cheeks, and moving on to the neck and around the mouth.
- Hold the skin taut and avoid any sores or moles. The person may be able to help by tightening his facial muscles. However this would not be possible for all men, for example if facial weakness is present.
- For some men the facial skin can be hypersensitive, and therefore great care should be taken.
- Rinse the razor after each stroke.
- When you have finished, rinse the face with clean water and dry, apply aftershave if used. Dispose of used equipment safely.

Dry shaving

- The skin should be clean and dry – a little talcum powder may help. Work with circular strokes, keeping the skin taut as for wet shaving.
- Assist the person to rinse his face when finished, apply aftershave if desired, and clean the razor ready for the next occasion.

Document your care in the care plan or nursing notes.

■ Activity   Find a willing male friend, relative or colleague and practise both a wet shave and a dry shave. Even if you shave yourself, you may find this more difficult than you expect. Ask your 'patient' to comment on your technique.

Summary

■ Facial shaving is important to many people. Nurses should assist if people are unable to self-care, thus maintaining self-esteem.

■ A gentle and careful technique should be used, using the person's preferred equipment.

ORAL HYGIENE

Maintaining oral hygiene is an important aspect of nursing care, as it can do much to enhance quality of life and promote health. Jones (1998) advocates that nurses should include mouth care as part of daily hygiene for people who are debilitated, but should also be promoting effective oral hygiene in people who are capable of self-care.

LEARNING OUTCOMES

By the end of this section you will be able to:

1. Discuss the rationale for the maintenance of good oral hygiene.
2. Identify factors that increase vulnerability to poor oral hygiene, and consider how those at risk can be identified.
3. Understand how oral hygiene can be carried out safely and based on best evidence.

Learning outcome 1: Discuss the rationale for the maintenance of good oral hygiene

Oral hygiene aims to maintain a healthy oral mucosa, teeth, gums and lips, by the use of toothpaste, brush or other cleansing agents. Good oral hygiene is an important part of personal hygiene care (Somerville 1999), and a dry mouth has been identified as a symptom causing people considerable distress (Kaye 1992).

■ Activity   What problems may arise if oral hygiene is poor, as in Miss Smith's case?

You may have considered:

■ Mouth and gum infections such as candidiasis (thrush), which is a fungal infection (Torrance 1990).
■ Poor appetite and therefore malnutrition (Peate 1993).
■ Halitosis leading to social withdrawal.

■ Systemic spread of infection in immunocompromised patients (Corbett 1997).

■ Loss of self-esteem and poor body image (Somerville 1999).

Learning outcome 2: Identify factors that increase vulnerability to poor oral hygiene, and consider how those at risk can be identified

Activity

You already know that Miss Smith's oral hygiene is poor. What might be the reasons for this? Now consider the other people in this chapter's scenarios – do you think any of them are at risk of poor oral hygiene too?

Miss Smith's poor mobility has affected her ability to carry out her usual hygiene care as she cannot get to the bathroom. Although she could clean her teeth at the kitchen sink she might not have been able to adapt her routine in this way, perhaps because of a mental health condition. She may not have been able to access a dentist or buy the necessary equipment to carry out oral hygiene. Her poor oral hygiene might have led to poor oral intake of food and fluids, thus worsening her mouth condition.

Bill and Laura are both at risk of oral hygiene problems. Bill has an ill-fitting denture, he can drink only small amounts and he is generally debilitated. Oral *Candida* infections are common in people who are debilitated (Ayliffe *et al.* 2001). Laura is lethargic and reluctant to eat or drink.

Ellen may be maintaining good oral hygiene but the community nurse for learning disabilities could take this opportunity to check that she is coping with her oral hygiene. Some people with learning disabilities can have oral hyper-sensitivity, making it uncomfortable to clean their teeth. The Department of Health (2001c), in *Valuing People*, acknowledges that people with learning disabilities often have poor oral health leading to chronic dental problems. Davies *et al.* (2000) identify a number of reasons for this, including fear of dental treatment (particularly where there is difficulty understanding the need for treatment), the need to be accompanied, difficult access to health care facilities and negative professional attitudes. It is part of the **health facilitator**'s role to provide support in overcoming these barriers and regular visits to the dentist must be included in Ellen's Health Action Plan. Tooth decay would adversely affect her quality of life, leading to pain, the need for dental treatment and poor food intake.

There are many factors that can lead to poor oral hygiene (Table 7.1). Looking at this table might prompt you to identify further risk factors for the people in the scenarios. For example Laura could be receiving anti-histamines to reduce her itchiness which will increase her mouth dryness, and drowsiness. Thurgood (1994) notes that most seriously ill people have mouth problems, which cause them further discomfort and distress.

People's ability to self-care for oral hygiene can change quickly so nurses need to regularly reassess both this and other risk factors. *The Essence of Care* (2001a) emphasises the importance of assessing individuals in relation to how their oral hygiene can be maintained with its best practice benchmark: 'All

Health facilitator

A member of the community learning disabilities team (often a nurse) who supports a person with learning disabilities to access the health care they need. See *Valuing People* (Department of Health 2001c).

Table 7.1 Factors predisposing to mouth problems (adapted from Thurgood 1994)

Drugs	Cytotoxic drugs (reduce autoimmune response) Corticosteroids (affect tissue healing) Antibiotics (alters oral bacterial balance, allowing infection by *Candida albicans*) Antihistamines, antispasmodics, anticholinergics, psychotropics, antidepressants and tranquillisers (reduce salivary production) Diuretics (increase fluid loss) Morphine (causes mouth dryness)
Treatments	Radiotherapy of head/neck (causes localized inflammation, affects ability to eat/drink normally) Oxygen therapy, particularly if given unhumidified at high flow rates (dries oral mucosa) Suction (can damage oral mucosa) Restricted oral intake, e.g. nil by mouth pre- or post-operatively (potential for dehydration and dry mouth)
Mental or physical health problems or disability	Diseases: diabetes, thyroid dysfunction, oral disease/trauma, cerebrovascular disease Mental health problems: confusion, depression Terminal illness Acute/chronic breathing problems Unconsciousness Lack of manual dexterity

patients/clients are assessed to identify the advice and/or care required to maintain and promote their individual oral hygiene' (p. 52). Further benchmarks of best practice advise that the care planned and the level of assistance provided should be based on this assessment and individual needs.

Assessment tools can be helpful for assessing the need for and frequency of mouth care. Several of these have been published (Dickinson *et al.* 2001; Freer 2000; Lockwood 2000; Regnard and Fitton 1989), and they incorporate scoring systems, indicating levels of risk. Factors commonly included in these assessment tools are current mouth condition, nutritional status and special risk factors, like those in Table 7.1 (e.g. certain medication, oxygen therapy). Table 7.2 gives an example of an oral assessment tool. The higher the score, the greater the risk of the person assessed developing oral problems, indicating the need for mouth care to be planned. Note that Bowsher *et al.*'s (1999) systematic review suggests that as yet, there is insufficient evidence to support oral assessment procedures, or how frequently mouth care should be carried out.

Learning outcome 3: Understand how oral hygiene can be carried out safely and based on best evidence

Bowsher *et al.*'s (1999) systematic review indicates that oral care is not always evidence based. For example, there is clear evidence against the use of hydrogen

Table 7.2 Oral risk indicator tool (University Hospitals of Leicester 2000) (cited in Beretta 2003)

Mental status		Food/fluid intake		Teeth/dentures/jaw	
Alert	0	Good	0	Clean and free from debris	0
Apathetic	1	Inadequate diet	1	Debris present	1
Sedated	2	Fluids only	2	Denture present top/ bottom (delete)	2
Unco-operative	3	No intake	3	Limited jaw mobility	3
Lips		**Tongue**		**Saliva**	
Smooth and moist	0	Pink and moist	0	Present and watery	0
Dry and cracked	1	Coated	1	Thick	1
Bleeding	2	Shiny/red	2	Insufficient/excess	2
Ulcerated	3	Blister/cracked	3	Absent	3
Mucous membranes		**Patient's age**		**Airway**	
Pink and moist	0	16–29	1	Normal	0
Red and coated	1	30–49	2	Humidified oxygen	1
White areas	2	50–69	3	Nebulized therapy	2
Ulcerated	3	70+	4	Open mouth breathing or non-humidified oxygen	3
				Et/oral intubation	4

Additional scores		Risk indicator	
High dose antibiotics	4	Score of 30+	high
Steroids	4	24–29	medium
Radiotherapy	4	Below 23	low
Diabetes	4		
Anaemia	4		
Cytotoxic drugs	4		
Immunocompromised	4		

peroxide mouthwashes, lemon and glycerin swabs, and using foam swabs for teeth cleaning, yet they can still be found used in practice. As with any other nursing practice, best available evidence should be used for oral hygiene. A variety of equipment may be needed, depending on the care identified as appropriate for the individual. Possible items are listed in Box 7.5.

Rationale for choice of equipment

A small, soft-bristled toothbrush has been identified as the most effective agent for removing plaque and debris from the mouth, teeth and tongue (Thurgood 1994). A trial comparing the ability of foam swabs and toothbrushes in removing plaque confirmed that toothbrushes perform substantially better (Pearson and Hutton 2002). Toothpaste is the most pleasant cleaning agent (Roth and

- Spatula and pen torch (to inspect the oral cavity)
- Small, soft-bristled toothbrush (for teeth cleaning)
- Foam sticks (for moistening oral mucosa)
- Mouthwash, e.g. chlorhexidine (to prevent dental plaque) or water (for teeth cleaning)
- Toothpaste
- Container for dentures, if needed
- Lip lubricant, e.g. soft paraffin, to prevent dry lips (Bowsher *et al.* 1999)
- Beaker and receiver (for mouth rinsing)
- Disposable gloves and plastic apron
- Towel, tissues, waterproof sheet.

Box 7.5 Equipment for oral care

Creason 1986). It should always be fluoridated, a low fluoride formulation being used for children (Jones 1998). Jones (1998) advises that toothpaste has a generally drying effect so it should be used sparingly. Sodium bicarbonate 1 per cent is often advocated if the mouth is filled with thick, sticky mucus, as it can break down mucin, but there remains insufficient evidence to support its use (Bowsher *et al.* 1999), and Jones (1998) warns that in a critically ill person, its application could affect electrolyte balance.

Most antiseptic mouthwashes have a very transient effect so they are of limited value (Jones 1998). However, those containing chlorhexidine gluconate, for example Corsodyl, if used for one minute, can reduce bacterial counts by up to 80 per cent (Schiott *et al.* 1970, cited by Jones 1998). This is therefore worthwhile in a very vulnerable person, for example immunocompromised, very sick or frail older people. Jones (1998) advises that for cleansing and moistening oral mucosa, pH-balanced swabsticks are preferable, but if foam swab sticks are used, they are best when coated with Corsodyl gel, as that is gentler to the delicate oral mucosa. Note that there are saliva substitutes available for people with dry mouths (Jones 1998).

Activity	Drawing on your practice experience, how could nurses approach promoting oral hygiene for each of the people in this chapter's scenarios?

Some suggestions:

- Bill may be able to carry out his own oral hygiene if equipment is placed within his reach. If possible he could sit at a sink to carry out his oral care, which will include cleaning his teeth and dentures. Due to the current poor condition of his mouth however, and if his condition worsens, he may need regular oral hygiene carried out for him in between teeth cleaning. This is discussed later.
- For Laura, her usual oral hygiene should be continued, using the sink in her cubicle. Drinking small amounts of fluid regularly will help to keep

her mouth moist. Young children under 7 years need their teeth to be cleaned by an adult (Kay 2000) to ensure that plaque is removed effectively. Thus if parents are unable to be present nurses should help with teeth cleaning.

■ As suggested earlier, for Ellen the opportunity to review her hygiene needs can be extended to check that she is managing to carry out her oral hygiene. She can be verbally encouraged and supported in carrying out her own oral hygiene in the bathroom.

■ For Miss Smith, equipment for oral hygiene will need to be provided and nurses should support her and encourage her to re-establish teeth cleaning, which can be done in the bathroom at the sink. She will need to be referred to a dentist, and this subject should be approached sensitively to gain her agreement.

Teeth cleaning should ideally be carried out after each meal but at least twice daily, especially at night. Cleaning of dentures should be carried out at least daily but ideally after meals too. Therefore if patients are unable to carry this out independently, nurses must provide the necessary equipment and assistance. Some people, who are more dependent and debilitated, require nurses to carry out oral hygiene on a regular basis by the bedside, the frequency of oral care being determined on an individual basis. This care, which may be necessary for Bill, is described below.

Oral hygiene procedure: key points

■ Position: After explaining the procedure and gaining consent, the person should be assisted into a sitting position, or, if unconscious, on their side to prevent inhalation of solutions or secretions.

■ Protect the person's chest with a towel, or the bed with the waterproof sheet. Provide a receiver for spitting into.

■ Assemble the equipment – any mouthwash solution should be freshly prepared, and renewed after 24 hours. If water is used for immuno-compromised people, it should be sterile.

■ Wash hands, and put on gloves and apron, if required. Ayliffe *et al.* (2001) recommend that gloves should be worn as some infectious agents (e.g. herpes, hepatitis B) can be present in the mouth or saliva. However oral hygiene is a hygienic procedure rather than an aseptic one; it does not breach body defences but instead enhances them (Ayliffe *et al.* 2001). Therefore gloves need not be sterile.

■ Lip crusting can be removed by gently sponging with warm water (Jones 1998). Observe for any breaks in the skin or signs of herpes simplex (cold sore), which would require treatment with acyclovir cream.

■ Remove the person's dentures, if worn. They should be brushed well to remove debris using denture paste – ordinary toothpaste is too abrasive – and rinsed well. Box 7.6 lists key points for effective denture care.

- Wash hands and wear gloves
- Remove dentures into a container and rinse to remove loose debris
- Use the person's special denture brush, scrub all surfaces, using denture paste or a little soap, to remove all debris, over a bowl of tepid water
- Rinse thoroughly
- When dentures are not being worn, store in a marked container filled with clean water
- Soaking plastic dentures 2–3 times per week in dilute hypochlorite will help to prevent oral candidiasis. Again, always rinse thoroughly before replacing in the mouth
- Dentures with a metal portion should only be soaked in dilute hypochlorite for about 20 minutes, because of the danger of corrosion.

Box 7.6 Denture care (adapted from Jones 1998)

- If the person has their own teeth, they should be brushed using the toothbrush and paste. Box 7.7 explains how teeth cleaning should be carried out. If people can clean their own teeth it is better to facilitate this.
- Gentle swabbing of the mucous membrane with foam sticks moistened with warm water or chlorhexidine mouthwash will remove debris and moisten the oral mucous membrane, helping to keep it intact (Jones 1998).
- Observe the condition of the mouth and particularly the tongue. If the tongue is coated, swab gently as above. A whitened appearance indicates a candidal infection (thrush), and this should be reported so that an antifungal infection agent can be prescribed.
- Assist the person to rinse the mouth thoroughly with the chosen mouthwash solution, or use a rinsed toothbrush to do this if they are unable. Suction can be used to remove excess fluid from the mouth if they are unconscious, or have dysphagia (swallowing difficulty), as it is essential to prevent choking or aspiration of fluid (Jones 1998). A conscious person who is nursed flat, for example after a spinal injury, can use a straw to suck fluid into the mouth to rinse and to spit through afterwards.
- Replace any dentures, top set first.
- Apply lip lubricant, if lips are dry. Use tissues to blot any excess water or lubricant.
- Leave the person comfortable, and dispose of equipment according to waste disposal policy.
- Document care given in the care plan or nursing notes.

Activity

With a friend or colleague, take turns to clean each other's teeth, using your own toothbrushes and the instructions in Box 7.7. Also, try moistening each other's mouths using foam sticks, dipped in water or mouthwash solution. How did it feel?

- Explain procedure and gain consent
- Wash hands, wear gloves and maintain privacy
- It may be best to work at the side of the person, cradling the head
- Remove any partial dentures into a bowl
- Start at the front of the mouth in the upper jaw
- Use a soft brush with a small amount of toothpaste pressed into the surface (to avoid it dislodging into the mouth and possible aspiration)
- Place the brush sideways against the teeth (see diagram below) overlaying the gum edges with bristles pointing towards the teeth roots.
- Use a side-to-side motion, moving the brush head just a fraction of an inch at a time, using light pressure to squeeze the gum tissue against the teeth
- Move around the upper teeth, replacing the brush section by section against the teeth
- Try to use the same action inside the upper jaw
- Repeat for the outer and inner surfaces of the lower jaw
- Finally, scrub the chewing surfaces of the upper and lower teeth with a forward and backward motion
- Ask the person to rinse the mouth with warm water to remove debris, paste, etc., or use foam sticks moistened with water to gently sweep away the debris and toothpaste
- Wash toothbrush well and leave it to dry in the air. Do not store in a sponge bag or container. Toothbrushes should be replaced every 6–12 weeks.

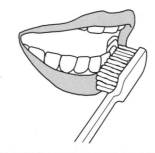

Box 7.7 Teeth cleaning (adapted from Jones 1998)

Summary

- ■ Effective oral care makes an important contribution to people's physical, psychological and social well-being.
- ■ Nurses should ensure that best evidence is used as a basis for assessing and implementing oral care.

LAST OFFICES

Last offices is the term given to the action of meeting the final hygiene needs of a deceased patient. There are a variety of points to consider when assessing the extent of the care required. The practice of preparing the body of a deceased patient for removal to the mortuary or undertaker's is the last caring act that nurses can perform for their patients, and it may be regarded as an expression of holistic care and respect. The management of people who are dying and their families is beyond the scope of this section, but recommended reading can be found at the end of the chapter.

LEARNING OUTCOMES

By the end of this section you will be able to:

1. Discuss the rationale for performing last offices.
2. Identify religious and cultural factors affecting the performance of last offices.
3. Understand the procedure for performing last offices and be prepared to carry it out safely.

Learning outcome 1: Discuss the rationale for performing last offices

Last offices are part of a long human tradition in the ritual of marking the transition between life and death (Quested and Rudge 2003). Relatives may find that viewing the body of their loved one, with a clean and cared-for appearance, helps them to accept the reality of death and aids the grieving process (Nearney 1998). It is also important that the body does not pose a risk to staff who come into contact with it. The first necessity after death has apparently occurred is for this to be confirmed, usually by a doctor, or senior nurse as locally agreed policy permits. The relatives, if not present, must also be informed as soon as possible. In cases where death is expected, relatives may be asked if they wish to be informed immediately if the death occurs at night or would prefer to wait until morning.

Places where people die

Bill is terminally ill and can be expected to die in the fairly near future, perhaps in the acute setting where he is currently cared for. However, depending on his condition following his blood transfusion, and on how he and his wife feel about him continuing to be cared for at home, he might be discharged with appropriate support. Alternatively he may be cared for in a hospice for his final days.

Activity | What difference might the care setting and the circumstances of a death make to what happens to the body after death?

If Bill dies in an acute care setting last offices will be carried out by nursing staff and his body will initially be moved to the hospital mortuary by porters, and at a later stage collected by an undertaker. However if he dies at home, care of his body after his death may be minimal prior to his body being removed by an undertaker. After death in a non-acute care setting, for example a care home or hospice, local policies impact on procedures, but again the body is likely to be removed by an undertaker. In some instances legal constraints will dictate what care may be given. For example, following an unexpected death or one that takes place within 24 hours of an operation, the Coroner's office must be informed, and a post-mortem may be required.

■ Activity   What hazards may a body present to those who handle it after death?

There may be leakage of body fluids or sharp objects such as cannulae attached to the body (see also Chapter 3 'Preventing cross-infection'). There will also be moving and handling issues. Therefore staff caring for a body after death should take appropriate measures to prevent problems arising.

Learning outcome 2: Identify religious and cultural factors affecting the performance of last offices

Regardless of the deceased person's cultural and religious background, there will be a need to maintain privacy and dignity for them and their relatives. Drawing the curtains around the bed in an open ward is the least requirement. Where possible, the body may be moved to a side room for greater privacy, and to minimise distress to other patients.

The patient's religious and cultural background must be considered at this point. Many of the world's major religions have very specific rules and rituals concerned with death, for example about who can touch the body. However, it is important not to assume that the patient or their relatives will wish these rules to be followed to the letter. As with all human activities, there are many shades of opinion and belief. Ascertaining these beliefs in advance, if possible, is part of sensitive, holistic care. Houley (2002) writes that as a student she witnessed a senior nurse placing an open bible in the hands of an older woman who had died. The woman followed the Islamic faith and her family, understandably, reacted with great distress. Such insensitivity is clearly indefensible.

■ Activity   Have you been involved in the death of a patient/client? Did the other patients/residents show awareness of what had occurred? What comments did they make? How can you respond?

In most settings other than the patient's own home there will be other patients/clients/residents around, and at least some of them will be aware of the event, and may ask, directly or indirectly, about the deceased person. It is important to answer questions sensitively and honestly, but without revealing confidential details.

■ Activity   Regarding Bill, who can be expected to die fairly soon, what would you expect his religious/cultural background to be?

From his name, you might assume that he will have a Western/Christian background, but such assumptions can be dangerous. Always ask, don't assume. And even among Christian religions there are variations, with different religious practices around the time of death.

Activity

> Do you know how to contact the local chaplain, rabbi, imam or other religious leaders, so that you can gain advice about any special requirements at the time of death and when carrying out last offices?

Nurses need to be aware of how to contact local religious leaders, as referring to, and liaising with them is an important contribution to people's spiritual support when in hospital. You may find there is a folder produced by the hospital chaplaincy with contact details and information regarding different religions. In many instances patients and their relatives, if they follow a particular religion, will have their own contacts.

Learning Outcome 3: Understand the procedure for performing last offices and be prepared to carry it out safely

Immediate care after death

In whatever setting a death takes place there are a few actions that should be carried out very soon afterwards:

- Closing the eyes, by gently applying pressure to the eyelids for about 30 seconds (Amene and Travis 2000).
- Lying the person down flat, leaving one pillow, and straightening the body and limbs into neutral positions (Nearney 1998).
- Inserting dentures, if usually worn (for example with Bill, we know he likes to wear his denture).
- Closing the mouth and supporting the jaw with a pillow, to ensure it remains closed.

This is because the body starts to become rigid soon after death, and all these actions become more difficult to perform later. In a hospital setting it is usual to leave the body for about an hour before full last offices are carried out. During this period relatives may visit and sit with the person, holding their hand if they wish. Therefore immediately after death the surrounding environment should be tidied up, equipment removed and the bedlinen attended to so that the person looks peaceful and comfortable. Houley (2002) writes that when she and her mother visited her grandmother after she had died they were horrified to find that her bloodstained nightdress had not been changed nor her teeth replaced. This upset them greatly as they felt that she would not have wanted to be seen like this. Relatives need to be given time and support and will, before they leave, need written information about what to do next (e.g. when and how to collect property, register the death, arrange the funeral).

Last offices procedure

Before commencing the procedure, you need to gather the equipment required. This will include items for washing the patient (see Box 7.1), cleaning the mouth (see Box 7.5) and for shaving a male patient if required.

■ **_Activity_**	What other items do you think might be needed in addition to those in Boxes 7.1 and 7.5?

If the patient is not to be dressed in their own nightclothes, a shroud (long white gown) might be required. Local hospital policies vary on this however; sometimes hospital nightclothes are used if patients' own are not available as some people consider shrouds, which were traditionally used, to be upsetting to relatives. The patient's property needs to be listed and packed ready for collection by the relatives, so the appropriate documentation (Property Book) will be needed. If the patient has a wound, a waterproof dressing is required. If there are tubes to be left in, spigots will be needed to plug the tubes. Additional name bands and identity labels may be needed according to the setting and local policy. A disposable receiver may also be required.

The procedure described below includes usual practice but always be guided by local policy and people's individual circumstances, and particularly religious and cultural requirements. For example in some instances a close relative of the deceased may wish to be involved, helping with washing or hair brushing for example. Note that when children die in hospital, care carried out after death may be quite different from that with an adult; you would need to be guided by experienced staff.

- Ensure privacy as previously described. Two nurses are usually required for this procedure due to the moving and handling required.
- Protect yourself against possible infection by the use of plastic apron and gloves (see Chapter 3 'Preventing cross-infection'). For patients with a communicable disease, the existing infection control measures should continue.
- Wash the patient as described in 'Bathing a person in bed', as culturally appropriate.
- Cover any wounds with waterproof dressings. Check local policy relating to removal of drains, tubes, cannulae or catheters. If a post mortem is to take place these should be left in unless advised otherwise but can be spigotted. If no post mortem is expected to be performed these tubes can usually be removed but always check if unsure.
- If leakage from any orifice seems likely to continue, insert packing, according to local policy, or an incontinence pad can be applied.
- Manually express the urinary bladder into a disposable receiver, if necessary and as per local policy.
- Place a clean sheet under the patient, using safe manual handling techniques.

- Remove and/or record the whereabouts of any jewellery as previously discussed with relatives (or patient). This should always be done in the presence of a witness. Jewellery left on the body should be secured with tape to prevent it being lost.
- Dress the patient in clean personal clothing or a shroud according to local policy and relatives' wishes.
- Shave a male patient as necessary.
- Brush hair.
- Clean the mouth and replace any dentures.
- If relatives have not yet viewed the body, this could be an appropriate point for them to do so.
- Attach identification labels to the patient according to local policy.
- Wrap the body in a clean sheet, securing it with tape.
- A body bag may be required if there are infection control issues. Consult local infection control policy or contact the infection control nurse for advice.
- Dispose of used equipment according to infection control principles and wash your hands.
- Make a list of and store property and jewellery according to local policy, in the presence of a witness.
- Arrange for the porters to collect the body, or the undertaker in a residential setting.

Activity   Find and compare the local policy on last offices with what you have read above.

As with any other clinical practices there will be a local policy, probably developed by a multidisciplinary group including the hospital chaplaincy, and which takes the local situation into account.

Summary

- Meeting the hygiene needs of a deceased patient in a safe and culturally sensitive way is an essential part of patient care.
- The extent to which last offices is carried out may vary according to the setting and will be influenced by local policy and the individual family.

CHAPTER SUMMARY

Giving personal care, with attention to the individual's dignity, privacy and personal needs, is a fundamental and essential skill for nurses, and this extends to the care of a patient's body after death. Further key principles include cultural sensitivity and prevention of cross-infection. It is important to assess carefully how hygiene needs can be met for each individual, maintaining and promoting independence where possible. People with physical and mental health problems may be able to regain self-care skills with appropriate aids, encouragement and support. Teaching people to manage personal hygiene and dressing can be an important part of rehabilitation, and should involve the multidisciplinary team, and an individualised approach.

REFERENCES

Amene, M. and Travis, S. 2000. Last offices. In Mallett, J. and Dougherty, L. (eds) *Royal Marsden Manual of Clinical Nursing Procedures*. London: Blackwell Science, 345–54.

Ayliffe, G.A.J., Babb, J.R. and Taylor, L.J. 2001. *Hospital-acquired Infection: Principles and prevention*, third edition. London: Arnold.

Bale, S. 1996. Caring for children with wounds. *Journal of Wound Care* **5**, 177–80.

Beretta, R. 2003. Assessment: the foundations of good practice. In Hinchliff, S., Norman, S. and Schoeber, J. (eds) *Nursing Practice and Health Care*. London: Arnold, 121–46.

Bowsher, J., Boyle, S. and Griffiths, J. 1999. Oral care. *Nursing Standard* **13**(37), 31.

Brawley, E.C. 2002. Bathing environments: how to improve the bathing experience. *Alzheimer's Care Quarterly* **3**, 38–41.

Briggs, M. 1997. Principles of closed wound care. *Journal of Wound Care* **6**, 288–92.

Christmas, M. 2002. Nursing with dignity Part 3: Christianity 1 *Nursing Times* **98**(11), 37–9.

Chur-Hansen, A. 2002. Preferences for female and male nurses: the role of age, gender and previous experience – year 2000 compared with 1984. *Journal of Advanced Nursing* **37**, 192–8.

Clegg, A. 2003. Older South Asian patient and carer perceptions of culturally sensitive care in a community hospital setting. *Journal of Clinical Nursing* **12**, 283–90.

Collins, F. 2001. Choosing bathing, showering and toileting equipment. *Nursing and Residential Care* **3**, 488–9.

Corbett, C.O. 1997. Mouth care and chemotherapy. *Paediatric Nursing* **9**(3), 19–21.

Coyne, I.T. 1995a. Parental participation in care: a critical review of the literature. *Journal of Advanced Nursing* **21**, 716–22.

Coyne, I.T. 1995b. Partnership in care: parents' views of participation in their hospitalized child's care. *Journal of Clinical Nursing* **4**, 71–9.

Davies, R., Bedi, R. and Scully, C. 2000. Oral health care for patients with special needs. *British Medical Journal* **321**, 495–8.

Department of Health 2001a. *The Essence of Care: Patient-focused benchmarking for health care practitioners*. London: DH.

Department of Health 2001b. *National Service Framework for Older People*. London: DH.

Department of Health 2001c. *Valuing People: A new strategy for learning disability for the 21st century*. London: DH.

Dickinson, H., Watkins, C. and Leathley, M. 2001. The development of THROAT: the holistic and reliable oral assessment tool. *Clinical Effectiveness in Nursing* **5**, 104–10.

Edwards, V. 1998. A multidisciplinary approach to foot care in diabetes. *Nurse Prescriber/Community Nurse* **4**(2), 53–5.

Foster, A. 1999. Diabetes care: getting your patients on a sure footing. *Nursing Times* **95**(37), 51–2.

Freer, S.K. 2000. Use of an oral assessment tool to improve practice. *Professional Nurse* **15**, 6357.

Getliffe, K. 2003. Catheters and catheterization. In Getliffe, K. and Dolman, M. (eds) *Promoting Continence: A clinical research resource*, second edition. London: Baillière Tindall, 259–301.

Gilchrist, B. 1990. Washing and dressing after surgery. *Nursing Times* **86**(50), Supplement, 71.

Gould, D. 1994. Helping the patient with personal hygiene. *Nursing Standard* **8**(34), 30–2.

Hancock, I., Bowman, A. and Prater, D. 2000. 'The day of the soft towel?: Comparison of the current bed-bathing method with the Soft Towel bed-bathing method. *International Journal of Nursing Practice* **6**, 207–13.

Hartley, J. 2003. Self-caring patients still want nurses to help them wash. *Nursing Times* **99**(44), 6.

Health Advisory Service 2000, 1998. 'Not because they are old': An independent inquiry into the care of older people on acute wards in general hospitals. London: Health Advisory Service 2000.

Henderson, V. 1960. *Basic Principles of Nursing Care*. Basel: S. Karger, for International Council of Nurses.

Holland, K. and Hogg, C. 2001. *Cultural Awareness in Nursing and Health Care*. London: Arnold.

Houley, C. 2002. A duty of dignity. *The Lamp* **59**(2), 22.

JBIEBNM (Joanna Briggs Institute for Evidence Based Nursing and Midwifery) 2002. Eye care for intensive care patients. *Best Practice* **6**(1), 1–6.

Jones, C.V. 1998. The importance of oral hygiene in nutritional support. *British Journal of Nursing* **74**, 76–8, 80–3.

Kawik, L. 1996. Nurses' and parents' perceptions of participation and partnership in caring for a hospitalized child. *British Journal of Nursing* **5**(7), 430–4.

Kay, J. 2000. Hygiene. In Huband, S. and Trigg, E. (eds) *Practices in Children's Nursing: Guidelines for hospital and community*. Edinburgh: Churchill Livingstone, 131–7.

Kaye, P. 1992. *A–Z of Hospice and Palliative Medicine*. Northampton: EPL Publications.

Laight, S.E. 1995. A vision for eye care: a brief study of the change process. *Intensive and Critical Care Nursing* **11**, 217–22.

Laight, S.E. 1996. The efficacy of eye care for ventilated patients: outline of an experimental comparative research pilot study. *Intensive and Critical Care Nursing* **12**, 16–26.

Lentz, J. 2003. Daily baths: torment or comfort at end of life? *Journal of Hospice and Palliative Nursing* **5**, 34–9.

Lockwood, A. 2000. Implementing an oral hygiene assessment tool on an acute ward for older people. *Nursing Older People* **12**(7), 18–19.

Nearney, L. 1998. Last offices, Part 1 (Practical Procedures for Nurses). *Nursing Times* **94**(26), 2p.

NHS Management Executive 1995. *Hospital Laundry Arrangements for Used and Infected Linen*. HSG(95)18. London: HMSO.

NICE (National Institute for Clinical Excellence) 2004. *Type 2 Diabetes: Prevention and management of foot problems*. London: NICE.

Peate, I. 1993. Nurse-administered oral hygiene in the hospitalised patient. *British Journal of Nursing* **2**, 459–62.

Pearson, L.S. and Hutton, J.L. 2002. A controlled trial to compare the ability of foam swabs and toothbrushes to remove dental plaque. *Journal of Advanced Nursing* **39**, 480–9.

Quested, B. and Rudge, T. 2003. Nursing care of dead bodies: a discursive analysis of last offices. *Journal of Advanced Nursing* **41**, 553–60.

Rader, J. 1994. To bathe or not to bathe: that is the question. *Journal of Gerontological Nursing* **20**(9), 53–4.

Rassool, G.H. 2000. The crescent and Islam: healing, nursing and the spiritual dimension. Some considerations towards an understanding of the Islamic perspectives on caring. *Journal of Advanced Nursing* **32**, 1476–84.

Regnard, C. and Fitton, S. 1989. Mouth care: a flow diagram. In Doyle, D., Hanks, G. and MacDonald, N. (eds) *Oxford Textbook of Palliative Medicine*. Oxford: Oxford University Press.

Renwick, P., Vowden, K., Wilkinson, D. and Vowden, P. 1998. The pathophysiology and treatment of diabetic foot disease. *Journal of Wound Care* **7**, 107–10.

Roper, N., Logan, W.W. and Tierney, A.J. 2000. *The Roper-Logan-Tierney Model of Nursing: based on Activities of Living*. Edinburgh: Churchill Livingstone.

Roth, P.T. and Creason, N.S. 1986. Nurse administered oral hygiene: is there a scientific basis? *Journal of Advanced Nursing* **8**, 33–4.

Simpson, C. 1998/9. Infection control. *Paediatric Nursing* **10**(10), 30–3.

Skewes, S.M. 1997. Bathing: it's a tough job! *Journal of Gerontological Nursing* **230**(5), 53–9.

Sloane, P., Rader, J., Barrick, A. *et al.* 1995. Bathing persons with dementia. *The Gerontologist* **35**, 672–8.

Somerville, R. 1999. Oral care in the intensive care setting: a case study. *Nursing in Critical Care* **4**(1), 7–13.

Tarling, C. 1997. Washing and bathing. In *The Guide to Handling of Patients: Introducing a Safer Handling Policy*, fourth edition. London: National Back Pain Association, 172–80.

Thaipisuttikul, Y. 1998. Pruritic skin diseases in the elderly. *The Journal of Dermatology* **25**, 153–7.

Thompson, J. 1999. Foot problems and care of feet: part two – common disorders. *Community Practitioner* **72**, 178–9.

Thurgood, G. 1994. Nurse maintenance of oral hygiene. *British Journal of Nursing* **3**(7), 351–3.

Torrance, C. 1990. Oral hygiene. *Surgical Nursing* **13**(4), 16–20.

Valk, G.D., Kriegsman, D.M.W. and Assendelft, W.J.J. 2003. Patient education for preventing foot ulceration. *The Cochrane Library*, Issue 2. Oxford: Update Software.

Walsh, K. and Kowanko, I. 2002. Nurses' and patients' perceptions of dignity. *International Journal of Nursing Practice* **8**, 143–51.

Whiting, L.S. 1999. Maintaining patients' personal hygiene. *Nursing Practice* **14**(5), 338–40.

Winkworth, J. 2003. Bathing is an intimate and valuable aspect of care. *Nursing Standard* **17**(21), 30.

Young, T. 1997. Diabetic foot ulceration. *Practice Nursing* **8**(9), 24–5, 27.

FURTHER READING: CARING FOR PEOPLE WHO ARE DYING

Bosanquet, N. and Salisbury, C. 1999. *Providing a Palliative Care Service. Towards an evidence base.* Oxford: University Press.

Clark, D. and Seymour, J. 1999. *Reflections on Palliative Care.* Buckingham: Open University Press.

Copp, G. 1999. *Facing Impending Death: Experiences of patients and their nurses.* London: NT Books.

Faull, C., Carter, Y. and Woof, R. 1998. *Handbook of Palliative Care.* London: Blackwell Science.

Field, D., Hockey, J. and Small, N. 1997. *Death, Gender and Ethnicity.* London: Routledge.

Goldmont, A. (ed.) 1994. *Care of the Dying Child.* Oxford: Oxford University Press.

Green, J. 1991. *Death with Dignity: Meeting the spiritual needs of patients in a multicultural society.* London: Macmillan.

Hockley, J. and Clark, D. 2002. *Palliative Care for Older People in Care Homes.* Buckingham: Open University Press.

Katz, J.S. and Peace, S. 2003. *End of Life in Care Homes. A palliative care approach.* Oxford: Oxford University Press.

Kemp, C. 1999. *Terminal Illness: A guide to nursing care*, second edition. Philadelphia: Lippincott.

Parkes, C.M., Laungani, P. and Young, B. (eds) *Death and Bereavement Across Cultures*. London. Routledge.

Sheldon, F. 1997. *Psychosocial Palliative Care*. Cheltenham: Stanley Thornes.

Thayre, K. and Peate, I. 2003. Coping with expected and unexpected death. In Hinchliff, S., Norman, S. and Schober, J. (eds) *Nursing Practice and Health Care*, fourth edition. London: Arnold, 291–314.

Young, M. and Cullen, G. 1996. *A Good Death*. London: Routledge.

Meeting elimination needs

Lesley Baillie and Vickie Arrowsmith

Elimination of urine and faeces is an essential bodily function and we usually become independent in it within the first few years of life. Elimination is then usually a private function, but when disability, or physical or mental health problems are present, independence in elimination is often affected. Assistance by nurses may then be needed so that potential problems can be avoided and actual problems can be managed. Wherever possible a return to independence in meeting elimination needs will be aimed for. Promoting dignity and privacy is integral to meeting people's elimination needs, and it requires great skill and sensitivity to carry out this care while preserving self-esteem in individuals. Many of the other chapters in this book are highly relevant to this care, particularly Chapter 2 'The nurse's approach' and Chapter 3 'Preventing cross-infection'.

This chapter includes:
- Assisting with elimination: helping people to use the toilet, bedpans, urinals and commodes
- Urinalysis
- Collecting urine and stool specimens
- Caring for people with urinary catheters
- Use of enemas and suppositories
- Promotion of continence and management of incontinence.

Recommended biology reading:
The following questions will help you to focus on the biology underpinning this chapter's skills. Use your recommended text book to consider the following:

- What are the components of the urinary system?
- Within the kidney, blood is filtered. What forces are involved in filtration?
- Where does filtration occur? Which substances are not filtered out and why?
- What is the role of the juxtaglomerular apparatus?

- What happens to the glomerular filtrate as it passes along the nephron?
- How and why does the concentration of urine vary?
- What factors affect renal function?
- Urine is stored in the bladder. How does the bladder expand as it fills up?
- What is micturition and how does it occur?
- What is cystitis? Why is it generally more common in females than in males?
- How can urinalysis be used to assess health?
- What factors can increase the risk of urinary tract infection?
- What are the signs of urinary tract infection?
- What are the different regions of the digestive tract and their functions?
- How does food move through the digestive tract?
- How are peristalsis and segmentation distinguished?
- What is the consequence of increased gut motility? When might this occur?
- What is the gastrocolic reflex?
- What do stools/faeces consist of?
- How do we defaecate?
- What is constipation?
- What factors increase the risk of constipation?
- How does the digestive tract respond to local infection or irritation?
- How does stress affect the digestive tract?

PRACTICE SCENARIOS

The following scenarios illustrate situations where assistance with elimination will be needed, and they are referred to throughout this chapter.

Adult

Multiple sclerosis

A disease characterised by progressive destruction of myelin sheaths of neurons in the central nervous system. It can cause loss of movement and sensation, and may affect elimination.

Miss June Edwards, aged 60, lives alone. She has a long history of **multiple sclerosis**, is a wheelchair user and has support from carers four times daily. In recent years she developed urinary incontinence and also had incomplete bladder emptying which led to recurrent urinary tract infections. After attempting different methods of managing this, including intermittent self-catheterisation, she now has an in-dwelling urethral catheter. Her catheter is changed every 12 weeks in line with manufacturers' recommendations and the catheter bag is emptied by her carers. She is also susceptible to constipation, which leads to the catheter bypassing. A bowel regime is established which includes evening laxatives, followed by morning suppositories and manual evacuation, three times per week. Occasionally an enema is required.

Child

James, aged 12 years, fractured his right tibia and fibula in a skateboarding accident. He has been admitted to the adolescent unit following a manipulation under anaesthetic and application of a full leg plaster cast. He has been in considerable pain both pre- and post-operatively. He is not allowed to bear weight on his right leg yet, and is confined to bed at present. His mother has stayed with him for most of the day but will be going home at night.

Learning disability

Ian is 25 years old and has a severe learning disability. He lives in a staffed group home where he is usually continent. However in unfamiliar surroundings he can become incontinent. He has been admitted to a surgical ward via Accident and Emergency (A&E) with abdominal pain, for monitoring and further investigations. A carer has accompanied him to hospital and the home is intending to supply a staff member as much as possible. However there may not be anyone able to stay overnight. Ian's **Health Action Plan** has been brought with him and the care staff have informed the community nurse for learning disability of his admission to hospital.

Health Action Plan
A personal action plan developed for each individual with a learning disability, containing details of their health interventions, medication taken, screening tests, etc. See *Valuing People* (Department of Health 2001a).

Mental health

John Avery is 58 years old. He has a long history of psychosis and during an acute psychotic episode, while admitted to an acute psychiatric ward, he was prescribed an atypical antipsychotic drug, clozapine, which is licensed for treatment of resistant schizophrenia only due to its known side effects. These include effects on white blood cell levels, thus causing vulnerability to infection. After six weeks there was a marked improvement in John's mental state but he developed urinary incontinence at night (nocturnal enuresis). He found this extremely embarrassing and distressing, never having been incontinent before. Unfortunately urinary incontinence is known to be another side effect of clozapine, the exact reasons for which are unknown. A urinalysis performed on admission had shown no abnormalities.

ASSISTING WITH ELIMINATION: HELPING PEOPLE TO USE THE TOILET, BEDPANS, URINALS AND COMMODES

LEARNING OUTCOMES

By the end of this section you will be able to:

1. Identify why a person might need help with elimination, and what equipment you could use to give assistance.
2. Discuss the important principles that you would need to consider when assisting with elimination.

Learning outcome 1: Identify why a person might need help with elimination, and what equipment you could use to give assistance

Reflect back on your practice experiences and write down all the reasons why a person might need help with elimination.

There are many situations where a person might need help with elimination, and part of the assessment of any newly admitted or referred person will be to identify any problems and whether assistance is required. An example of when help would be needed is when a person has impaired mobility. This might be someone, like James, who is temporarily confined to bed following orthopaedic surgery or someone, like June, who has a neurological disorder, for example. People who are very weak or unwell, for example bleeding severely, or confused, will also need help with elimination.

What equipment is available to assist with elimination? There may be examples of equipment in the skills laboratory or within your practice setting.

You may have listed the following:

■ **The toilet**: Whenever possible a person should be helped to reach the toilet. This is a more familiar environment in which to eliminate (particularly helpful if people are confused and/or disorientated), and it is more private. To eliminate in a ward, behind closed curtains, may not feel very private at all. Noise and smell may be obvious, and this potential embarrassment could lead to the person ignoring the need to defaecate, which can lead to constipation if the 'call to stool' is ignored repeatedly (Edwards *et al.* 2003). You might need to walk with the person, who may need to use sticks, a frame or crutches (see Chapter 5, section on 'Assisting with mobilisation and preventing falls'), and this could be part of this person's programme of mobilisation. If a patient is unable to walk, you would use the wheelchair to take them to the toilet.

■ **The commode**: If a patient is very ill or weak it may be unwise for them to leave the bedside. When making decisions about this it is important to check the care plan, and seek advice if you are unsure. If a patient is able to get out of bed, a commode is preferable to using a bedpan, as it promotes a more conducive position for elimination and will usually feel more comfortable. A commode has a pan underneath, which can be removed after use, and either macerated (if disposable) or put into the washer-disinfector if reusable. There are many types of commode available but those that are a good size, easy to manoeuvre, and have arms that are easy to remove are preferable (Ballinger *et al.* 1996). Tarling (1997) discusses types of commodes and their advantages and disadvantages, with particular reference to moving and handling issues.

■ **Bedpans/urinals/potties**: Some people, like James, may have to stay in bed for medical reasons. If a bedpan must be used, you will need to choose between a standard bedpan which the patient will need to sit up on, and a flat 'slipper' pan, which a patient can roll on to – essential when someone is unable to sit up. To pass urine there are both male and female urinals available. Male patients sometimes find passing urine sitting or lying down difficult so if assistance can be given for them to stand instead this is usually preferred. Female urinals are particularly useful for women who have to lie flat (for example following back surgery) or where change in position is difficult, due to pain for example. There are now a wide variety of female urinals available (see McIntosh 2001; Vickerman 2003). For a young child, a potty will be used. If the child is in hospital for a long time, the family may wish to bring the child's own potty in as this can decrease anxiety.

■ **Reusable equipment**: Equipment can be reusable, in which case it may be made from stainless steel or plastic. After use it needs to be put in the washer-disinfector. This first cold rinses, then hot rinses, then disinfects, which includes heating to 80°C for one minute, before being cooled. Disadvantages of this system are that it is not always effective (up to 22 per cent of bedpans need to be reprocessed) and the cycle is slow (Johnson 1989).

■ **Disposable equipment**: Disposable equipment is made from paper pulp and so the bedpans and potties need to be placed onto a plastic support. After use, the disposable equipment is put into a macerator which processes them quickly. The plastic supports should be washed with hot water and detergent. Johnson (1989) found that nurses preferred the disposable system, which was also assessed as being cheaper once capital costs were considered.

Learning outcome 2: Discuss the important principles that you would need to consider when assisting with elimination

Activity | If you are assisting someone with elimination, what do you think would be important principles of care?

Box 8.1 lists important principles which you could have identified. Adhering to these can enable this practical skill to be a therapeutic action by nurses (see Chapter 1). These principles will now be discussed.

- Approachability and communication
- Privacy and dignity
- Promptness
- Prevention of cross-infection
- Observation
- Prevention of accidents
- Promotion of independence and patient/parent participation
- Promotion of hygiene and comfort.

Box 8.1 Principles to follow when assisting with elimination

Approachability and communication

People who have needed help with their elimination invariably describe it as embarrassing and even distressing. The authors have known patients admit to reducing their fluid intake (thus increasing their risk of complications such as a urinary tract infection), so that they need not call for a bedpan or commode so often. In Koch and Kelly's (1999) study, women with multiple sclerosis talked of feelings of 'humiliation' at having to ask for help with elimination. If a nurse does not appear approachable, then people may not feel that they can ask for help. This could lead to discomfort (emotionally and physically), or even to incontinence, retention of urine or constipation. Chapter 2 discusses in detail the nurse's approach to patients/clients. You will need to be aware of non-verbal communication such as proximity to people, body language, and facial expression/eye contact.

If people have communication difficulties, nurses need to observe for non-verbal cues (such as restlessness), and sometimes a picture board (which could include a picture of a toilet) can be used for people to indicate their need to eliminate. The staff from Ian's home who are familiar with his needs and how he communicates should ensure that nurses in the admitting ward know how Ian will communicate his need to go to the toilet, which may be through a signing system including gestures. The nurses will also need to understand that if they ask Ian if he needs to go to the toilet, they should give him enough time to answer, as processing information may take much longer for people with learning disabilities. Verbal communication when assisting with elimination should include clear and appropriate use of language, taking developmental stage into account. Young children often have particular terms that they use in relation to elimination, and nurses need to know these if parents will not be readily available.

Privacy and dignity

These important principles (discussed in Chapter 2) are included in the bench-marking statements of best practice in *The Essence of Care* (Department of Health 2001b). If not maintained, people may feel embarrassed and degraded, and self-esteem is thus affected. These principles are identified in the Code for

Professional Conduct (Nursing and Midwifery Council 2002). To maintain privacy and dignity always ensure that bedside curtains are pulled shut properly, or the toilet door closed, and that patients are covered up while on the bedpan or commode. Note that some people may only want a nurse of the same sex to help them (Chur-Hansen 2002). Nurses should approach each person as an individual, being sensitive to non-verbal cues and, without making assumptions, being aware of possible cultural issues. For example within some South Asian cultures modesty is very important (Holland and Hogg 2001). Nurses should also speak privately and quietly when assisting with elimination.

Promptness

This is an important principle as people with certain types of incontinence (urge incontinence) will not be able to wait (see section later in this chapter). Also if patients are not able to attempt to open their bowels when they feel the need, faeces are pushed back into the sigmoid colon or remain in the rectum, where water continues to be reabsorbed. This leads to faeces becoming harder and more painful and difficult to pass, which may lead to constipation (Edwards *et al.* 2003). Nurses should try to prioritise meeting elimination needs, remembering that patients are in a powerless position, dependent on nurses for help with this basic need. When patients have finished eliminating, again nurses should respond promptly, to avoid discomfort and maintain safety. Patients should be provided with a call bell and told how to use it.

Prevention of cross-infection

When helping people with elimination, cross-infection is a high risk. Patients in an in-patient setting are often particularly vulnerable to infection due to their medical conditions, and some microorganisms are resistant in nature (see Chapter 3). Equipment used to assist with elimination must be cleaned adequately. Commodes used for more than one patient must be cleaned after each and every usage (Pratt *et al.* 2001). Non-disposable urinals and bedpans should be disinfected by thermal disinfection (exposure to hot water or steam) (Ayliffe *et al.* 2001). Block *et al.* (1990) found that a third of reusable bedpans may be contaminated with (mainly Gram-negative) bacteria after having been through a cleaning cycle. However newer washer-disinfectors have demonstrated better cleaning efficacy (Dempsey *et al.* 2000). Careful handwashing is the most important measure when assisting with elimination. Ayliffe *et al.* (2001) found that after handling bedpans nurses' hands often showed *Staphylococcus aureus* and/or Gram-negative bacilli but that handwashing was effective in removing these organisms.

Urine is normally sterile, but is often contaminated while voiding by bacteria present around the urethral opening (Gould 1994). Urine provides an excellent medium for bacterial growth, especially Gram-negative bacteria (*Pseudomonas, Klebsiella, Escherichia coli, Proteus*), which can survive only when water and inorganic ions are present (Gould 1994). Urine passed into a bedpan or urinal should therefore be disposed of quickly, as standing at room temperature allows any bacteria present to divide rapidly, doubling approximately every 30 minutes (Gould 1994), thus becoming a reservoir of infection. When a patient has diarrhoea, which could be infected, prevention of cross-infection is essential. As well as prompt disposal of the diarrhoea and handwashing, it is likely that nurses would need to employ source isolation techniques, including nursing the patient in a single room and use of gloves and aprons (see Chapter 3).

Observation

When assisting with elimination there are many useful observations which you can make, such as an assessment of the patient's ability to move, or about the condition of their skin. These are listed with explanations in Table 8.1.

Prevention of accidents

To prevent damage to either yourself, colleagues or patients, you need to do a moving and handling risk assessment, and this should be documented.

Table 8.1 Observations to make when assisting with elimination

Observation	Explanation
Ability to move	Ability to lift onto a bedpan, transfer to a commode or toilet, or stand to use a urinal. Whether any apparent discomfort/pain, breathlessness or weakness when moving
Skin condition	Redness or broken areas on sacrum or buttocks. Soreness of groin, perineum, penis or vulva
Self-care ability	Physical/mental ability to remove or adapt clothing, before and after elimination, and to carry out hygiene afterwards
Amount and frequency of urine output	A fluid input/output chart may be maintained if there are concerns about fluid balance. Urine will be measured in a jug and recorded in millilitres. Nappies can be weighed: $1\,g = 1\,mL$. Poor overall urine output could occur in dehydration or shock. No urinary output could mean retention of urine. Frequent small amounts of urine might indicate a urinary tract infection (UTI). Monitoring of frequency and amount may be part of a bladder re-education programme
Appearance of urine	See 'Urinalysis', next section. Very dark, concentrated urine might indicate dehydration, and smoky offensive urine might indicate UTI. Presence of blood may be due to kidney trauma or disease
Appearance of stools	Consistency and frequency of stools – hard and infrequent which could indicate constipation, or frequent and loose, termed diarrhoea, which could be infected. A stool chart to record frequency, appearance and consistency might be maintained. If infection is suspected, a stool specimen will be collected and sent (see later section)

Questions to consider might be:

■ Can the patient move onto the bedpan unaided or with assistance from one nurse or two?
■ Can the patient weight bear and transfer onto a commode or toilet unaided, or with one nurse or two nurses, or is a hoist necessary?

Tarling (1997) advises that if two nurses are needed to support a standing patient, a third will be needed to adjust clothing and clean the patient. Moving and handling in relation to toileting is covered in detail by Tarling (1997). Falls in bathrooms, often associated with transferring to the toilet, are not uncommon in older people (Aminzadeh *et al.* 2000). If patients are using bedpans in bed you need to ensure that they do not topple over. Balancing on a bedpan can be difficult, and it may be safer for the bed or trolley side rails to be up so that they can be held onto for support. You need to be aware that some organisations require an assessment to be carried out before bed side rails are used as they can be hazardous. You also need to be sure about your reasons for using them (i.e. not using them as a form of restraint).

Using the commode by the bedside is potentially hazardous. You must ensure that brakes are on securely, and that there are no fluids on the floor or other slippery substances. You need to consider: is the person safe to leave, or are they confused and likely to try to stand up alone, leading to a fall? A fall risk assessment scale can help to identify people who are at risk of falls. Find out if such risk assessment tools are used in your local practice setting. Chapter 5 looks at causes and prevention of falls.

Promotion of independence and patient/parental participation

Cerebrovascular accident
Cerebral damage caused either by decreased blood flow or haemorrhage. Effects vary but often causes paralysis down one side of the body (hemiplegia), speech and swallowing difficulty, and elimination difficulties. Commonly termed a 'stroke'.

The Essence of Care (Department of Health 2001b) includes benchmarks of best practice for 'self-care' and these highlight the importance of assessing people's self-care abilities and facilitating their skills and knowledge to promote self-care ability. You therefore need to assess ability and promote independence while also maintaining hygiene and safety. Learning how to use the toilet unaided, after a **cerebrovascular accident** (CVA) for example, may take some time, and both short- and long-term goals may be necessary. Teaching people how to manage transfers safely (for example from chair to commode), how to remove clothing, and, as with James, walk to the toilet on crutches, are situations where education is needed.

For people with learning disabilities, independence will be promoted if they are well orientated to their environment and where the toilet is and are taken to the same toilet by the same route each time. It will be helpful for the ward nurses to take Ian with his carers to show them where the toilet is and to show Ian how the facilities work. For example Ian may be used to a toilet with a pull handle and separate taps, while the ward might have a toilet with a button to press for flushing and a mixer tap. Ian's carers will know the best way of explaining this to him. Ian may then be able to find his own way to the toilet and use it independently. These steps could also be helpful for people who have dementia.

With children, when their family is present, it should be assessed as to what involvement they want in the care. Are the parents comfortable and confident to assist, and to what extent? Nurses need to ensure that parents know where equipment is kept, and that they are aware of any special requirements, such as the need to measure and record urine output. Kawik (1996) found that there is an assumption that parents will be involved in care, but the extent and scope of involvement is often not negotiated. When children with complex health care needs are admitted to hospital settings parents have found that they are expected to provide 24-hour care without this being negotiated by staff (Kirk 2001). A review by Coyne (1995a) indicated that there is a wide variation in the level of care which parents are willing to undertake, and that nurses should work in partnership with parents. A subsequent small study conducted by Coyne (1995b) suggested that parents all expected to carry out everyday care such as bathing and toileting, but more technical skills (which included measuring urine) were considered to be the nurse's job. James, at 12 years old, may be happy for his parents to assist him with elimination but this should not be assumed.

Promotion of hygiene and comfort

You need to consider how hygiene can be promoted for people whose elimination needs are met by their bedside, ensuring that you enable them to wash hands, and their perineal and genital area where necessary. Unfortunately Pritchard and Hathaway (1988) found that nurses often overlooked offering handwashing facilities to bedfast patients after the use of bedpan or urinal. When taking people to the toilet, always ensure that they are able to wash their hands at the sink afterwards. Always leave access to toilet tissue, and if people are unable to wipe themselves, then you must either do this for them, or give assistance to people who are learning or relearning this skill. With female patients always wipe the vulval area from front to back to prevent transmission of bowel bacterial flora (such as *E. coli*) from the anal area to the urethra (Nazarko 1995). Females have a short urethra (4 cm), which can easily lead to contamination by such bacteria if care is not taken. Within Asia, the left hand is traditionally reserved for washing underneath after using the toilet, the right hand being used for eating and other activities (Holland and Hogg 2001). These rules may also be important to some Asians living in Britain so nurses should be aware of this. Also Muslims prefer to wash their genitals with running water after using the toilet (Akhtar 2002).

At all times make sure that the patient does not become cold – it may be necessary to cover their legs with a blanket for example – and ensure that anyone using a bedpan is comfortably supported with pillows. Remember that psychological comfort will be promoted by your attitude and approach (see Chapter 2).

Summary

- Many health problems lead to people needing help with elimination.
- Various items of equipment are available to assist people who are unable to go to the toilet. Nurses need to assess which is appropriate for each individual.
- There are a number of important principles which need to be followed when helping people with elimination to ensure that care is therapeutic, effective and safe.

URINALYSIS

Urinalysis is the testing of urine for the presence of a variety of substances. This gives valuable and immediate information about an individual's kidneys, urinary tract and liver, and often influences subsequent management decisions (Rowell 1998).

LEARNING OUTCOMES

By the end of this section you will be able to:

1. Understand the process of urinalysis.
2. Show insight into the meaning of the results of a urinalysis, and what action to take if abnormal results are obtained.
3. Identify when urinalysis should be performed.

You should be able to access urinalysis equipment either in the skills laboratory or your practice setting.

Learning outcome 1: Understand the process of urinalysis

Activity

You may have already seen the reagent strips which are used to test urine. If not, ask whether you can look at them, in the skills laboratory, or in a practice placement. Find the expiry date on the bottle, and note the substances that are tested for and the timings for reading the results, on the side of the bottle.

It is important that reagent strips are in date, and are stored and used properly (Rowell 1998), otherwise results may not be accurate. The full range of substances which can be tested in a urinalysis are: leucocytes, nitrite, urobilinogen, protein, pH, blood, specific gravity, ketones, bilirubin and glucose. You may find that the reagent strips that you have looked at include this full range, but there are strips available which test for only a selection or even just one substance, such as blood.

Conducting a urinalysis

Bayer (1998), who produce the reagent strips, give detailed explanations as to how to conduct a urinalysis accurately. Key points are summarised in Fig. 8.1, with some additional explanatory notes and rationale given below.

First voided morning urine is best for a urinalysis as it is most concentrated. It should be voided directly into a clean container or preferably a sterile one. Ideally the urine should be tested immediately, or within 4 hours. Otherwise you can refrigerate the specimen, but you must let it return to room temperature before testing. It is particularly important to use fresh urine when testing for bilirubin and urobilinogen as these compounds are relatively unstable when exposed to room temperature and light. Bayer (1997a) advises that to test for nitrite it is best to use a first morning sample (when urine will have been in contact with bacteria, if present, for at least 3 hours).

When testing urine always observe the appearance of the urine sample first. Bayer (1997 a,b) explains the appearance of normal urine and the cause of some abnormalities. Normal fresh urine is pale to dark yellow or amber in colour, and clear. If the urine is red or red-brown this could be from a food dye, eating beetroot, a drug, or the presence of haemoglobin. If there are many red blood cells present, the urine will be cloudy as well. A strongly yellow sample could indicate **jaundice**. The smell of the urine should also be noted. Freshly voided, non-infected urine should be virtually odourless, but if urine is infected it may smell offensive.

The strips must be read accurately as per the timings given on the bottle. However, Rowell (1998) reports that reading of the reagent strips may not always be done reliably. Nurses on a busy ward may not wait the correct amount of time before reading the result, and lighting and colour vision may affect readings, leading to a lack of uniformity. There is an electronic reader available which can help to minimise reader error – the Clinitek 50 analyser – which also prints the results. This should lead to greater uniformity and consistency in readings. The print-out includes the time and date, and asterisks abnormal readings. A small-scale study by Rowell (1998) found use of the Clinitek 50 to be quick, clean and reliable, and well accepted by staff.

Jaundice

A condition characterised by yellowness of skin, whites of eyes, mucous membranes and body fluids due to the presence of bile pigment resulting from excess bilirubin in the blood.

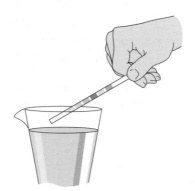

Requirements
- Reagent strip and bottle
- Freshly voided urine in a clean (preferably sterile) container

Procedure
- Observe urine for colour, consistency and smell
- Immerse all reagent areas in fresh urine and remove immediately
- Run the edge along the rim of the container to remove excess urine
- Hold the strip horizontally to prevent mixing of the chemicals from adjacent areas and prevent soiling of hands with urine
- Compare the test areas with the corresponding chart on the bottle or bench reader at the specified time

Figure 8.1 Conducting a urinalysis: key points (Bayer 1998).

Learning outcome 2: Show insight into the meaning of the results of a urinalysis, and what action to take if abnormal results are obtained

If you look on the side of the urinary reagent bottle you will find the key as to what each colour is testing for. It is clearly indicated which are the normal results, and which are the abnormal. Abnormal results should be reported. Table 8.2 indicates the significance of abnormalities and suggests some possible actions. A nursing dictionary will help you with some of the technical terms included.

Table 8.2 Clinical significance of test results (adapted from Bayer 1997b, 1998, with kind permission)

Significance of positive results	Commonest causes of abnormalities, and possible action to take
Glucose Not normally detectable in urine. Found when its concentration exceeds the renal threshold	• In people with raised blood glucose concentration: diabetes mellitus or glucose infusion • In people without raised blood glucose concentration: pregnancy or renal glycosuria **Action**: If positive, a blood glucose measurement should be performed, and further action may follow
Bilirubin Presence in urine indicates an excess of conjugated bilirubin in plasma. Note that stale urine may give a false negative result	• Liver cell injury: e.g. viral or drug-induced hepatitis, paracetamol overdose, late-stage cirrhosis • Biliary tract obstruction: e.g. by gallstones, carcinoma of the head of pancreas, biliary atresia in infants **Action**: Should always be reported as further investigations will be needed
Ketones Indicates accumulation of acetoacetate secondary to excessive breakdown of body fat. Some drugs e.g. L-dopa, may give a false positive result	• Fasting, particularly with fever and/or vomiting. Most often seen in children • Diabetic ketoacidosis • Ketotic hypoglycaemia in young children **Action**: Urgent action is needed if the person is known or suspected to have diabetes
Specific gravity A measure of total solute concentration in urine. In health varies widely according to the need to excrete water and solutes	• High values are found in dehydration, or in impaired kidney function, e.g. chronic renal failure • Low values are found in people with intact renal function and high fluid intake, diabetes insipidus, chronic renal failure, hypercalcaemia, hypokalaemia
Blood May be haematuria (intact blood cells) or haemoglobinuria (free haemoglobin – excreted from plasma or liberated from red cells in the urine)	• Haematuria: Due to kidney disorders, e.g. glomerulonephritis, polycystic kidneys, tumours • Due to urinary tract disorders, e.g. stones, tumours, infection, benign prostatic enlargement • Haemoglobinuria: Severe haemolysis, e.g. sickle cell disease crisis. Breakdown of red cells in urine (especially when urine is dilute and testing is delayed) **Action**: Should be reported. Follow-up will depend on other tests and clinical picture

(continued)

Table 8.2 (*continued*)

Significance of positive results	Commonest causes of abnormalities, and possible action to take
pH In health, the pH of uncontaminated urine ranges from 4.5–8.0. Note: a high pH will be found if testing stale urine, therefore such specimens should not be used	• Low values: Found in acidaemia as in diabetic ketoacidosis. Also starvation or potassium depletion • High values: Found in stale urine, alkalaemia (except when due to potassium depletion), e.g. due to vomiting and consumption of large amounts of antacids, renal tubular acidosis, urinary tract infection with ammonia-forming organisms **Action**: Depends on other test results.
Protein A range of proteins can be detected but the reagent is most sensitive to albumin, so a negative result does not rule out presence of other proteins	• Albuminuria may be found in acute and chronic glomerulonephritis, urinary tract infection, glomerular involvement in systemic lupus erythematosus, nephrotic syndrome, pre-eclampsia, fever, heart failure and postural (orthostatic) proteinuria **Action**: Transient results are seldom important but persistent positive results need investigating for underlying cause. Other test results and clinical picture should be considered
Urobilinogen Urinary excretion of urobilinogen reflects the combined effects of production of bilirubin, conversion of bilirubin to urobilinogen in the gut, and reabsorption into the bloodstream. Note that false negatives are found in stale urine	• Increased secretion: May be due to increased production, e.g. in red blood cell disorders such as sickle cell disease, or due to decreased uptake by the liver, e.g. in viral hepatitis and cirrhosis • Decreased secretion: May be due to biliary tract obstruction, e.g. gallstones, carcinoma of pancreas, or due to sterilisation of the colon by unabsorbable antibiotics, e.g. neomycin, which prevents bacterial conversion of bilirubin to urobilinogen **Action**: Urgent investigation is needed
Nitrite Most organisms that infect the urinary tract contain an enzyme system which catalyses the conversion of dietary nitrate (which is normally present in urine) to nitrite (which is not found in urine unless there is a urinary tract infection)	• Presence indicates urinary tract infection due to nitrite-producing organisms • However absence does not exclude infection, as some organisms are unable to convert dietary nitrate to nitrite. False negatives are also found if there is insufficient dietary nitrate, or urine has not been in the bladder long enough (4 hours is ideal) for the conversion to take place. **Action**: Specimen should be sent for microscopy and culture
Leucocytes Will be present when some of the leucocytes that have entered inflamed tissue from the blood are shed in the urine	• Indicates a urinary tract infection, especially when it is accompanied by acute inflammation of the urinary tract **Action**: Specimen should be sent for microscopy and culture

When to collect a urine specimen for microscopy and culture

An important reason for urinalysis is to check for a urinary tract infection (UTI) and therefore whether to send a urine specimen for microscopy, culture and sensitivity (MC & S). Studies have confirmed that urinalysis can help to screen out the unnecessary ordering of urine cultures (Moore *et al.* 2001; Reilly *et al.* 2002). This laboratory test examines the urine under the microscope, cultures the urine to see whether bacteria grow, and then checks what antibiotics the bacteria are sensitive to. The prevalence of UTI increases with age but typical symptoms (such as pain, **frequency** and pyrexia) may not be present in older people (O'Meara 1999). Urine should first be assessed visually and if obviously infected (cloudy and offensive) or blood-stained, then it should be sent for MC & S. However if urine is visually inspected and found to be clear this does not totally rule out a UTI (Bullock *et al.* 2001). A urinalysis will show whether there are leucocytes, nitrites, protein or blood present. A positive nitrite test indicates infection but a few cases may be missed. Positive tests for leucocytes, blood or protein may also suggest UTI. If all four tests (for nitrites, leucocytes, blood and protein) are negative it is highly likely that there is no infection, and therefore sending urine for MC & S is not indicated (Bayer 1997a). This systematic assessment of urine helps to avoid the unnecessary sending of urine specimens (McNaughton and Cavanagh 1998) (see flowchart from Bayer 1997a, Fig. 8.2).

Frequency

Passing urine more frequently than about seven times in 24 hours.

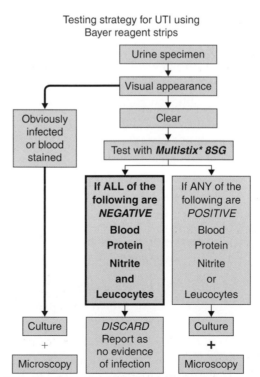

Figure 8.2 Flow chart from Bayer (1997a) showing when to send urine for microscopy and culture. (Reproduced with kind permission.)

Learning outcome 3: Identify when urinalysis should be performed

For each of the people in the scenarios at the start of the chapter, identify why you would want to do a urinalysis, and how the urine should be collected.

A urinalysis is a simple and non-invasive procedure which gives many clues as to the health and well-being of a person, thus a nursing assessment of a newly referred or admitted patient/client should always include a urinalysis. Urinalysis will also be performed for other people who may be at risk of developing health problems that can be indicated through a urinalysis. Examples include: during pregnancy (when presence of protein or glucose may be particularly significant), or after an abdominal injury (to screen for blood which might indicate kidney damage).

When John was first admitted, a urinalysis would have been performed as part of a general health screen. He should be reassured that this is routine and nothing to be worried about and given a clean container in which to pass the urine the morning after admission. When he developed urinary incontinence, he should have been asked for a further morning specimen to rule out urinary tract infection, which can predispose to, or compound, urinary incontinence. Remember that taking clozapine has rendered him more vulnerable to infection.

Both James and Ian have been newly admitted, and a urinalysis will give insight into their physical well-being. A urinalysis will be a useful indicator as to whether Ian's abdominal pain is caused by a urinary tract problem. James, although confined to bed, should be able to pass urine into a clean bottle for testing. When collecting a specimen from Ian, it would probably be best for the nurses to ask his carers to help as he is used to them and they know best how to communicate and explain the procedure to him. They may prefer to take him to the toilet in which a receptacle has been placed. June's urine is also likely to be tested if the district nurse observes signs of a UTI, and then a catheter specimen of urine (see Box 8.3) would be collected and tested.

Summary

■ Urinalysis is a non-invasive and frequently performed practical skill which can provide very useful information about people's health status.

■ To obtain an accurate result, the steps in a urinalysis must be carried out carefully with an appropriately collected specimen.

■ It is important to understand the significance of abnormal results and subsequent action to take.

COLLECTING URINE AND STOOL SPECIMENS

In this section common types of urine specimen and the collection of a stool (faeces) specimen are discussed. It is often necessary to obtain specimens such as these from patients/clients as they can provide important diagnostic information, which will impact on management and care. General principles relating to specimen collection were considered in Chapter 3 'Preventing cross-infection', and you are recommended to look at these in full again. For quick reference purposes key points can be found in Box 8.2.

LEARNING OUTCOMES

By the end of this section you will be able to:

1. Discuss the collection of a catheter specimen of urine.
2. Discuss the collection of a midstream specimen of urine, and how this can be adapted for different age groups and in different situations.
3. Discuss the collection of a 24-hour specimen of urine.
4. Discuss the collection of a stool specimen.

Learning outcome 1: Discuss the collection of a catheter specimen of urine

A catheter specimen of urine (CSU) is often taken for bacteriological examination to find out if treatment is required when symptoms of a urinary tract infection (UTI) are present in a person who has been catheterised. Symptoms of UTI include frequency of micturition, pain on micturition (dysuria), fever and sometimes loin or supra-pubic pain. However a person with a catheter may not display these symptoms and in an older and/or confused person the symptoms can be still less apparent. As discussed earlier in the chapter, the district nurse may need to collect a CSU from June if a UTI is suspected. Urine is nearly always

- Use of sound infection control principles (hand hygiene, personal protective equipment) to prevent cross-infection
- Clear explanations
- Maintenance of patient/client privacy, dignity and comfort
- Avoid contamination of the specimen
- Prompt transportation to the laboratory, or refrigerate for up to 24 hours
- Clear labelling
- Correct and comprehensive accompanying information
- Documentation in patient/client notes of the date and time of the specimen collection.

Box 8.2 Collection of specimens: key points

infected after 5 days following catheterisation (Mead 1998a). However it is important to distinguish between bacteriuria and a 'clinical infection'. Bacteria can colonise the urinary tract without invading the surrounding tissues (bacteriuria), often do not cause clinical symptoms and may not be susceptible to treatment. On the other hand clinical infection involving invasion of surrounding tissues, often producing symptoms in infected people, requires treatment.

Whatever the classification of the infection, if a specimen is considered necessary then nurses must use aseptic technique and sterile equipment. This is to reduce the risk of further contaminating the specimen and potentially introducing different bacteria to those from the patient. This is particularly important since the treatment is based on the results of the bacteriological examination of the urine. Urine should be obtained from the special sampling port on the drainage system; the catheter and drainage system should never be disconnected to take a specimen. You should adhere to manufacturers' instructions concerning the number of times the port may be punctured safely. Urine should never be taken from the catheter bag because the bag acts as a reservoir where microorganisms can multiply. It is thus likely to contain greater numbers of microorganisms than urine accessed via the port. The bag can also be heavily contaminated from environmental sources. Box 8.3 outlines the key principles to follow when taking a catheter specimen of urine.

Equipment
- Alcohol swab, receiver, syringe (20 mL) and needle (21 g bore), specimen pot and request form. A gate clamp may be required.

Key points
- Adhere to general points outlined in Box 8.2.
- Locate the sample port on the catheter bag tubing. Some drainage bags have a latex port which requires a needle and syringe to aspirate the urine. Others have a needleless port and a syringe can be attached directly to this to withdraw the urine.
- If there is no urine present in the catheter tubing, clamp the tubing below the sample port until sufficient urine collects. Never clamp the actual catheter, as this could damage it.
- Swab the sample port with alcohol swab and allow the port to dry. Insert the needle into the port at an angle of 45 degrees to prevent going straight through the tubing.
- For needleless sampling ports follow the same procedure, but attach the syringe directly to the sampling port.
- Withdraw the required amount of urine, remove the top from the specimen pot and fill the pot with urine. Dispose of the needle and syringe into a sharps box immediately. Replace the cap on the pot.

Box 8.3 Collection of a catheter specimen of urine: equipment and key points

Learning outcome 2: Discuss the collection of a midstream specimen of urine, and how this can be adapted for different age groups and in different situations

The midstream specimen of urine (MSU) is collected if a UTI is suspected in a non-catheterised patient, and is obtained using a clean procedure. It is a useful aid in diagnosis and the aim is to collect the midstream, which is not contaminated by microorganisms outside the urinary tract. How MSUs should be collected has been the subject of much research but the evidence base for best practice remains unclear. It appears that the specimen is best collected as soon as possible after waking, when urine is normally available and in concentrated form. People have often been asked to undertake perineal cleansing with sterile swabs and saline prior to giving an MSU, to prevent contamination. However, a study conducted in Canada (Mousseau 2001) concluded that contamination of urine specimens from women with acute dysuria who cleaned the perineal area prior to collection did not differ from those who did not. It is theorised that the first part of the stream flushes away microorganisms from the first part of the urethra, and that the urine does not flow over the perineum as long as there is sufficient urine in the bladder to produce a good stream. If there is insufficient urine in the bladder the specimen should be collected later. The equipment required and key points of the procedure are listed in Box 8.4.

Note that if a urine specimen is being collected because of suspected tuberculosis (TB) or cancer of the urinary tract, then an early morning specimen is preferable because it is more concentrated and it is most likely to contain the tubercle bacillus or malignant cells (Beynon 1997). Usually, three consecutive early morning specimens are required.

Activity

Read through Box 8.4. As you can see, co-operation and understanding by the person would be needed. Look at the practice scenarios and consider to what extent you might achieve understanding and consent from John, Ian and James.

Equipment
- A toilet or commode as appropriate
- A specimen pot and laboratory request form
- Disposable gloves.

Procedure
- Adhere to key points in Box 8.2.
- Explain to the person to start passing urine as usual, then catch some urine (about 20 mL: about 2.5 cm up the pot) in the specimen pot, and then finish voiding into the toilet or commode. Wear gloves and assist the person if necessary.

Box 8.4 Midstream specimens of urine: equipment and procedure

You are more likely to gain informed consent and co-operation from any patient or client if you explain the procedure and its importance carefully and confidentially. You should respect the person's right to privacy and dignity throughout the whole episode of care. Remember that what may be a simple and routine procedure in your eyes may feel quite different to the person concerned.

Given the approach just discussed it is likely that John would be able to produce the specimen with little assistance. Ian may have difficulty understanding and co-ordinating what is expected of him if he has not been asked for a urine specimen before. However he may have become used to giving urine samples through health screening at his GP's surgery as part of his Health Action Plan. One approach would be for his carer or a nurse to take him to the toilet about 30 minutes after a drink (assuming he is not being kept nil by mouth), and try to collect the specimen in a clean receptacle in the toilet or, if possible, catch the midstream in a pot for him, while wearing gloves. This approach can also be used for people who are confused.

James at 12 years old would almost certainly be able to understand the instructions for collecting an MSU. However it is difficult for anyone to produce an MSU and being confined to bed makes this even more difficult. Additionally the pain James experiences complicates matters, making the collection even more problematic. Adaptations will need to be made, for example, placing a waterproof pad beneath James to soak up any possible spillage, helping to diminish fears of wetting the bed. Allowing James plenty of time and not rushing is also important. You should remember that many young people feel sensitive about their changing bodies and their rights to privacy and dignity must be upheld.

Collecting MSUs from children younger than James poses particular problems, although toilet-trained children may be able to manage it (de Sousa 1996). Disposable nappies are not suitable for urine collection because manufacturers have adopted gel-based absorption (Vernon *et al.* 1994). Methods described in the literature for collecting urine samples from infants include pads (sterile urine collection packs), attaching an adhesive urine bag and clean catch (see Box 8.5). All these methods have advantages and disadvantages. Liaw *et al.* (2000) describe a study comparing these methods used by parents, who were instructed to wash their hands and the infant's perineum prior to the procedure. The pads were checked every 10 minutes until wet (but not soiled) and then urine was aspirated with a syringe. The adhesive bag was also checked every 10 minutes. The clean catch method involved the infant being left without a nappy and a sterile bottle kept handy to catch the urine.

The three methods were found to be equally effective but the pad method was preferred by parents. Parents disliked the clean catch method and found the bag often leaked and was difficult to remove, leaving red marks. A pilot study reported by Farrell *et al.* (2002) compared specimen collection using the pads versus urine bags and concluded that pads may affect bacterial count and that larger scale studies are needed. As you can see, there is no ideal method for

General principles
- Appropriate explanation to child and family.
- Parents may be able to collect the specimen, or help.
- Use the child's familiar terminology for passing urine (Campbell and Glasper 1995).
- Normal social hygiene, e.g. washing genitalia with soap and water and drying carefully is considered sufficient prior to specimen collection (MacQueen 2000).

Clean potty specimen
- Can be used for a potty trained toddler.
- Wash the potty in washing up liquid and hot water.
- Give the child a drink, and offer the potty about 30 minutes later.

A clean catch specimen
- Used for a toddler who is not toilet trained or a baby.
- Give the infant a drink, apply a clean nappy and remove it 30–60 minutes later.
- Try to catch the urine in a sterile gallipot inside a potty (Vernon 1995).
- Alternatively ask the parent to try to catch a specimen in a container, perhaps with the baby lying in the cot or up playing.

Adhesive bag
- Used for an infant or toddler who is not toilet trained.
- Uses a single-use, sterile adhesive urine bag.
- Remove the nappy, and apply the bag firmly.
- With females, stretch the perineum taut during application to ensure a leak-proof fit.
- With males, place the penis and the scrotum inside the bag.
- Check the bag regularly so that it can be removed as soon as a specimen is produced.

Box 8.5 Collecting a urine sample from an infant or young child

collecting an uncontaminated urine sample from a non-toilet-trained child or infant and you should be guided by local policy.

You should also be aware of supra-pubic aspiration, which is a less usual method used to obtain urine from an infant (de Sousa 1996). It is performed by a doctor and involves aspiration of bladder contents through a needle.

Learning outcome 3: Discuss the collection of a 24-hour specimen of urine

Sometimes it is necessary to collect the total volume of urine passed within a 24-hour period. This is then analysed within the laboratory so that the 24-hour

Equipment
- A toilet, commode, urinal, bedpan, potty or collection bags (as appropriate for the individual)
- A jug, a 24-hour urine collection container, gloves.

Procedure
1. Assess the person's ability to participate in the collection. When the person next passes urine, it is discarded. This marks the beginning of the 24-hour period for collection.
2. Label the container with the person's details (name, ward and hospital number), and the time and date the collection started.
3. Put a sign on the bed or door of the room belonging to the person indicating that a 24-hour urine collection is in place, the date and time it started and when it will finish.
4. Every time the person passes urine it is collected and poured into the container, which is stored in the sluice. The person may be able to do this independently or may need assistance. Check the person's understanding and ability.
5. Ask the person to empty his or her bladder just before the end of the 24-hour collection period, and advise that this ends the collection period.
6. Remove the sign from the door or bed.
7. Clean or discard the jug used.
8. Record the completion time and ensure that the urine collection and laboratory request forms are dispatched correctly as soon as possible.

Note: if one sample of urine becomes contaminated or is accidently discarded, the test must be discontinued and restarted.

Box 8.6 24-hour urine collection: equipment and key points

excretion of a variety of key metabolites (e.g. protein, creatinine) can be assessed (Laker 1994). Box 8.6 outlines the equipment needed and the procedure. Campbell and Glasper (1995) note that a 24-hour urine collection in infants and children is somewhat challenging. For infants and small children, collection bags are required, which can include collection tubes so that the bag will not need frequent removal, causing irritation. All children and parents, but especially older children, will need a clear explanation.

Learning outcome 4: Discuss the collection of a stool specimen

Activity

When do you think it might be necessary to collect a stool specimen? Thinking about a 'normal' stool will help you begin to answer this question.

You may have identified that a stool specimen is collected if a person has complained of abnormal stools, or you have observed an abnormality when assisting a person. Normal stools are brown, soft and formed, and you should note the amount, particularly if diarrhoea (liquid stools) are present because patients can lose a lot of fluid this way. There are many causes of diarrhoea, but these include gastrointestinal infection. Infection is particularly likely if the stool is offensive, and has an abnormal colour such as green. In these instances the stool is sent for MC & S, to detect the causative microorganism and identify any antibiotics to which it is sensitive.

Normal frequency of passing stools varies from person to person but if frequency is altered this can be a reason to collect a specimen. Altered consistency, might also be a reason, for example lots of mucus can indicate disease such as **ulcerative colitis**, whereas fatty offensive smelling and floating stools sometimes indicate gallbladder disease. Stool specimens are also sent for examination for occult (hidden) blood, if rectal bleeding is suspected but not obvious. However if the colour of a stool is different to that normally seen this too can be suggestive of disease and will indicate that a specimen should be taken. Bright red fresh blood should always be reported and may indicate the presence of **haemorrhoids** or other disease. Stools that are black and tarry in consistency can indicate digested blood from the alimentary tract (termed malaena). Sometimes stool specimens are sent for examination for parasites. Additionally if a person experiences pain or discomfort associated with defecation, or flatus is a problem, then a stool specimen might be taken.

The key points in the collection of a stool specimen are outlined in Box 8.7. There are stool specimen collectors available which have a spoon

Ulcerative colitis
Ulceration of the mucosa of the colon, causing offensive, watery stools with mucus and pus. Can cause haemorrhage and perforation.

Haemorrhoids
Dilated blood vessels in the rectal mucosa. Lay term is 'piles'.

Equipment
- A bedpan, gloves, apron, a sterile stool specimen pot or a sterile specimen pot and a spatula, a specimen bag and the laboratory request form.

Procedure
1. Adhere to general points in Box 8.2. Note that infection control procedures are essential throughout.
2. Ask the person to use a bedpan or commode to catch the specimen. If possible the patient should be helped to a toilet rather than use a commode. A disposable bedpan can be placed under the toilet lid.
3. When the stool is available, take the bedpan to the sluice, open the sterile container and using a spatula, fill the container about a third full with faeces, and then secure the lid.
4. Refrigerate the specimen if it cannot go to the laboratory immediately. In infections such as amoebiasis, the stool must be fresh and warm (Mead 1998b), thus special arrangements for collection must be made with the laboratory.
5. Remember to complete the stool chart if a record being kept.

Box 8.7 Collection of a stool specimen: equipment and key points

attached to the lid. Although these are easy to use when collecting the specimen, they can be difficult for laboratory staff to handle without getting contaminated. Also pots should not be overfilled as the contents may ferment and build up sufficient pressure to force off even a tightly fitting lid (Gould and Brooker 2000).

Summary

- Explaining the procedure and its importance carefully, while maintaining dignity, privacy and respect for people, is of prime importance when collecting specimens.
- It is essential to be certain about the purpose for collecting the specimen so that it is collected appropriately.
- Great care should be taken when collecting urine and stool specimens to prevent contamination of the specimens, thus invalidating results.
- Precautions to prevent cross-infection must be adhered to when collecting urine and stool specimens.
- It is essential to label specimens accurately, and to document their collection in patients' notes.

CARING FOR PEOPLE WITH URINARY CATHETERS

Urinary catheterisation involves the insertion of a hollow tube into the bladder for the purpose of evacuation or instilling fluids. The catheter may be inserted intermittently, or left *in situ* (termed 'in-dwelling') and emptied intermittently via a catheter valve. In these instances, the bladder then retains its function as a reservoir. In many cases an in-dwelling catheter is continuously drained within a closed system into a bag, in which case only a small volume of urine will be present at the base of the bladder. Some people are taught to self-catheterise intermittently, termed 'intermittent self-catheterisation', often as a means of managing incontinence in those with neurological disorders such as multiple sclerosis. This method was tried for June's bladder management before a long-term in-dwelling catheter was inserted. For a child with a neurogenic bladder, parents may undertake intermittent catheterisation. Teaching a person to self-catheterise requires specific skills and knowledge which will not be covered in this chapter, but the topic is covered comprehensively by Getliffe (2003).

Urinary catheters are usually passed along the urethra, but sometimes a supra-pubic catheter is passed directly through the mid supra-pubic region of the anterior abdominal wall into the bladder. This is a surgical procedure, performed under anaesthesia, and may be used for people who need a long-term urinary catheter or after certain surgical procedures and in pelvic/urethral trauma or disease. The principles of care for people who have supra-pubic catheters are the same as for those with urethral catheters (Macauley 1997).

LEARNING OUTCOMES

By the end of this section you will be able to:

1. Identify the main indications for urinary catheterisation.
2. Show awareness of a range of equipment commonly used for catheterisation.
3. State the main complications associated with urinary catheterisation.
4. Understand the principles underpinning urethral catheterisation.
5. Discuss the care required for people who have in-dwelling urinary catheters.

You may be able to access a urinary catheter in the skills laboratory. An opened one would be particularly useful. If not, see if you can look at equipment in your practice setting.

Learning outcome 1: Identify the main indications for urinary catheterisation

 Activity | Make a list of the reasons you can think of why people are catheterised. Thinking back to your practice experience will give you some clues.

You may have identified the following:

A neurogenic bladder
A neurogenic bladder commonly results from lesions of the central nervous system e.g. CVA, spinal injury, multiple sclerosis. Effects include urinary retention, overactive, underactive or uncoordinated detrusor activity.

Cytotoxic
Drugs that have a destructive effect on cells and are used to treat cancer.

■ To relieve retention of urine.
■ Before pelvic surgery and certain investigations, to minimise the risk of damage to the bladder.
■ To measure urine output accurately post-operatively and in very ill patients (for example major trauma, shock).
■ To empty the bladder during labour.
■ To empty the bladder where **neurogenic bladder** dysfunction exists.
■ To introduce fluids into the bladder for irrigation purposes.
■ To introduce drugs as direct therapy, for example **cytotoxic** drugs.
■ To facilitate bladder healing.
■ Following certain pelvic, urethral or bladder neck surgery.

You will notice that incontinence is not given as a primary reason for catheterisation in the list above. This is because long-term catheterisation is rarely free of complications and should, therefore, only be considered when other options have failed, or are no longer appropriate. The major complications of catheterisation are considered in more detail later in this section.

Learning outcome 2: Show awareness of a range of equipment commonly used for catheterisation

Activity

In the skills laboratory there may be a sterile or non-sterile (for demonstration purposes) urinary catheter complete with packaging material. See Fig. 8.3 for examples. If you are able to access such 'real' equipment take note of the following:

- The manner in which it is packaged, batch number, expiry date
- Size
- Length
- Balloon capacity
- The catheter material.

If you have access to a non-sterile catheter try inflating and deflating the balloon using a syringe and water. Some catheters are manufactured pre-filled with water for inflation and you should take note of the manner in which these operate.

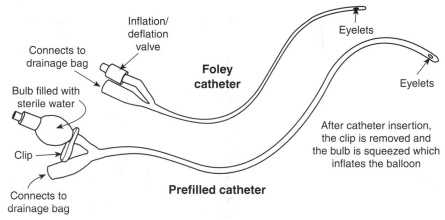

Figure 8.3 Examples of urinary catheters. (From a photograph of a Biocath™ Foley catheter kindly provided by Bard Limited. Trademark of C.R. Bard, Inc. or an affiliate.)

Now read through the following points and relate them to your observations.

Packaging

Catheters are packaged to enable ease of insertion into the bladder, and with only the exception of self-catheterisation, strict aseptic technique is employed. The way in which the catheter is packaged, including double wrapping, assists in the maintenance of sterility. Note also that there is a batch number and expiry date on the packaging. These are important and will need to be entered into patients' documentation.

Catheter size

You will have noted the size of the catheter. The size is measured in relation to its external diameter, and is measured in Charriere (Ch) or French gauge units (Fg). One Ch unit equals 0.3 mm, and the catheters range in size from 6–8 (for paediatric use) to 30 Ch. A size 12 Ch catheter is 4.0 mm in diameter. The size most commonly used for women is 12–14 Ch and for men, 12–16 Ch (Macauley 1997). The key general rule to follow is that the smallest size catheter should be used that will allow free urinary outflow (Pratt *et al.* 2001). Large catheters are associated with complications including urethral irritation, urethral trauma, bladder spasm, urinary bypassing, pressure necrosis and increased risk of infection (Getliffe 1996; Laurent 1998).

Catheter length

Catheters are usually manufactured in three lengths: standard catheters (sometimes referred to as 'male-length') are 40–44 cm, female catheters are 30–40 cm, paediatric catheters are 30 cm (Robinson 2001). The standard catheter is often used for women, particularly if obese, because it allows easier access to the junction of the catheter and the drainage bag (Macauley 1997).

Balloon

The foley catheter is the design most frequently used for in-dwelling urethral catheterisation (Getliffe 2003). It has a rounded tip with two drainage eyes and an integral balloon, which, when inflated, holds the catheter *in situ*. There are two channels, one for drainage and the other for inflating the balloon. The balloon sits at the sensitive base of the bladder and can potentially cause irritation, spasm and mechanical damage to the bladder. Retention balloons come in various sizes: 3–5 mL for children, 10 mL is recommended for adults, but larger 30-mL balloons are sometimes used after some urological procedures (Macauley 1997; Pratt *et al.* 2001). Inflation valves are colour coded according to the Charriere size (Robinson 2001). Catheters for intermittent use are usually a simple tube design and do not have an inflatable balloon as there is no requirement for them to be retained in the bladder. Some supra-pubic catheters do not have a balloon, but are secured by a flange and held in place by skin sutures.

Material

Catheters are available in different materials and the choice of which type is used will depend upon the clinical experience of the practitioner, patient assessment and the length of time it is envisaged the catheter will remain *in situ* (Pratt *et al.* 2001). For short-term use, plastic, latex (up to 7–10 days) and Teflon-coated latex (up to 28 days) are commonly used, and these materials are considerably cheaper than long-term catheter materials. Some patients are allergic to latex, and screening is advisable if latex is to be used (Woodward 1997). Plastic catheters have been found to exert low toxicity because of the inert nature of plastic. Also, the rate that this material absorbs water is low, and so the catheter retains the widest internal diameter, making these catheters a common material of choice for drainage of post-operative blood clots and debris. However, plastic catheters can remain rigid at body temperature and have been associated with bladder spasm, pain and leakage of urine (Blannin and Hobden 1980, cited by Macauley 1997). The Department of Health (2003) recommends that in-dwelling

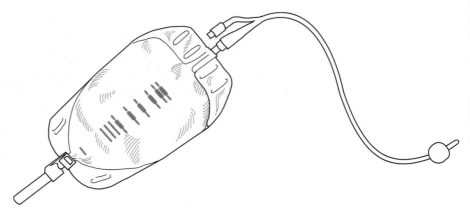

Figure 8.4 A urinary catheter attached to a leg bag. (From a photograph of Biocath™ Foley catheter attached to Uriplan™ Leg Bag kindly provided by Bard Limited. Trademark of C.R. Bard, Inc., or an affiliate.)

catheters used for long-term use should have low allergenicity. Silicone, silicone elastamer-coated latex and hydrogel-coated catheters are suitable products (Laurent 1998). The cost of the catheter should not be the primary factor in the selection process but nurses should be aware of the different costs when selecting.

Urine drainage bags and catheter valves

In-dwelling catheters are normally used in conjunction with an attached collection bag to allow periodic emptying. This is known as a closed system. Figure 8.4 shows a catheter attached to a leg bag, which would be secured to the patient's leg with straps. Figure 8.5 shows a urinary catheter attached to a bed bag supported on a stand, which will be suitable for when the person is in bed. A catheter valve (see Fig. 8.6) may provide an alternative for some patients but an adequate bladder capacity is required. Unless a committed carer is available, the user also requires good manual dexterity for manipulating the valve, and sufficient cognitive function to understand the need to release the valve regularly to prevent over-distension (Fader *et al.* 1997). Catheter valves are also unlikely to be suitable if the person has uncontrolled detrusor over-activity, ureteric reflux or renal impairment (Fader *et al.* 1997).

When selecting a bag, factors to consider are capacity, length of inlet tube and type of outlet tap for emptying. Bags vary in capacity from 350–750 mL and up to 2 L for use overnight or post-operatively. Some bags are specially designed for wheelchair users. Outlet taps are usually of a lever type design or push-across mechanism, but other designs are available. The manual dexterity of patients and carers needs to be considered. There are a number of catheter supports available for people with restricted mobility. These supports aim to provide firm support to prevent tugging, without restricting movement or impeding drainage.

Whatever equipment is used it is important to document details of the catheter and drainage system used in the patient's records carefully. You should

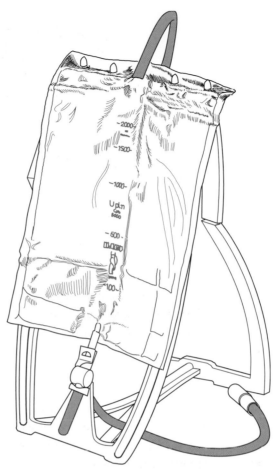

Figure 8.5 A bed bag on a stand. (From a photograph of Uriplan™ Bed Bag on Uristand™ kindly provided by Bard Limited. Trademark of C.R. Bard, Inc., or an affiliate.)

also provide the person with adequate information in relation to the rationale for insertion, the insertion itself, and details of maintenance and removal of catheter.

Activity | What sort of drainage bag might be suitable for June?

Following discussion with June you may decide to use a leg bag. The length of the inlet tube selected would depend upon whether June found it most comfortable to position the bag on her thigh, knee or calf. At night, June's carers will be able to attach a night bag on a stand, directly to the leg bag. For most patients, body-worn bags are preferable because their attachment to the person's leg or suspended from the waist allows maximum freedom and at the same time can be concealed beneath clothing. This reduces discomfort and promotes dignity for people like June who find themselves in the difficult and sometimes embarrassing situation of needing a urinary catheter permanently *in situ*.

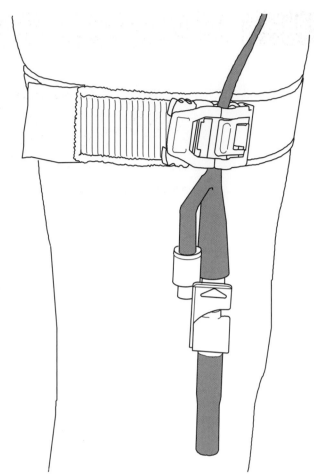

Figure 8.6 A urinary catheter strapped to the leg, with a valve in place, for emptying (From a photograph of Biocath™ Foley catheter, with Flip-Flo™ catheter valve, secured with a ComfaSure™ catheter retainer strap, kindly provided by Bard Limited. Trademark of C.R. Bard, Inc., or an affiliate.)

Did you know?

Prior to the use of closed drainage systems almost all patients developed urinary tract infections within 96 hours (Kass 1957, cited by Macauley 1997). As closed drainage systems have been shown to reduce this rate of infection, they are now accepted as good practice (Macauley 1997). However, there is consistent evidence that a significant number of hospital-acquired infections are related to urinary catheterisation, and these cause significant morbidity and even mortality. It has been estimated that 1 in 8 people in hospital has an in-dwelling catheter and 4 per cent in the community, and problems with infection affect about 50 per cent of patients (Laurent 1998). Therefore care for people with catheters must aim to prevent infection, as well as promoting comfort and understanding. But catheterisation is best avoided if at all possible (Ayliffe *et al.* 2001; NICE 2003; Pratt *et al.* 2001).

Activity Figure 8.7 shows a diagram of a closed urinary drainage system. Where do you think bacteria could enter into the system?

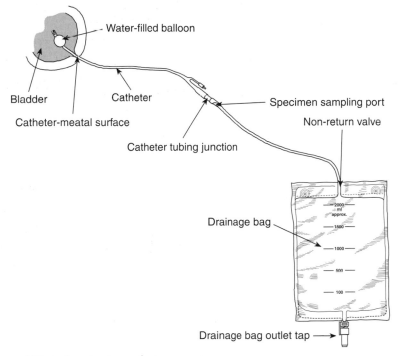

Water-filled balloon

Bladder   Catheter

Catheter-meatal surface

Catheter tubing junction

Specimen sampling port

Non-return valve

Drainage bag

Drainage bag outlet tap ⟶

Figure 8.7 A closed urinary drainage system.

Compare your answers with the following list. Potential ports of entry include:

■ The catheter tip at catheterisation.
■ The urethral meatus around the catheter. Bacteria are also believed to enter the bladder at the time of catheterisation via the peri-urethral space. Coagulase-negative staphylococci or micrococci can normally be found in the anterior urethra, and these are a common cause of infection immediately following catheterisation (Ayliffe *et al.* 2001).
■ The junction between the catheter and the tubing to the catheter bag. Some systems now have a tamper-evident seal at the junction between the catheter and the connection tube aimed at preventing bacteria entering at this principal site of infection entry.
■ The specimen sampling port.
■ The drainage outlet.

Early infections are often endogenous, but cross-infection (exogenous infection) occurs later in patients with in-dwelling catheters (Ayliffe *et al.* 2001).

Learning outcome 3: State the main complications associated with urinary catheterisation

Activity

Look back over this section and see if you can name one major complication associated with catheterisation and try to identify some others.

You probably identified that infection is a major complication of catheterisation. Encrustation and eventual blockage are also major problems associated with urinary catheterisation (Burr and Nuseibeh 1997; Laurent 1998). Other complications include urethral strictures, pressure necrosis, spasm, discomfort and pain (Winn 1996).

With a catheter *in situ* the bladder's normal closing mechanism is obstructed and the natural flushing mechanism of micturition is lost. Additionally the close proximity of the catheter to the bowel presents a risk of infection, because bacteria can be mechanically transferred across skin surfaces from anus to urethral meatus (Meers *et al.* 1995). Bacteria having entered the urinary system may cling to the surface of the catheter. This creates a living biofilm that is almost impossible to remove and that is highly resistant to antibiotics (Getliffe 2002). The bacteria can cause the urine to become more alkaline than usual and encrustation on the catheter surface then occurs, which can lead to blockage. This in turn may lead to retention of urine or to leaking, and pain. These outcomes are distressing for patients, and can result in loss of comfort and dignity (Laurent 1998).

When tissue is invaded by bacteria, problems include local infection, which may result in foul-smelling urine, or systemic infection leading to pyrexia. You should be aware that catheterising patients places them in significant danger of acquiring a urinary tract infection. Additionally, the longer a catheter is in place the greater the danger. The risk of acquiring infection has been shown to increase by 5 per cent for each further day of catheterisation and after 10 days, 50 per cent of patients have bacteria in their urine (Garibaldi *et al.* 1974, cited by Wilson 2001). Of patients with a UTI, 1–4 per cent develop bacteraemia and of these 13–30 per cent die (Pratt *et al.* 2001). Therefore an in-dwelling urethral catheter should only be used when there is no suitable alternative and after considering alternative methods of management. Additionally patients must be reviewed frequently and the catheter removed as soon as possible.

Learning outcome 4: Understand the principles underpinning urethral catheterisation

Activity

Before reading the following section refer to Chapter 3 for an explanation and discussion of non-touch technique. It is important that you understand these principles as they underpin the procedure of urinary catheterisation. You should note that catheterisation is a skilled aseptic procedure and should only be carried out by health care personnel who are trained and competent to carry it out (Pratt *et al.* 2001).

In addition to using a non-touch technique, there are a number of other factors to take into account when catheterising a patient. In many NHS Trusts additional training must be undertaken by trained nurses to perform male urethral catheterisation. However, many of the principles are synonymous with female urethral catheterisation. Supra-pubic catheterisation is usually a medical procedure, and is not considered here. It is important to note that catheterisation is an invasive procedure and the effects on patients may be many: physical, psychological and social.

Appropriate and effective communication and sensitivity are essential when catheterisation takes place (see Chapter 2). Care should be taken to explain where the catheter is inserted, and why the procedure is necessary, ensuring that verbal consent is gained. This could be difficult with a person who is confused. For children, parents can support and comfort them during the procedure; sedation may be necessary (Mohammed 2000). Also, catheters should not be changed unnecessarily or as part of routine practice.

Once the catheter has been inserted, dietary advice, including fluid intake and avoidance of constipation, is an important part of patient education (Getliffe 1996). Further explanations and instructions concerning why and how the catheter has been inserted, its maintenance requirements and discussion of removal will be required if the person goes home with a urinary catheter *in situ*. Patients and carers should also be educated about techniques to prevent infection (Department of Health 2003). The district nurse (as in June's case) will probably be involved. Box 8.8 outlines the equipment needed and key points when undertaking female urethral catheterisation.

Learning outcome 5: Discuss the care required for people who have in-dwelling urinary catheters.

Activity

For June, think about what specific care might be needed in relation to catheter care.

You may have thought of the following:

■ Maintaining hygiene
■ Emptying of the catheter bag
■ Appropriate positioning of the catheter bag
■ Adequate fluid intake.

These issues will now be discussed.

Maintaining hygiene

The main aim of cleansing is to remove secretions and encrustation and prevent infection. Where possible patients should be encouraged to attend to their own meatal and perineal hygiene needs, thus reducing the risk of cross-infection while promoting self-care and dignity. Maintaining routine daily hygiene is all that is needed, with the meatus being washed with soap and water (NICE 2003).

Equipment

- A catheterisation pack if available, or a dressing pack and sterile receiver, sterile gloves, an appropriate catheter, sterile sodium chloride, catheter bag and stand or holder, sterile single patient use lubricant or anaesthetic gel, syringe and sterile water of appropriate size and amount to inflate the balloon, disposable waterproof absorbent pad, specimen pot (if required), a good light source.

Note: A second nurse may be needed to help position the patient, who needs to be preferably flat with her legs apart to allow good access and visibility.

Procedure

1. Non-touch technique should be strictly adhered to throughout (see Chapter 3 sections on 'Hand hygiene', 'Use of gloves and aprons' and 'Non-touch technique').
2. Place the disposable pad under the patient's buttocks.
3. Open the catheter bag and arrange at the side of the bed, ensuring the attachment tip remains sterile.
4. Open the catheterisation or dressing pack, and open the catheter on to the sterile field but do not remove it from its internal wrapping.
5. Draw up the sterile water to inflate the balloon (unless catheter is pre-filled).
6. Pour sodium chloride into the gallipot.
7. Open sterile gloves, wash hands and apply gloves.
8. Place sterile towels over patient's thighs and between legs.
9. Cleanse the perineal area with the sodium chloride, and then using non-dominant hand, separate labia minora and cleanse the meatus.
10. Carefully locate the urethra and insert single-patient-use lubricant gel to minimise urethral trauma and infection (NICE 2003). Some gels contain anaesthetic too. Inserting the gel directly into the urethra opens up and lubricates the length of the urethra. Lubricating the tip of the catheter only is ineffective as the lubricant is quickly wiped away on insertion. Wait for the time recommended by the manufacturer, usually 5 minutes.
11. Place a receiver with the catheter on the sterile towel between the patient's legs.
12. Expose the tip of the catheter by pulling off the top of the wrapper at the serrations.
13. Hold the catheter so that the distal end remains in the receiver and gradually advance it out of its wrapper in an upward and backward direction along the line of the urethra.
14. Advance the catheter 5–7 cm or until urine flows out of the catheter.

15. Advance the catheter a further 5 cm. Never force the catheter. If resistance is encountered stop and seek medical advice.
16. Inflate the balloon with the correct amount of sterile water, generally 10 mL for adults and 3–5 mL for children (NICE 2003). Incorrectly filled balloons can inflate irregularly and irritate the bladder mucosa (Wilson 1997).
17. Attach the urinary drainage bag, and make the patient comfortable.
18. Send a urine specimen if indicated and measure and record the urine collected.
19. Document the catheterisation in the patient's notes, including date of insertion, catheter size and amount of water used to inflate the balloon.

Box 8.8 Female urethral catheterisation: equipment and procedure

However, for people unable to maintain their own hygiene, nurses should carry this out, wearing gloves, and with a gentle and sensitive manner. Vigorous cleansing may increase the risk of infection (Pratt *et al.* 2001).

In both male and female patients, cleansing of the perineum and the area surrounding the catheter–meatal junction is essential after faecal incontinence, and should be carried out using clean wipes (Wilson 2001). For female patients, it is important to clean from front to back, thus preventing possible movement of bacteria from the anal area and perineum to the catheter–meatal junction. The catheter should be gently wiped in one direction, away from the vulva. In male patients the foreskin should be retracted before cleansing and the same principles of cleaning the catheter away from the catheter–meatal junction should be adhered to. The foreskin must be replaced afterwards. With a suprapubic catheter, once the wound has healed around the catheter, simple cleansing with soap and water is usually sufficient to maintain hygiene.

Emptying the catheter bag

Activity

You may recall that microorganisms can be introduced into the drainage system at the junction between the catheter and bag or via the drainage tap. Bearing this in mind try to work out the equipment you would need, and how you would use it, to safely empty a catheter bag.

Compare your answer with Box 8.9.

Unless hands are thoroughly washed between patients and a clean container used to collect the urine, microorganisms are readily transferred to the next patient. Although disinfection of hands with 70 per cent alcohol is rapid and effective, hands that are visibly soiled or potentially grossly contaminated with dirt or organic material must be washed with soap and water (see Chapter 3 section on 'Hand hygiene').

The urinary drainage bag should be emptied frequently enough to maintain urine flow and prevent reflux, and to prevent it becoming so heavy that its

Equipment

- Non-sterile gloves and apron, a heat disinfected or disposable container, e.g. a urinal or jug, paper towel to cover, alcohol swab.

Procedure

1. Explain the procedure to the patient. Some patients may prefer to be screened.
2. Wash hands and put on apron and gloves.
3. If the drainage bag is on a stand it may not need removing. If it is hanging on the bed, you may need to access it by removing the bag and placing it over the jug.
4. Clean the outlet port with alcohol swab and allow it to dry.
5. Open the port and drain the urine into the receptacle.
6. Close the port and wipe with alcohol swab.
7. Reposition bag.
8. Cover the container and take to sluice for disposal. Measure the urine first if a fluid balance chart is being kept.
9. The container should be disinfected, or macerated if disposable.
10. Remove gloves and apron and wash hands.

Box 8.9 Emptying a catheter bag: equipment and procedure

weight pulls on the catheter and causes urethral trauma. There is no evidence that bags need to be changed at specific intervals, but in addition to being changed when full, bags should also be changed when damaged or blocked with deposits.

In June's case she lives at home where the risks of cross-infection are low and bags can be reused for up to one week if rinsed with water and allowed to dry between use. However in hospital and other institutional settings patients should have a new bag each time it requires changing, including from day to night bag. Disconnection of the catheter from the drainage bag significantly increases the risk of introducing bacteria into the system and should therefore be avoided if possible (Wilson 2001).

According to recent advice, bags should be changed when clinically indicated and/or in line with the manufacturers' recommendations (NICE 2003; Pratt *et al.* 2001). But the key principle and the way in which to prevent bacteria or other harmful organisms entering the system, is to leave the closed system alone as much as you can. The National Institute for Clinical Excellence (2003) recommends that the connection between the catheter and the drainage system should not be broken except for sound clinical reasons.

Appropriate positioning of the catheter bag

Catheter bags should be positioned to avoid reflux and facilitate the use of gravity, and positioned clear of floors or other sources of contamination

(NICE 2003). Drainage bags should always be positioned below the level of the bladder and the catheter and the inlet tubing secured in a downward position (Macauley 1997). This is because reflux urine is associated with infection, so bags must be positioned to prevent back flow of urine. Where it is difficult to maintain the level of the bag below the bladder, for example when moving and handling, then clamp the urinary drainage bag tube and remove the clamp as soon as dependent drainage can be resumed (Pratt *et al.* 2001). The catheter itself should never be clamped as this can easily be damaged.

The catheter in females should be secured to prevent movement of the catheter within the urethra, which may introduce infection (Ayliffe *et al.* 2001). A variety of straps, 'net' sleeves, holsters and sporrans are available to suspend the drainage bag. Adding antiseptic or antimicrobial solutions into drainage bags is not recommended as clinical trials have shown these to be ineffective (Pratt *et al.* 2001).

Adequate fluid intake

If the patient's condition allows, encourage oral fluids. This has traditionally been believed to result in dilute urine containing fewer nutrients thus discouraging the growth of bacteria in the drainage bag and encrustation of components. In addition, it is thought that the larger volume of urine will maintain a constant flow through the drainage system and make it more difficult for bacteria to multiply in the drainage bag (Wilson 2001). Getliffe (2003) however asserts that there is no clear evidence that drinking large quantities of fluid will prevent infection, but in practice it remains seen as sensible to promote good fluid intake to prevent dehydration and constipation.

Catheter removal

■ Activity Taking into account what you have learned about the risks of urinary catheterisation, when do you think a catheter should be removed?

As mentioned above, the risk of infection increases with each additional day of catheterisation. Therefore urinary catheters should be removed as soon as possible (Department of Health 2003; NICE 2003). Ayliffe *et al.* (2001) advise that this should be within 5 days whenever possible.

■ Activity Imagine that June's catheter has become blocked and requires changing. Think about how you would prepare June, or any other patient, for catheter removal before inserting a new catheter.

A clear explanation should be given, emphasising that the procedure is not normally painful but that there may be a feeling of discomfort. Box 8.10 outlines equipment and key points for removing a catheter.

If a catheter is removed at the end of an episode of care, without insertion of a new catheter, Noble *et al.* (1990) suggest that the catheter should be removed

Equipment
- Disposable gloves and apron.
- A syringe of sufficient volume to remove the water from the balloon.
- The water capacity of the balloon is written on the catheter itself.
- A disposable absorbent pad.
- A receiver and a yellow waste bag.
- A specimen pot, a 20 mL syringe, needle and alcohol swab, if a catheter specimen of urine is required.

Procedure
1. Preparation: Give explanation, ensure privacy and position the person comfortably. For a female the knees and hips should be slightly flexed and apart.
2. Wash and dry hands and apply gloves and apron.
3. Obtain a specimen of urine from the sampling port if indicated (see Box 8.3).
4. Place the disposable pad under the patient's buttocks and then place the receiver between the thighs.
5. Check the balloon volume, and attach an appropriately sized syringe to the balloon port of the catheter. Withdraw the water from the balloon via the syringe.
6. Ask the patient to breathe in and out, and as they exhale, the catheter is gently withdrawn and placed in the receiver. If problems are encountered, stop and seek medical advice.
7. Remove gloves and apron and wash hands.
8. The patient should be made comfortable and because frequency may be experienced the nurse should ensure that a toilet or commode is close by. If the patient needs help with mobility, ensure a call bell is nearby.
9. Document the date and time of catheter removal in the clinical notes and record the amount of urine in the catheter bag.
10. The patient may be encouraged to increase fluid intake to 'flush' out the bladder.
11. Monitor whether the person is passing urine satisfactorily. A chart may be kept so that frequency and amount can be monitored. Also ask the patient to inform a nurse if any unusual symptoms are experienced, e.g. dysuria (pain when passing urine).

Box 8.10 Removal of a urethral catheter: equipment and procedure

at midnight rather than the traditional time of first thing in the morning. This increases the length of time before passing urine, leading to a greater initial volume and a faster return to normal voiding, decreasing levels of anxiety. It is important to ensure that urine is passed satisfactorily after catheter removal.

Additionally in those people who do not have a new catheter inserted observe for problems such as incontinence, frequency and retention. A person who is confused may well need prompting to pass urine (see section on promoting continence, later in this chapter). Some people, particularly men who have had prostate surgery, will need to perform pelvic floor exercises to help them to regain control (see section on pelvic floor exercises later in this chapter). In some patients who have a long-term catheter for specific medical reasons, like June, removing the catheter altogether is unlikely to be an option. It will, however, need changing periodically depending upon clinical need, such as any problems experienced, and/or in line with manufacturers' recommendations (Pratt *et al.* 2001). Removal of the old catheter is a procedure that needs to be undertaken with care.

Summary

- Urinary catheterisation is experienced by many patients/clients and may be a short-term or long-term measure.
- Catheterisation is an invasive procedure and there are many complications associated with it, infection being particularly common. Therefore catheterisation should only be performed if there is a clear indication, strict asepsis should be maintained, and the catheter should be removed as soon as possible, using the correct technique.
- Nurses should be aware of the different types of equipment available, and make appropriate choices in relation to types of catheter and drainage bag.
- The closed system should not be broken except for good clinical reasons.
- Care should be taken to reduce physical and psychological discomfort for people with urinary catheters.

Getliffe (2003) has reviewed the literature extensively and covers catheterisation in depth. Further reading from this source is recommended.

USE OF ENEMAS AND SUPPOSITORIES

An enema is a liquid which is inserted into the rectum, while a suppository is a medicated solid formulation, usually torpedo-shaped, and is inserted into the rectum, where it will dissolve at body temperature. As will be discussed below, there are a number of indications for these procedures. However, if being given for constipation, it should be remembered that preventing constipation, for example through increasing dietary fibre, fluids and physical exercise, is preferable to the use of suppositories or enemas.

LEARNING OUTCOMES

By the end of this section you will be able to:

1. Identify the reasons for administering an enema or a suppository.
2. Show awareness of the precautions to be taken into account prior to administering an enema or a suppository.
3. Understand the principles to follow when administering suppositories and enemas.

Learning outcome 1: Identify the reasons for administering an enema or suppository

Activity

> An enema may be prescribed as a treatment for constipation, to prepare the bowel for investigations or surgery, or to administer medicines. When do you think an enema would be described as an evacuant enema and when as a retention enema?

If the purpose of the enema is to retain the solution for a specified period of time, this is generally referred to as a retention enema. It is primarily used for its local effect, for example a steroid enema may be administered to people with ulcerative colitis, for its anti-inflammatory effect. If the enema is to be expelled within a few minutes, along with faecal matter and flatus, this is called an evacuant enema. Thus this type of enema would be used for constipation or to empty the bowel prior to surgery or investigations of the gastrointestinal tract.

As explained above, June has had problems with constipation due to her impaired mobility (see Chapter 5) and her loss of sensation is a further factor, so suppositories, and occasional enemas, have become an established part of her care. James, being in hospital and confined to bed is experiencing reduced exercise alongside a changed diet. His usual bowel elimination habits are also altered and these factors make him susceptible to constipation. Additionally, medication alone or a number of medicines taken together can cause constipation. For example, codeine and its derivatives are known to cause constipation (www.bnf.org). These are common analgesics which might well be prescribed for James, making him more at risk of constipation. Many nursing guidelines, especially in respect of the care of older people, fail to acknowledge this (Annells and Koch 2002).

Suppositories are often administered for evacuant purposes too. However they are also a commonly used route to administer medication, and may be administered as a local treatment, as for haemorrhoids.

Activity

> Examples of drugs that are commonly prescribed rectally include paracetamol (for its analgesic and/or anti-pyretic effect) and anti-convulsants. What do you think are the advantages and disadvantages of this route of drug administration?

You might have thought of the following advantages:

- The rectum is an alternative route for when people cannot take the drug orally because they are vomiting, unable to swallow (as an unconscious person or someone who has had a CVA) or is nil by mouth for other reasons such as pre-operatively. For example, the rectal route would be appropriate for a child with a high temperature who must have their temperature reduced to prevent the risk of a **febrile convulsion** but is vomiting so cannot be given the anti-pyretic orally.

- The rectum is very vascular and drugs are absorbed rapidly via this route, as they avoid liver metabolism (Addison *et al.* 2000). For example, if a person is fitting, they cannot take the drug orally. Rectal absorption will be more rapid than by intramuscular injection, which could also be dangerous to administer safely to a person who is fitting. Note that faecal impaction can inhibit absorption of drugs via the rectal route, and therefore constipation should be prevented in people who might require emergency use of the rectal route.

Febrile convulsion
A convulsion (fit) that may occur in a young child who has a rapid elevation of temperature.

Disadvantages you thought of might include:

- Administration of enemas and suppositories is more invasive and embarrassing than oral administration, and involves some discomfort, undressing and movement, i.e. into the correct position.
- Schmelzer and Wright's (1996) review of the literature notes that there have been a number of traumatic and even fatal side effects of enemas reported, including inflammation, electrolyte imbalance and perforation of the colonic mucosa. Newer, pre-packaged enemas aim to prevent many of these potential problems. Nevertheless medication is only administered rectally if it is clearly indicated, and an enema would only be used if there is no alternative.
- Faecal impaction and diarrhoea are contraindications (Kay 2000).
- In addition, Kay (2000) notes that due to sexual taboos about anal penetration, there is reluctance to administer drugs rectally. She advises that, particularly with older children and adolescents, great sensitivity should be shown. Guidelines from the Royal College of Nursing (2003a) recommend that enemas and suppositories should only be administered to children and young people to manage constipation in exceptional circumstances.

Learning outcome 2: Show awareness of the precautions to be taken into account prior to administering an enema or a suppository

Prior to administering an enema or suppository the nurse should carefully assess the appropriateness of this route.

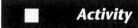

    Can you think of any physical problems which might be contraindications?

Anal fissure

A painful crack in the mucous membrane of the anus, generally caused by hard faeces.

Rectal prolapse

Protrusion of rectal mucosa through the anus.

Contraindications might include: recent colorectal or gynaecological surgery, malignancy or other pathology of the perineal area, and a low platelet count, as this would predispose to bleeding. Thus the nurse should check with both the patient and the case notes for any previous ano-rectal surgery or abnormalities. Further checks should also be made visually immediately prior to administration. The peri-anal region should be checked for abnormalities including haemorrhoids, **anal fissure** and **rectal prolapse**.

Digital rectal examinations and manual removal of faeces – should they be done?

It is sometimes recommended that a digital rectal examination (DRE) is carried out to check for faecal impaction, and for abnormalities such as blood, pain or obstruction. Manual removal of faeces, using a lubricated, gloved finger inserted into the rectum, is sometimes part of a patient's bowel regime, as it is for June. However, there has been increasing concern about nurses carrying out these procedures, particularly as there have been cases of professional misconduct involving the inappropriate use of DREs and manual evacuation of faeces in frail older people (Willis 2000). The issues have particularly concerned lack of consent to DRE by patients. These procedures are invasive and should only be carried out if necessary and after individual assessment (Royal College of Nursing 2003b).

Many organisations are now developing policies and guidelines on these procedures and the Royal College of Nursing has published a document to guide nurses, which covers all aspects in detail including issues of consent (Royal College of Nursing 2003b). A further document discusses these issues specifically in relation to children and young people (Royal College of Nursing 2003a). It is strongly advised that you, as a student, only carry out a DRE if it is agreed under local policy, the patient has explicitly consented to the procedure, and you are under the supervision of the registered nurse. Consent to DRE or manual removal of faeces (which is necessary for a small number of people with neurological disorders such as spinal injury) should be clearly documented in the nursing records (Willis 2000).

Learning outcome 3: Understand the principles to follow when administering suppositories and enemas

Choice of enemas/suppositories

This is straightforward if you are administering prescribed medication. However, when giving an enema or suppositories for evacuation purposes, there can be a choice of products. Local drug policies may vary as to whether these need to be prescribed. Often they can be administered at a registered nurse's discretion.

Activity Find out what types of enemas and suppositories are available to evacuate the bowel. There may be examples in the skills laboratory, or you can look at them in your practice setting.

Suppositories may be of the type that will simply soften the stools, or they may have a stimulant effect. Trounce (2000) recommends that glycerol suppositories are satisfactory, and others offer no advantage. There are microenemas available containing only 5 mL of solution which act as a colon stimulant. For more vigorous bowel cleansing (for example prior to a bowel investigation) a larger phosphate enema may be used. It is important to check the manufacturer's instructions when using these as there are a number of contraindications, and they are unsuitable for older or debilitated patients (Addison *et al.* 2000). They can be given for occasional constipation, but should not be given regularly. They are also not recommended in children under 3 years, and should only be given to children aged 3–12 years with medical direction.

Administration

The procedure will need careful explanation to the patient, or child and family, including the likely effects. Addison *et al.* (2000) advises that consent must be obtained, otherwise the procedure can constitute assault and lead to legal proceedings. There are exceptions to this, however, for example in a life-threatening situation such as when an unconscious person is fitting. Note that some patients may prefer to insert a suppository themselves. If so, the nurse must carefully explain the procedure and be on hand to give assistance if required. Privacy and sensitivity when administering enemas and suppositories are very important. Kay (2000) recommends that for a child, a chaperone, preferably a parent, should be present.

If the enema or suppositories are being given to evacuate the bowel, the patient/client will need to have their bowels open quite rapidly after administration. As discussed previously, if possible the person should be helped to the toilet. The more familiar environment of the toilet will be particularly helpful for someone who is confused and disorientated, or for a person with a learning disability. Otherwise, a commode is preferable to using a bedpan as it promotes a more conducive position for elimination. Safety and hygiene needs must be taken into consideration; see first section in this chapter ('Assisting with elimination') for detailed discussion.

Schmelzer and Wright's (1996) study of enema administration used in-depth interviews with 24 nurses who were highly experienced in enema administration. They found that the use of interpersonal skills to gain co-operation was emphasised. The nurses suggested honesty, asking about previous experiences of enema administration, describing expected sensations, warning about discomfort, showing patients equipment, and teaching relaxation techniques. With children, the nurses used distraction, including singing and looking at colourful pictures. Schmelzer and Wright (1996) suggest that enema technique has evolved through trial and error rather than systematic research, and their thorough review of the literature identifies much conflicting advice,

Equipment

- An absorbent under pad, tissues, lubricating gel, the enema or suppository/ies, gloves and apron.
- Ensure that a good light source is available and that privacy can be maintained.

Procedure

1. If the enema or suppository/ies are being given as medication they will be prescribed and therefore the checking and documenting procedures as per the local drug policy should be adhered to (see Chapter 4).
2. Maintain infection control procedures throughout: handwashing, use of gloves and aprons, and correct waste disposal (see Chapter 3).
3. Give explanations, encouragement, reassurance and feedback, and maintain privacy (Schmelzer and Wright 1996).
4. Some enemas need to be warmed before administration – check the manufacturer's instructions. Warming can be done by placing the enema in a jug of warm water. The temperature should be slightly higher than body temperature, feeling warm to the wrist (Schmelzer and Wright 1996).
5. Position the person on the left side to allow easy flow of the fluid into the rectum by following the anatomy of the patient. Place the under-pad under the patient's buttocks, and ask them to lie at the edge of the bed with knees flexed, and covered by a blanket. This position will aid the passage of the nozzle of the enema through the anal canal. This position may need adapting for someone with a physical disability.
6. Examine the perianal area.
7. Only perform digital rectal examination if: (a) the procedure is specifically indicated (e.g. the need to check for faecal impaction, on which suppositories would have minimal impact), (b) if it is agreed under local policy that it can be performed by nurses, and (c) if explicit consent has been given by the patient. A digital examination involves lubricating the index finger and gently inserting it into the rectum to check whether there is faecal impaction.
8. **Enemas**: Expel any air from the enema container, because if introduced into the colon this can cause distension and discomfort. Then lubricate the nozzle of the enema. Some enemas have a pre-lubricated tip. Part the buttocks and gently insert into the anal canal. Squeeze the fluid gently into the rectum from the base of the container in order to prevent backflow. Some enemas include one-way valves which prevent backflow. Then slowly withdraw the container nozzle to avoid reflux emptying of the rectum. Clean the perianal area and make the patient comfortable.

9. **Suppositories**: Lubricate the end of the suppository with the gel. Insert the suppository blunt end foremost into the anal canal. This allows the lower edge of the contracting sphincter to close tightly around the anus. Inserting the blunt end foremost also makes it easier to retain the suppository and aids patient comfort (Abd El Maeboud *et al.* 1991). Wipe the patient's perianal area.

10. If the enema or suppository/ies were given to empty the bowel, ask the patient to retain it inside for as long as possible (Schmelzer and Wright 1996). Often the patient will find it more comfortable to remain lying down. An enema, however, can be very difficult to hold onto for long as the effect is likely to be rapid. The person should be assisted to the toilet or other receptacle as necessary.

11. Medication administered as a suppository should be retained by the patient. With a retention enema, the patient should remain lying down for the amount of time prescribed on the manufacturer's instructions. A call bell must be near at hand.

12. Document that the enema/suppository/ies have been administered in the nursing notes or prescription chart if a medication. If the enema or suppositories were given to empty the bowel you will need to note the result.

Box 8.11 Administration of enemas and suppositories: equipment and procedure

and many areas which need additional research. For example, they found that most nursing texts suggest positioning patients on their left side due to the anatomy of the colon, but there are some research articles to support the right side.

Based on the evidence available, principles to follow for safe administration of suppositories/enemas can be found in Box 8.11.

Summary

- Suppositories or enemas may be given to administer medication or to evacuate the bowel.
- Careful assessment should precede administration as there are contraindications.
- Preparation of the patient/client should include explanation and gaining consent, correct choice of enema/suppositories and other equipment, maintenance of dignity and privacy, and correct positioning of the person to prevent damage to the wall of the rectum.
- If the enema or suppositories were given to evacuate the bowel, assistance to reach the toilet, or other receptacle if necessary, must be given.

PROMOTION OF CONTINENCE, AND MANAGEMENT OF INCONTINENCE

The Department of Health defines **incontinence** as 'the involuntary or inappropriate passing of urine and/or faeces that has an impact on social functioning or hygiene. It also includes nocturnal enuresis (bedwetting)' (Department of Health 2000, p. 7). In children, incontinence is considered to be the involuntary discharge of urine or faeces in a child over 5 years. **Primary enuresis** describes a state when bladder control has never been achieved, while **secondary enuresis** occurs if the child has a period of bladder control for at least a year, and then relapses. In children the term **encopresis** is usually used for the passage of a normal consistency stool in a socially unacceptable place (Lukeman 2003).

Continence care is one of the eight aspects of care chosen for best practice benchmarking in *The Essence of Care* (Department of Health 2001b), highlighting that it is a fundamental aspect of patient care. This section focuses on developing understanding of the causes and effects of incontinence and practical issues of management, but not specialist interventions; incontinence is a huge topic to which whole books are devoted.

LEARNING OUTCOMES

By the end of this section, you will be able to:

1. Identify the causes and prevalence of urinary and faecal incontinence.
2. Show insight into the potential psycho-social and physical effects of incontinence.
3. Demonstrate understanding into how incontinence might be assessed.
4. Identify appropriate nursing interventions for the promotion of continence.
5. Discuss how incontinence can be managed.

Learning outcome 1: Identify the causes and prevalence of urinary and faecal incontinence

Continence is a complex skill, which relies on hormonal, muscular and neurological control, and requires elaborate interplay between the individual and the environment (Nazarko 1997). Children achieve continence by learning a complex sequence of events, and being able to co-ordinate both voluntary and involuntary actions (Stanley 1996). Achieving bladder control depends on the child's neuromuscular and cognitive development, the manner in which potty training is undertaken, the personality of the child and the emotional environment of the family (Campbell and Glasper 1995). The age at which bladder control is achieved varies widely in different countries, but in the UK bladder control is usually expected by the age of 4–5 years. Continence relies on being able to recognise the need to eliminate faeces and/or urine, being able to identify an appropriate place in which to eliminate and being able to wait until arriving there. When any of these fail, incontinence results.

| **Activity** | Reflect back on patients/clients that you have been in contact with. From your experience, what are the causes of urinary and faecal incontinence? |

Causes are diverse and varied – see Table 8.3 for a summary of causes and types. Medication can also play a part in causing incontinence, for example diuretics

Table 8.3 Summary of causes and types of incontinence

Urinary incontinence (adapted from Colley 1996)

Type	Description	Causes
Stress	Urine leakage associated with, for example, coughing, sneezing or exercise	Weakness of the sphincter mechanism. Most common in women, e.g. after childbirth. Can occur in men after a prostatectomy
Urge	Leakage occurring with urgency – little or no warning of the need to void. Symptoms of frequency and nocturnal enuresis may accompany	Detrusor instability (motor urgency) due to, e.g. bladder neck obstruction, or hypersensitive detrusor muscle (sensory urgency) due to infection or bladder stones for example
Overflow	Urinary leakage caused by incomplete bladder emptying	May be due to: • Outflow obstruction: e.g. by faecal impaction • An atonic or hypotonic bladder (one which does not produce adequate detrusor contraction for micturition) e.g. in diabetic neuropathy • Detrusor-sphincter dyssynergia (lack of co-ordination between detrusor contraction and relaxation during bladder emptying), e.g. in spinal injury
Functional	Bladder emptying when the person is unable to reach the toilet, adjust/remove clothing, and use it appropriately	Physical impairment (e.g. lack of mobility or dexterity) or mental impairment such as confusion. An unconducive environment and unsupportive carers also contribute

Faecal incontinence (Jensen 1997)

Group 1	People with intact anal function, e.g. CVA, diarrhoea, faecal impaction	
Group 2	People with compromised anal sphincter function, e.g. congenital malformation or obstetric trauma	

appear to predispose to urge incontinence (Roe and Williams 1994), and as you read, John's incontinence was caused by clozapine.

According to McCreanor *et al.* (1998), stress and urge incontinence are the two main types of urinary incontinence, and may occur together – 'mixed' incontinence. Nazarko (1997) notes that the environment in a nursing home may not promote continence as the corridors can be long and confusing, and the message portrayed may be that incontinence is expected. Schnozzle *et al.* (1998) identify that in nursing homes immobility and dementia are the primary risk factors for incontinence. The problem is compounded as impaired mobility is associated with constipation, which in turn increases the risk of UTI and urge incontinence (Nazarko 1997), and constipation can also lead on to overflow faecal incontinence. For an immobile person such as June these are potential problems.

In people with a learning disability, for example Ian, a combination of factors may affect the learning and maintenance of continence; these include physical, psychological, social and environmental factors (Stanley 1996). People with learning disabilities can take time to orientate themselves to an unfamiliar environment, and incontinence can result if they don't know, or can't remember, where the toilet is. When Ian is admitted to hospital, the nurses will need to understand this and try to orientate him to the ward. People with a physical disability may not be able to independently reach and use the toilet, and if carers do not assist effectively, functional incontinence results. Robinson (2000) cites a nursing home resident saying 'When I have to go and I'm sitting in the wheelchair, and I'm wheeling my chair, and I can't do it fast enough, I wet my pants'. This is an example of probable urge incontinence, compounded by functional incontinence. People with a learning as well as a physical disability may not be able to communicate that they need to be taken to the toilet, especially if staff are not familiar with their method of communicating this need, which may be through signing or symbols.

To accurately assess the underlying cause and therefore possible management of incontinence, a thorough assessment is necessary. This is considered in learning outcome 3.

Prevalence

Box 8.12 shows some statistics about the prevalence of incontinence from the Department of Health (2000).

Activity   Why might it be difficult to accurately identify the prevalence of incontinence?

People may be too embarrassed or ashamed to report their incontinence. This is unfortunate as it has been claimed that 70 per cent of incontinence sufferers can be cured while the remaining 30 per cent can benefit from proper management (Chester 1998). Chester (1998) claims that incontinence is a taboo subject and that

Urinary incontinence

Women living at home	15–44 years: between 1 in 20 and 1 in 14
	45–64 years: between 1 in 13 and 1 in 7
	Aged 65 years plus: between 1 in 10 and 1 in 5
Men living at home	15–64 years: over 1 in 33
	Aged 65 years plus: between 1 in 14 and 1 in 10
Both sexes living in institutions	1 in 3 in residential homes
	Nearly 2 in 3 in nursing homes
	1/2 to 2/3 in wards for older people or older people with mental health problems
Children	1 in 6 of children over 5 years
	1 in 7 of children aged 7 years
	1 in 11 of children aged 9 years
	1 in 50 of teenagers

Faecal incontinence

Adults	1% of adults living at home
	17% of older people
	25% of adults living in institutions
Children	4–5 years: 1 in 30 children
	5–6 years: 1 in 50 children
	7–10 years: 1 in 75 children
	11–12 years: 1 in 100 children

Box 8.12 The prevalence of incontinence (Department of Health 2000)

while people are willing to discuss their struggle against cancer or alcoholism, they will be much less likely to talk about their incontinence. Mason *et al.* (2001) found that women with stress incontinence following childbirth were reluctant to seek help although they were inconvenienced and troubled by it. Alternatively, people may not report their incontinence because they are unaware that there might be help available. Also people's definitions of incontinence vary so they may not interpret their problem as incontinence. Bush *et al.* (2001) found that almost half of the women they surveyed believed urinary incontinence was normal. A study involving nursing home residents found they considered that urinary incontinence was an inevitable part of ageing (Robinson 2000). However urinary incontinence is not a disease or a normal result of ageing, but a symptom of an underlying condition. Young people and children may view incontinence as a condition of older people, causing reluctance to seek help (Mahoney 1997).

Learning outcome 2: Show insight into the potential psycho-social and physical effects of incontinence

You have read that John was both distressed and embarrassed about his urinary incontinence.

 Activity

> Consider for a minute the situation for Ian, who is usually continent at home but is now in the unfamiliar environment of a hospital ward. It is night time and no carer from his unit has been able to stay. He knows that he needs to go to the toilet, but he does not know where it is, and cannot communicate with the nurses to ask where the toilet is. Consequently he is incontinent. How might Ian feel?

You probably identified both physical effects, such as discomfort, and psychological distress too. There are also many social consequences of incontinence and all these effects have been documented (see Table 8.4). Nurses need to be

Table 8.4 Possible psycho-social and physical effects of incontinence

Effect	Source
Increase in falls	Smith 1998, Brown *et al.* 2000
Increase in UTIs	Smith 1998
Skin problems	Robinson 2000, Department of Health 2000
Adverse effect on psychological status and socialisation	Smith 1998, Robinson 2000
Embarrassment	Cochran 1999, Koch and Kelly 1999
Depression, isolation and adverse effects on self-esteem	Chiverton *et al.* 1996
Distress	Koch and Kelly 1999
Adverse effect on relationships, employment and social activities	Norton 1997, Department of Health 2000
Trigger older people's admission to care homes	Department of Health 2000
Leads to children being bullied	Department of Health 2000
Added workload for carers of people with learning disabilities	Stanley 1997
Greater likelihood of admission to long-term care for people with learning disabilities	Stanley 1997
Social undervaluing of people with learning disabilities	Stanley 1997
Adversely affects quality of life and choices on leaving school for children with learning disabilities	Rogers 1998
Catastrophic reactions in people with early or middle-stage Alzheimer's disease	Hutchinson *et al.* 1996

sensitive to how incontinence can affect people and consider this during their assessment and care for people with continence problems.

Learning outcome 3: Demonstrate understanding into how incontinence might be assessed

As discussed under learning outcome 1 there are many possible underlying causes of incontinence. The key to continence promotion is an effective assessment (Nazarko 1999). Without careful assessment, people may employ inappropriate self-help strategies, such as fluid intake reduction (Koch *et al.* 2000; Robinson 2000). Temporary causes of incontinence, such as UTI, confusion, medication, faecal impaction, impaired mobility and depression, should be identified. In John's case, staff investigated further the side effects of clozapine and discovered that incontinence was a recognised side effect but it was also important that their assessment included a urinalysis. Mason *et al.* (2001) found that women with urinary incontinence following childbirth wanted health professionals to be proactive about asking them if they had bladder problems because the women were reluctant to broach the subject. The Department of Health in *The Essence of Care* (2001b) advises that a trigger question should be asked at all initial contacts with patients; for example 'Does your bladder or bowel ever cause you a problem?' If the answer is 'Yes' then an initial bladder or bowel continence assessment should be offered.

Activity

Assessment includes interviewing, observation and measurement. Keeping these in mind, think about how a nurse might assess incontinence. Have you seen any specific assessment documents used in practice for assessment of incontinence?

Box 8.13 identifies some key points, and these are expanded below.

Many practice settings have a specific incontinence assessment tool that will help nurses to identify both the cause and possible management of incontinence. Examples of these are given by Getliffe and Dolman (2003). The Department of Health (2001b) advises that the assessment should be carried out by a 'suitably trained individual' and should include a review of symptoms and their effect on quality of life, physical examination (for example perineum), urinalysis, and assessment of manual dexterity and environment. If a UTI is suspected, following the urinalysis, a urine specimen should be sent for microscopy and culture.

Nazarko (1999) suggests that the following questions will be useful when interviewing people:

- What is the patient's problem?
- What is causing the problem?
- What solutions are available?
- Who is the best person to provide those solutions?
- What outcome does the patient want?
- How can we meet the patient's needs?

- Use of an assessment tool will promote a systematic approach
- Referral to a continence advisor may be needed

Interviewing

- Sensitive, empathetic approach
- Careful and appropriate use of language
- Involvement of carers

Observation

- Physical factors, e.g. obstructive symptoms
- Psychological factors, e.g. confusion
- Environmental factors, e.g. access to toilet

Measurement

- Urinalysis
- Charting frequency and amount

Box 8.13 Assessment of continence: some key points

Interviewing skills

When using interviewing skills to assess incontinence, approach and terminology used need careful consideration. Woodward (1996) reports that people often see incontinence as a taboo subject and need permission from nurses to discuss it, but nurses must remain sensitive to people's need for privacy and dignity. Cochran (1999) found that the term 'incontinence' was not a term used by older people and that it is preferable to ask 'Do you have bladder control problems?' or 'Do you leak?' Woodward (1996) also stresses the importance of terming questions clearly in understandable terms, for example the term 'frequency' may not be understood; it is preferable to ask: 'How often do you go to the toilet to pass urine during the day?'

Cognitive impairment

For cognitively impaired adults who may be unable to give a clear history, Thompson and Smith (1998) give useful hints for assessing incontinence, emphasising the importance of observing for clues to indicate frequency and severity, and involving carers in assessment. Nurses can observe clients voiding, noting signs of pain, obstructive symptoms, such as hesitancy, intermittent stream, dribbling after voiding and straining to void, urge symptoms, and functional barriers, such as being unable to undress.

Learning disability

Shaw (1998) asserts that continence problems in people with a learning disability have often gone untreated, as there is an assumption that they cannot acquire the skills for continence, and an accurate assessment (including urology referral) has not been done. However the white paper *Valuing People* (Department of Health 2001a) makes it clear that people with learning disabilities must have equal access to all services and the responsibility lies with primary care to ensure that people with learning disabilities can access services, like those for promoting continence. The **health facilitator** must empower their client to access such services and, where appropriate, continence will be addressed in the individual's Health Action Plan.

Health facilitator
A member of the community learning disabilities team (often a nurse) who supports a person with learning disabilities to access the health care they need. See *Valuing People* (Department of Health 2001a).

A proper assessment means that signs of detrusor instability can be identified and treated with medication, prior to commencing bladder training (Shaw 1998). People with a physical disability and a communication difficulty may know when they want to go to the toilet, but carers will not be able to recognise this need if a method of communication has not been established. Thus Stanley (1997) explains that incontinence in people with a learning disability should be assessed by carrying out a functional analysis, considering the person, their situation or environment, and the significant people in their life. Stanley (1997) emphasises that this individualistic approach is complex, and requires careful observation and a good knowledge about the person and their life; a number of structured instruments are available to help the assessment. Assessment of children with learning disabilities must take into account developmental level, assessing motor, cognitive and language development (Rogers 1998).

Assessing faecal incontinence

For faecal incontinence assessment, Jensen (1997) advises that history taking should address the duration of faecal leakage, current bowel management, and type, frequency, amount and duration of the faecal incontinence and how it affects lifestyle. She also suggests that physical factors (such as mobility and dexterity), environmental factors (such as access to the toilet) and psychological factors (such as motivation and cognition), should be assessed.

Referrals

Some people with urinary and/or faecal incontinence require a more specialist assessment and so need to be referred to the continence service, to see a continence specialist nurse for example. Specialist investigations are sometimes necessary, such as urodynamics.

The Department of Health (2000) recommends that everyone should have access to integrated continence services managed by a director of continence services (normally a specialist continence nurse or physiotherapist). This has been reinforced by targets set in the *National Service Framework for Older People* (Department of Health 2001c).

Activity | Find out about the continence services in your area, and how referrals are made.

Learning outcome 4: Identify appropriate nursing interventions for the promotion of continence

After assessment, appropriate interventions can be planned. Complete remission may not be achievable, but at least a reduction in incontinence leading to a more controllable situation may be possible (Steeman and Defever 1998). Emphasis in this section is on selected nursing interventions to promote continence. However it is useful to be aware that treatment for incontinence can include surgery and pharmacology (Steeman and Defever 1998), and biofeedback (Jensen 1997). Intermittent catheterisation is also used to maintain continence by some people and can be taught to people or their carers. As you read earlier, this approach was tried for June but unfortunately was not successful.

Activity From previous experience, write down any methods that nurses can use to promote urinary and faecal continence.

Promotion of urinary continence

How continence is promoted obviously depends on the underlying cause and that is why an understanding of causes and careful assessment is important. The Department of Health (2000) recommends general advice about healthy living, including diet and drinking appropriate fluids. Smith (1998) reports that enthusiasm and commitment of staff can be very helpful in promoting continence, and also emphasises that nurses should refer patients and liaise with the multidisciplinary team as appropriate. Physiotherapists can help with mobility and balance, enabling quicker transfers. Occupational therapists help with making the environment and dressing and undressing easier. Clothing adaptations, such as replacing trouser zips or buttons with Velcro, can be helpful. Vickerman (2003) asserts that many people are rendered incontinent by a poorly adapted environment and goes on to explain that the heights of chairs, beds and toilets should be assessed and adjusted, as well as considering lighting, signs, floor coverings, grab rails and provision of commodes and hand-held urinals.

Two specific interventions, which you may have identified, are: pelvic floor exercises and bladder re-education.

Pelvic floor exercises

Pelvic floor exercises (PFEs) aim to strengthen the pubococcygeal muscle, resulting in increased urethral closure pressure and stronger reflex contractions when there is a sudden rise in intra-abdominal pressure, such as when sneezing (Dolman 2003). It is thought that strengthening pelvic floor muscles improves a person's ability to hold on until reaching the toilet, and so they may be useful in urge incontinence too. Hay-Smith *et al.*'s (2003) review of PFEs for urinary incontinence in women concluded that they appear to be an effective treatment for women with stress or mixed incontinence but their use in urge incontinence is unclear, with more trials needed. Dougherty's (1998) literature review on

PFEs gives specific detail about all aspects of this complex subject, and Dolman (2003) also covers the topic in depth.

A PFE protocol needs to be clear and specific, addressing the frequency, how many to be done, the duration of each contraction, and the rest phase between repetitions (Dougherty 1998). The PFE regimen may be prescribed for a set period of weeks, followed by a maintenance plan. Clients should also be advised to squeeze these muscles if they feel the need to cough or sneeze, so that it becomes almost an automatic reaction in circumstances where stress incontinence might occur.

Bladder re-education

This involves re-educating the bladder to an improved pattern of voiding and has a number of variations, suitable for different client groups. When these programmes are in use for clients it is essential that all staff are fully aware, and are motivated towards them, so that they are implemented consistently.

- **Bladder training**: This aims to gradually extend the interval between voiding, with voiding being initiated by the clock, rather than desire to void (Anders 1999). For example, the person might initially be asked to go to the toilet every hour, and then this is gradually extended by half an hour at a time. Education of patients and carers, use of a continence chart and continuous encouragement are all important elements. Carers need to praise to build up confidence and reinforce behaviour, and to be patient and understanding. There is some evidence to support its success with urge incontinence (Roe *et al.* 2003) but more evidence is needed.
- **Timed voiding**: This is often used for people with a neurogenic bladder, such as those with spinal cord lesions, and for people with a physical/mental disability. It entails voiding at fixed times, which can include techniques to trigger voiding, such as tapping over the supra-pubic region, or running water.
- **Habit retraining**: This involves developing an individualised toileting schedule (Anders 1999). Initially a person might be encouraged not to use the toilet between fixed 2-hourly intervals unless they need to. A record of voiding and incontinent episodes is kept so that the schedule can be adjusted, with voiding intervals lengthened if the person is dry, and reduced if incontinence occurs.
- **Prompted voiding**: This involves prompting a person to void at regular intervals, but only taking them to the toilet if their response is positive. Evidence for this method was reviewed by Eustice *et al.* (2003), who concluded that it appears to be beneficial for older people in the short term but more research is needed. Prompted voiding has been used with people with learning disabilities, and might be an appropriate strategy for Ian, in the unfamiliar environment of the hospital ward. Ian's carers would be able to advise about this. It is also used with cognitively impaired adults, where

the underlying cause of incontinence is often functional and/or urge incontinence (Thompson and Smith 1998). However, this is not without difficulty, depending on the client variables: degree of confusion, physical mobility, and affective response (Hutchinson *et al.* 1996). As dementia progresses, timed voiding with a toileting schedule will be more suitable than prompted voiding (Hutchinson *et al.* 1996). Smith (1998) outlines a number of tips when using prompted voiding with people with dementia:

- Have the word 'toilet' on the door with a picture
- Increase environmental safety, e.g. hand rails
- Use simple verbal or behavioural clues
- Use pleasant distraction such as singing
- Keep to a routine and, where possible, a familiar nurse
- Use easy to remove clothes
- Stay pleasant and avoid hurrying or confrontation.

Behavioural techniques

Behavioural techniques to promote continence in people with learning disabilities must include assessing the client's baseline ability, then performing a task analysis, identifying a sequence of manageable steps to be learnt and what prompts will be needed at each stage (Stanley 1997). These techniques are explained in more depth by Stanley (1997). Smith and Smith (2003) examine continence training for people with learning disabilities in detail.

Continence promotion for children

Management of enuresis and encopresis with children are considered in detail by Lukeman (2003). Rogers (1998) gives useful suggestions in relation to toilet training in children with learning disabilities. Preparation for toilet training could include using a doll and a potty, and books. The family will need to be supported in developing a routine which fits with school and home, and any success must be praised. Day time wetting alarms (which raise the child's awareness of being wet) and star and reward charts may help to motivate. Rogers (1998) advises that lack of success should lead to abandonment of the programme, and then retrying three months later. A systematic review indicated that simple behavioural methods like star charts and waking children at night to urinate can be effective for some children but further trials are needed (Glazener and Evans 2002a). The same reviewers concluded that alarms are an effective treatment for nocturnal enuresis in children (Glazener and Evans 2002b).

Promotion of faecal continence

The range of treatments for faecal incontinence is sparse – most focus on surgery and there is little nursing research into this problem (Norton 1997). However one study found biofeedback to have a high success rate in treating faecal incontinence with 43 per cent regarding themselves as cured and 24 per cent as improved (Norton and Kamm 1999). This technique can be used by specialist nurses or physiotherapists. It involves techniques used to bring under conscious control bodily processes usually considered to be beyond voluntary command (Jensen 1997). Medication, such as loperamide, may help to slow bowel transit and solidify the stool. Norton (1997) highlights that staff attitude to faecal incontinence is crucial, and that much is preventable amongst older dependent people, with proper attention to diet, fluids, mobility, medication and establishment of bowel habit.

Diet and activity

Jensen (1997) advises that mild faecal incontinence may be eliminated by changes to diet and activity level. Clients should thus be encouraged to take regular, well-timed meals, which include adequate fibre and fluids, in order to promote a soft, well-formed stool. Mild exercise optimises gastrointestinal function.

Developing a pattern

People with intact sensation and normal sphincter function should be encouraged to try to establish a regular pattern for defaecation to maximise the potential benefit from the gastrocolic reflex; they should also be encouraged to respond promptly to the need to defaecate (Jensen 1997). Thus where help is needed from the nurse, such as taking the patient to the toilet, the nurse should respond promptly to requests. When normal sensation and sphincter function is compromised (such as in people who have spinal injuries), a programme to establish stimulation by using suppositories or enemas will be needed. Doughty (1996) reviews such programmes in detail. Clearly such a regime has been established for June.

Learning outcome 5: Discuss how incontinence can be managed

Incontinence should be managed in a manner that is unobtrusive, reliable and comfortable. Thus incontinence aids should preserve hygiene, psychological and social comfort as far as possible (Steeman and Defever 1998). As discussed earlier, urethral catheterisation is rarely an appropriate means of managing urinary incontinence as it may lead to catheter-related problems such as urinary tract infection (see section 'Caring for people with urinary catheters'). It can also jeopardise subsequent bladder retraining, in people who have had a CVA for example (Hodges 1997). However for some people, such as June, long-term catheterisation will be the most appropriate solution. Generally these include people who do not completely empty the bladder due to neurological disease or injury, people with bladder outlet obstruction for whom surgical repair is not possible, and those with chronic incontinence, often with associated confusion or debility, who cannot be managed any other way (Getliffe 2003).

If you find that a patient/client has been incontinent, what would your priorities of care be?

Priorities of care

The person will need to be attended to quickly, in order to prevent skin damage, relieve discomfort and restore dignity. Many of the principles discussed earlier related to dealing with a person's elimination needs are relevant, in particular: approachability and communication, privacy and dignity, punctuality, prevention of cross-infection, observation, hygiene and comfort. The nurse's approach when dealing with incontinence is absolutely crucial to the level of distress experienced. Nurses dealing with John's urinary incontinence should be discreet and matter-of-fact in changing his bed while reassuring him that the cause would be investigated. In a study of patient dignity a patient is quoted as saying: 'if you have [soiled the bed] they'll come in and they're really discreet and they'll just go about their business, clean you up and that before it's noticed by anyone else … I had pooed myself and hadn't really noticed until sometime later … She was friendly, just talking and everything. She was saying, "Oh don't worry love … I'll have it fixed in two seconds and you can just go back to sleep".' (Walsh and Kowanko 2002, 149). In faecal incontinence, in particular, prompt changing of soiled pads or clothing is essential to help to prevent odours and skin excoriation (Norton 1997). This also applies to the soiled nappies of infants and toddlers, which should also be changed promptly.

How skin is cleaned is very important, and if incontinence cannot be prevented, then a suitable method of containment is needed, for example pads, or for a man with urinary incontinence, possibly a penile sheath.

Skin cleansing

Le Lievre (1996) identified that nurses' skin care of patients with incontinence is not always based on sound research. This may be because skin care relating to urinary incontinence has been little addressed in the literature (Vinson and Proch 1998). Box 8.14 lists some key points about skin cleansing for people who have been incontinent, and these are further discussed below.

Nurses need to be aware of the potential skin problems that may result from incontinence. Jeter and Lutz (1996) explain that the presence of moisture from urine and sweat increases friction and shear, skin permeability and microbial load, while the frequent washings that may result lead to physical and chemical irritation. If a patient has been incontinent of both urine and faeces, their interaction can result in the formation of ammonia, leading to a rise in pH and an increase in the activity of faecal enzymes that damage the skin (see Figure 8.8). Thus Gibbons (1996) emphasises the importance of changing a soiled product promptly in cases of faecal incontinence to prevent skin excoriation. Super-absorbent pads aim to prevent mixing of urine and faeces by keeping skin dry (see section on 'Pads').

- If super-absorbent body worn pads are used, skin cleansing is not necessary at every pad change.
- Gloves and an apron should be worn for cleansing.
- Cleansing with plain water is sufficient for urinary incontinence.
- Faecal incontinence must be dealt with promptly and skin cleaned. If soap is used, rinse off thoroughly. Skin cleanser is preferable.
- Cleanse from front to back, and least soiled area to most soiled area
- Start with the labia with females, and the tip of the penis with men.
- Cleanse the anal area last.
- Dry skin carefully. Do not use talcum powder.
- Consider use of barrier creams/barrier films for particularly vulnerable skin.

Box 8.14 Skin cleansing after incontinence: a summary of key points

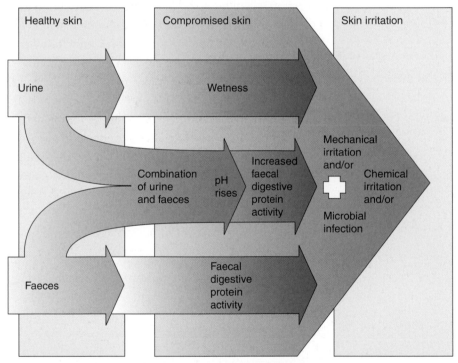

Figure 8.8 Diagram showing how incontinence affects skin. (Reproduced with permission from Paper-Pak UK Ltd.)

Washing with soap and water can cause drying of the skin or even contact dermatitis and eczema (Spiller 1992). Vinson and Proch (1998) conclude that soap and water may not provide adequate skin care. Soap, which is designed to remove dirt and grease, also removes natural skin lipids and water-holding substances and weakens the epidermis. Skin is normally slightly acidic, but bars of soap are alkaline and are therefore unsuitable for use on skin assessed as at risk of breaking down, as if the skin becomes more alkaline it becomes more permeable

(Jeter and Lutz 1996). If soap and water are used, the skin should be thoroughly rinsed with clean water and then dried gently. However, studies have indicated that when specially formulated skin cleansers are used to cleanse the skin of people who have been incontinent, their skin is more likely to remain healthy than when soap and water is used (Byers *et al.* 1995; Whittingham and May 1998; Cooper and Gray 2001).

Le Lievre (1996) makes a number of recommendations for skin care. These include assessment of present skin condition, adequate fluid and nutritional input, daily social cleansing of skin, and use of either unscented soap which is washed off thoroughly, or preferably wash cream. When pads are changed, skin should be patted dry gently. If only urinary incontinence occurs and pads containing super-absorbents are used, then skin washing at each pad change is not necessary; however the skin should be washed as soon as possible after faecal incontinence (Le Lievre 1996).

Norton (1997) recommends the use of barrier creams for preventing and treating milder cases of excoriated skin due to faecal incontinence, and stoma care products to promote healing where skin is broken. These creams are also suitable for nappy-wearing babies and toddlers during diarrhoeal illnesses, when there is increased risk of skin excoriation.

Talcum powder should be avoided as it can create a warm moist environment for infection (Gibbons 1996). Cleaning with moist toilet tissue may be more comfortable for a person who has been faecally incontinent than dry paper (Norton 1997). The anal area should always be cleaned last. There are products, such as no-sting barrier films, which can be applied to protect vulnerable skin in incontinent patients, and these have been shown to improve skin condition (Williams 1998). Skin should be cleaned and dried prior to application.

Pads

Pads for managing incontinence can be divided into three types: under-pads, all-in-one body worn products, and pads worn with elasticated pants (see Figure 8.9). The Department of Health (2000) advises that all types of pads should be available as part of the integrated continence services, and individual choice should be considered in their selection.

Choice of product

There is a vast array of incontinence pads produced by a variety of companies and all are suitable for both urinary and faecal incontinence. However there is a lack of high-quality research into the effectiveness of these products, making evidence-based selection difficult (Dunn *et al.* 2002). Disposable pads containing super-absorbents can keep the skin in a near normal state, but there are also pads containing pulp only, which encourage skin hydration and permeability. Such pads allow mixing of urine and faeces, causing further enzyme activity and potential skin damage (Le Lievre 1996). A systematic review by Shirran and

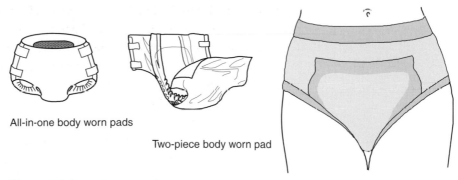

All-in-one body worn pads

Two-piece body worn pad

Figure 8.9 Incontinence pads.

Brazzelli (2003) concluded that although available evidence did not provide a sound basis for practice, disposable pads may cause less skin problems than non-disposable pads, and super-absorbent pads may perform better than pads containing pulp only. Although most pads used are disposable, washable pads are also produced. Reusable pants with a sewn-in absorbent pad resemble normal underwear better and are suitable for light incontinence. There are various types to meet different individuals' manual dexterity, such as those with poppers or Velcro fastenings. However an evaluative trial of ten such products found that all were disappointing in relation to leakage (Clarke-O'Neill *et al.* 2002). Gibbons (1996) suggests that faecal collectors can be used for patients who have persistent diarrhoea. Box 8.15 summarises key points in the choice and use of incontinence pads.

In a multi-sited study, carers' comments indicated that a successful pad should be leak-free, not too bulky, and keep the skin dry (Medical Devices Agency 1998). They also said that pants should not rip easily, keep their shape, and not be too tight around the tops of the legs. Choice of product should take into account comfort, easy removal for toileting, client preference and adequate protection in relation to amount of urine lost (Thompson and Smith 1998). Pads are produced for all situations, ranging from light to severe and night-time use:

- Light would be suitable for when there is only occasional voiding of a few drops of urine.
- Moderate for when there is frequent voiding of small to moderate amounts of urine.
- Severe for uncontrolled daily voiding of moderate to large amounts.

Different shaped pads are available for men and women. It is important to read manufacturers' instructions for the optimal fitting of these pads as correct fitting of the product is essential to contain urine and faeces, and will reduce skin contact with excreta to the minimum (Gibbons 1996). As urine is broken down into its constituents – ammonia and urea – on contact with air, fitting the pads closely ensures that urine and air are not mixed. Additional features, which some pads have, are wetness indicator strips, and adhesive strips for extra security.

Choice of pad
- Disposable, super-absorbent pads are preferable.
- Body worn pads (either all-in-ones, or pad and pants) should be used rather than under-pads.
- Choose the correct pad for the individual client, considering gender, size, and extent and frequency of incontinence.

Fitting
Always follow manufacturer's instructions for fitting, but the following general principles normally apply:

- Maintain privacy, dignity and prevention of cross-infection during pad changes.
- If using pants, ensure the seams are on the outside, and pull up to mid-thigh.
- Fold the pad lengthways and create a cupped shape.
- Place the pad from front to back with largest area at the back.
- Ensure pad is smoothed out both front and back, and fitted into the groin well.
- If using pants, pull up, or if all-in-ones, seal the tapes firmly, lower tapes should be sealed first.
- Check pad is as close to the body as possible.

Box 8.15 Choice and use of incontinence pads: key points

Misuse of under-pads

According to Norton (1996) under-pads are one of the most misused of all items used by nurses for managing incontinence. She states that one good-quality body worn pad is usually more effective than using several under-pads, which are costly and of little benefit to patients. Under-pads need changing immediately to prevent urine break down and excessive skin hydration, they are not in close contact with the body so the urine rapidly becomes cold, thus waking the patient at night, and finally, they do not contain super-absorbents so excessive skin hydration results. Thus under-pads should be used only as a procedure pad when a clean (not sterile) field is needed, for extra chair/bed protection, for example after administration of an enema, or where a body worn pad is not practical or possible as with a very obese person, or for persistent diarrhoea in bed.

Additional points

When changing a pad, it should never be referred to as a 'nappy' which is demeaning. Nurses should take care not to show annoyance or embarrass patients (see Chapter 2). It is important to ensure that people have a clean pad at mealtimes and before going out anywhere. When changing the pad maintain privacy by shutting curtains, and change any wet or soiled clothing. To prevent

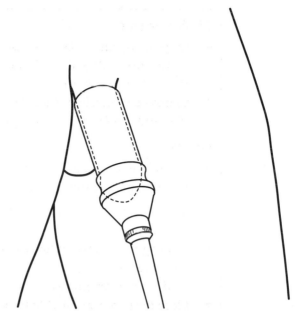

Figure 8.10 Penile sheath.

cross-infection use of gloves, hand hygiene and correct waste disposal are essential (see Chapter 3).

Penile sheaths

Penile sheaths (see Fig. 8.10) that channel the urine into a collection bag are available. These are a widely established means of managing urinary incontinence in male patients although there is a lack of research into their use (Doherty 1998). Use of sheaths avoids the disadvantages and complications of long-term in-dwelling urethral catheters, and the inconvenience of pads (Medical Devices Agency 1995). They are sometimes used by men who manage their continence using intermittent self-catheterisation, to avoid leakage in-between (Doherty 2000). Many people are allergic to latex (Le Lievre 1996) so use of a silicone sheath avoids this risk, and a clear sheath as opposed to an opaque one allows observation of the penile skin.

Sheaths are most suitable for men who have a moderate to severe degree of incontinence and/or have frequency and urgency, and are not able to get to the toilet easily (Medical Devices Agency 1995). However the Medical Devices Agency report that assessment for suitability should include assessing manual dexterity of the user (or carers), independence/availability of the carers and skin condition of the user. Penile sheaths are also inappropriate for people who have retention of urine (Pomfret 2000). Sheaths may be two-piece or one-piece. The two-piece sheath requires application of an adhesive strip to the penis before rolling the sheath on, while the one-piece sheath has an integral adhesive coating. The adhesive can cause skin problems in some people (Le Lievre 1996). One-piece sheaths have been rated more highly than two-piece, but acceptability of different products

- Assess client for suitability and give a clear explanation.
- Choose appropriate size and type of sheath. Be prepared to try others if it is found to be unsuitable.
- Maintain principles of preventing cross-infection throughout.
- Wash and dry penis and surrounding area.
- Trim (but do not shave) pubic hair if necessary.
- If using a two-part sheath, apply adhesive strip to penile shaft in a spiral manner.
- Roll the sheath on to the penis, leaving a space between the cup of the sheath and the end of the penis.
- Gently squeeze the sheath to ensure adhesion.
- Attach to a urinary drainage bag.
- Remove by gently rolling off (preferably in the bath) every 24 hours, and wash and dry skin before reapplying.

Box 8.16 Fitting a urinary sheath: key points

has been found to be highly individualised (Medical Devices Agency 1995). Thus men for whom a sheath might be an acceptable containment strategy should be encouraged to try out different products before deciding on one for long-term use.

Box 8.16 summarises some important points about fitting a penile sheath but further details are given below. A clear explanation should be given to patients about the sheath. Doherty (1998) notes that a positive attitude is necessary for successful use and that initially there may be problems but these can be overcome. Application of a urinary sheath is an intimate procedure, which may be embarrassing for both patient and nurse (Doherty 1998). The nurse should also be aware that a patient with reduced or absent sensation will not be able to feel if the sheath is too tight or a sore is developing, so the patient and his carers need to be observant for any such problems. In many cases patients can manage the system themselves. Hands should be washed prior to application, and any cuts should be covered with a plaster. Gloves can be worn if wanted but they are not essential.

Steps to ensure effective use of urinary sheaths are outlined in some detail by Doherty (1998). These include: choice of correct size by measuring the circumference of the penis at its widest point and measuring the length; if it is too tight it could cause sores and discomfort, while if it is too big it will lead to leakage as urine will seep under the sheath. Doherty (1998) notes, however, that penile size can vary and that sheath measurement should allow for expansion, although both latex and silicone are flexible materials. The penis and surrounding area should then be washed and dried; powder, cream or spray deodorants should not be used as they will inactivate the adhesive. If necessary, pubic hair should be trimmed but should not be shaved. A piece of paper/card, sometimes supplied by the manufacturer, can be held over the penis to keep back pubic hair while the sheath is applied.

When fitting the sheath, roll it over the penis, leaving a small space between the end of the penis and the cup of the sheath to allow for changes in the size of the penis while wearing. If the patient is uncircumcised, ensure that the foreskin remains over the glans and is not retracted. Pomfret (2000) suggests the sheath should be rolled back one turn prior to application to an uncircumcised penis in order to form a space of 1–2 cm between the end of the penis and the outlet of the sheath. Once the sheath is in place, gently squeeze it to ensure adhesion, and then attach it to a urine drainage bag. Never apply sticky tape as it is inflexible and could lead to restriction of the blood supply leading to sores or gangrene. Ensure that the tubing is not kinked, thereby allowing collection of urine and pressure on the sheath, weakening the adhesive, and that the urine bag is kept lower and is well supported. Drainage bags should be chosen carefully according to individual need. For example there are leg bags, thigh bags and bags specifically for wheelchair users; more detail about these can be found in Doherty (2000).

■ Activity   Can you think of any patients for whom this method of dealing with urinary incontinence might be particularly unsuitable?

Patients with any sore of the penis should not have a sheath applied. Patients with a small or retracted penis are not suitable (Medical Devices Agency 1995), unless a device such as a flange and belt is used. Patients who are confused, and do not understand what the sheath is, are likely to try to pull it off.

Support for people with continence problems

People with continence problems can benefit from support and advice, but may often be unaware of what support is available, and where it can be accessed. It is important that nurses are aware of the resources available so that they can advise people with continence issues. There are many local self-help support groups which can be very beneficial to participants. They give people the opportunity to meet informally, and share ideas and experiences, and the Department of Health (2001b) recommends that this support is actively promoted. 'Incontact' is one such organisation which helps people to set up groups. Many Disabled Living Centres (DLCs) hold the PromoCon Continence Resource Package, which is composed of a range of products, fact sheets and other relevant information. DLCs display materials to promote continence alongside other equipment for easier living. Many organisations have developed information leaflets for people who have continence problems, for example the Stroke Association, Alzheimer's Disease Society, and also Help the Aged.

■ Activity   Try to find out about advice and support within your area. Find out where your nearest DLC is, and if possible, arrange to visit so that you can see the resources available.

Summary

■ Nurses within almost any setting are likely to encounter people with continence issues, and therefore an understanding of the underlying causes and the wide-ranging effects on people is important.

■ Nurses should have knowledge about specialist services, e.g. the continence advisor and support organisations, so that they can advise and refer people accordingly.

■ Promoting continence and managing incontinence requires careful assessment of each individual, and knowledge about appropriate strategies and products. Care for people with continence problems should be based on the best evidence available.

CHAPTER SUMMARY

This chapter focused on assisting people with elimination, and has emphasised that to achieve quality care requires a sensitive and empathetic approach, effective communication skills, and a sound, evidence-based knowledge. Implementing measures to prevent cross-infection, while assisting people with elimination, are also paramount. Urinalysis and specimen collection were dealt with in some detail, as these are very common investigations but if not carried out with care they can lead to misleading results, and therefore, inappropriate treatment. Administration of suppositories and enemas is a relevant skill for nurses in most settings, and must be carried out with care and understanding. Urinary catheterisation is invasive and potentially harmful, but is nevertheless often necessary as a short- or long-term measure. An understanding of this procedure, and particularly how potential complications can be reduced, is also important. As stated, continence is a huge topic, and may require specialist involvement. Here, the practical skills in dealing with continence have been explored, and it is expected that students wishing to extend their knowledge will access the referenced material. To conclude, nurses need to value the care given in relation to patients/clients' elimination needs as, if effective, it can do much for comfort, well-being and self-esteem.

REFERENCES

Abd-el-Maeboud, K.H., el-Naggar, T., El-Hawi, E.M.M. *et al.* 1991. Rectal suppositories and mode of insertion. *The Lancet* **338**, 798, 800.

Addison, R., Ness, W., Abulafi, M. *et al.* 2000. How to administer enemas and suppositories. *Nursing Times NT Plus: Continence* **96**(6), 3–4.

Akhtar, S.G. 2002. Nursing with dignity Part 8: Islam. *Nursing Times* **98**(16), 40–2.

Aminzadeh, F., Edwards, N., Lockett, D. and Nair, R.C. 2000. Utilization of bathroom safety devices, patterns of bathing and toileting, and bathroom falls in a sample of community living older adults. *Technology and Disability* **13**(2), 95–103.

Anders, K. 1999. Bladder retraining. *Professional Nurse* **14**, 334–6.

Annells, M. and Koch, T. 2002. Older people seeking solutions to constipation: the laxative mire. *Journal of Clinical Nursing* **11**, 603–12.

Ayliffe, G.A.J., Babb, J.R. and Taylor, L.J. 2001. *Hospital-Acquired Infection. Principles and Prevention*, third edition. Oxford: Butterworth-Heinemann.

Ballinger, C., Pain, H., Pascoe, J. and Gore, S. 1996. Choosing a commode for the ward environment. *British Journal of Nursing* **5**, 485–6.

Bayer 1997a. *Technical Information Bulletin Number 8. Urinary Tract Infection*. Newbury: Bayer.

Bayer 1997b. *Urine Analysis: The essential information*. Newbury: Bayer.

Bayer 1998. *A Practical Guide to Urine Analysis*. Newbury: Bayer.

Beynon, M. 1997. Urological investigations. In Fillingham, S. and Douglas, J. (eds) *Urological Nursing*, second edition. London: Baillière Tindall, 30–56.

Block, C., Baron, O., Bogokowoski, B. *et al.* 1990. An in-use evaluation of polypropylene versus stainless steel bedpans. *Journal of Hospital Acquired Infection* **16**, 331–8.

Brown, J.S., Vittinghoff, E., Wyman, J.F. *et al.* 2000. Urinary incontinence: does it increase risk for falls and fractures? *Journal of the American Geriatrics Society* **48**, 721–5.

Bullock, B., Bausher, J.C., Pomerantz, W.J. *et al.* 2000. A clear urine specimen on visual inspection cannot totally exclude a diagnosis of urinary tract infection. *Evidence-Based Nursing* **4**(55), 106, e60.

Burr, R.G. and Nuseibeh, I.M. 1997. Urinary catheter blockage depends on urine pH, calcium and rate of flow. *Spinal Cord* **35**, 521–5.

Bush, T.A., Castellucci, D.T. and Phillips, C. 2001. Exploring women's beliefs regarding urinary incontinence. *Urologic Nursing* **21**, 211–18.

Byers, P.P.I., Ryan, P.A. and Regan, M.B. 1995. Effects of incontinence care cleansing regimens on skin integrity. *Journal of Wound, Ostomy and Continence Nursing* **22**, 187–92.

Campbell, S. and Glasper, E.A. 1995. *Whaley and Wong's Children's Nursing*. London: Mosby.

Chester, R. 1998. *Towards Continence*. London: Counsel and Care.

Chiverton, P.A., Wells, T.J., Brink, C.A. and Mayer, R. 1996. Psychological factors associated with urinary incontinence. *Clinical Nurse Specialist* **10**, 229–33.

Chur-Hansen, A. 2002. Preferences for female and male nurses: the role of age, gender and previous experience – year 2000 compared with 1984. *Journal of Advanced Nursing* **37**, 192–8.

Clarke-O'Neill, S., Pettersson, L., Fader, M. *et al.* 2002. A multicentre comparative evaluation: washable pants with an integral pad for light incontinence. *Journal of Clinical Nursing* **11**, 79–87.

Cochran, A. 1999. Response to urinary incontinence by older persons living in the community. *Continence* **19**, 15–24.

Colley, W. 1996. Charting new waters. *Nursing Times* **92**(24), 59–60, 62, 64.

Cooper, P. and Gray, D. 2001. Comparison of two skin care regimes for incontinence. *British Journal of Nursing* **10**, Tissue Viability Supplement: S6, S8, S10.

Coyne, I.T. 1995a. Parental participation in care: a critical review of the literature. *Journal of Advanced Nursing* **21**, 716–22.

Coyne, I.T. 1995b. Partnership in care: parents' views of participation in their hospitalized child's care. *Journal of Clinical Nursing* **4**, 71–9.

de Sousa, M.E. 1996. The renal system. In McQuaid, L., Huband, S. and Parker, S. *Children's Nursing*. London: Churchill Livingstone, 211–37.

Dempsey, K.M., Chiew, R.F., McKenzie, J.A. and Mitchell, D.H. 2000. Evaluation of the cleaning and disinfection efficacy of the DEKO-190; a ward-based automated washer/disinfector. *Journal of Hospital Infection* **46**(1), 50–4.

Department of Health 2000. *Good Practice in Continence Services*. London: DH.

Department of Health 2001a. *Valuing People: A new strategy for learning disability for the 21st century*. London: DH.

Department of Health 2001b. *The Essence of Care: Patient-focused benchmarking for health care practitioners*. London: DH.

Department of Health 2001c. *National Service Framework for Older People*. London: DH.

Department of Health 2003. *Winning Ways: Working together to reduce healthcare associated infection in England and Wales*. London: DH.

Doherty, W. 1998. The clear advantage urinary incontinence sheath for men. *British Journal of Nursing* **7**, 730, 732–4.

Doherty, W. 2000. Urinary sheaths and drainage bags from Manfred Sauer. *British Journal of Nursing* **9**, 514–17.

Dolman, M. 2003. Mostly female. In Getliffe, K. and Dolman, M. (eds) *Promoting Continence: A clinical research resource*, second edition. London: Baillière Tindall, 53–79.

Dougherty, M. 1998. Current status of research on pelvic muscle strengthening techniques. *Journal of Wound, Ostomy, and Continence Nursing* **25**, 75–83.

Doughty, D.B. 1996. A physiologic approach to bowel training. *Journal of Wound, Ostomy and Continence Nursing* **23**, 46–56.

Dunn, S., Kowanko, I., Paterson, J. and Pretty, L. 2002. Systematic review of the effectiveness of urinary continence products. *Journal of Wound, Ostomy and Continence Nursing* **29**(3), 129–42.

Edwards, C., Dolman, M. and Horton, N. 2003. Down and away: an overview of adult constipation and faecal incontinence. In Getliffe, K. and Dolman, M. (eds) *Promoting Continence: A Clinical Research Resource*, second edition. London: Baillière Tindall, 185–225.

Eustice, S., Roe, B. and Paterson, J. 2003. Prompted voiding for the management of urinary incontinence in adults (Cochrane Review). In *The Cochrane Library*. Issue 3. Oxford: Update Software.

Fader, M., Pettersson, L., Brooks, R. *et al.* 1997. A multicentre comparative evaluation of catheter valves. *British Journal of Nursing* **6**, 359, 362, 364, 366–7.

Farrell, M., Devine, K., Lancaster, G. and Judd, B. 2002. A method comparison study to assess the reliablity of urine collection pads as a means of obtaining urine specimens from toilet-trained children for microbiological examination. *Journal of Advanced Nursing* **37**, 387–93.

Getliffe, K. 1996. Which catheter? A guide to catheter selection. *Professional Nurse* **12** (2) insert 2 p.

Getliffe, K. 2002. Managing recurrent urinary catheter encrustation. *British Journal of Community Nursing* **7**, 574–80.

Getliffe, K. 2003. Catheters and catheterization. In Getliffe, K. and Dolman, M. (eds) *Promoting Continence: A clinical research resource*, second edition. London: Baillière Tindall, 259–301.

Getliffe, K. and Dolman, M. 2003. Normal and abnormal bladder function. In Getliffe, K. and Dolman, M. (eds) *Promoting Continence: A clinical research resource*, second edition. London: Baillière Tindall, 21–51.

Gibbons, G. 1996. Skin care and incontinence. *Community Nurse* **2**, 37.

Glazener, S.M.A. and Evans, J.H.C. 2002a. Alarm interventions for nocturnal enuresis in children (Cochrane Review). In *The Cochrane Library*, Issue 4. Oxford: Update Software.

Glazener, S.M.A. and Evans, J.H.C. 2002b. Simple behavioural and physical interventions for nocturnal enuresis in children (Cochrane Review). In *The Cochrane Library*, Issue 4. Oxford: Update Software.

Gould, D. 1994 Controlling infection spread from excreta. *Nursing Standard* **8**(33), 29–31.

Gould, D. and Brooker, C. 2000. *Applied Microbiology for Nurses*. London: Macmillan.

Hay-Smith, E.J.C., Berghmans, L.C.M., Hendriks, H.J.M. *et al.* 2003. Pelvic floor muscle training for urinary incontinence in women (Cochrane Review). In *The Cochrane Library*, Issue 3. Oxford: Update Software.

Hodges, C. 1997. Continence care: choosing carefully. *Nursing Times* **93**(35), 48, 50, 52.

Holland, K. and Hogg, C. 2001. *Cultural Awareness in Nursing and Health Care: An introductory text*. London: Arnold.

Hutchinson, S., Leger-Krall, S. and Skodal Wilson, H. 1996. Toileting: a biobehavioural challenge in Alzheimer's dementia care. *Journal of Gerontological Nursing* **22**(10), 18–27.

Jensen, L.L. 1997. Faecal incontinence: evaluation and treatment. *Journal of Wound, Ostomy and Continence Nursing* **24**, 277–82.

Jeter, K.F. and Lutz, J.B. 1996. Skin care in the frail, elderly, dependent incontinent patient. *Advances in Skin Care* **9**(1), 29–34.

Johnson, A. 1989. Bedpans: disposable or reusable? *Nursing Times* **85**(41), 72–4.

Kawik, L. 1996. Nurses' and parents' perceptions of participation and partnership in caring for a hospitalised child. *British Journal of Nursing* **5**(7), 430–4.

Kay, J. 2000. Administration of medicines. In Huband, S. and Trigg, E. (eds) *Practices in Children's Nursing: Guidelines for hospital and community.* Edinburgh: Churchill Livingstone, 29–38.

Kirk, S. 2001. Negotiating lay and professional roles in the care of children with complex health care needs. *Journal of Advanced Nursing* **34**, 593–602.

Koch, T. and Kelly, S. 1999. Identifying strategies for managing urinary incontinence with women who have multiple sclerosis. *Journal of Clinical Nursing* **8**, 550–9.

Koch, T., Kralik, D. and Kelly, S. 2000. We just don't talk about it: men living with urinary incontinence and multiple sclerosis. *International Journal of Nursing Practice* **6**, 253–60.

Laker, C. 1994. Urological investigations. In Laker, C. (ed.) *Urological Nursing.* London: Scutari Press, 37–65.

Laurent, C. 1998. Preventing infection from indwelling catheters. *Nursing Times* **94**(25), 60–6.

Le Lievre, S. 1996. Incontinence dermatitis. *Primary Health Care* **6**(4), 17–19, 21.

Liaw, L.C.T., Nayar, D.M., Pedler, S.J. and Goulthard, M.G. 2000. Home collection of urine for culture from infants by three methods: survey of parents' preferences and bacterial contamination rates. *British Medical Journal* **320**, 1312–13.

Lukeman, D. 2003. Mainly children: childhood enuresis and encopresis. In Getliffe, K. and Dolman, M. (eds) *Promoting Continence: A clinical research resource,* second edition. London: Baillière Tindall, 107–34.

MacQueen, S. 2000. Specimen collection. In Huband, S. and Trigg, E. (eds) *Practices in Children's Nursing: Guidelines for hospital and community.* Edinburgh: Churchill Livingstone, 261–7.

Mahoney, C. 1997. The impact of continence problems on self esteem. *Nursing Times* **93**(52), 58, 60.

Mason, L., Glenn, S., Walton, I. and Hughes, C. 2001. Women's reluctance to seek help for stress incontinence during pregnancy and following childbirth. *Midwifery* **17**, 212–21.

McCreanor, J., Aitchison, M. and Woods, M. 1998. Comparing therapies for incontinence. *Professional Nurse* **13**, 215–19.

McIntosh, J. 2001. A guide to female urinals. *NTplus* 97(6), VII–X.

McNaughton, M. and Cavanagh, S. 1998. Changing urine testing protocols through audit. *Nursing Times* **94**(1), 42–3.

Macauley, M. 1997. Urinary drainage systems. In Fillingham, S. and Douglas, J. (eds) *Urological Nursing,* second edition. London: Baillière Tindall, 90–130.

Mead, M. 1998a. Midstream urine testing. *Practice Nurse* **15**(7), 408.

Mead, M. 1998b. Stool culture. *Practice Nurse* **16**(3), 170.

Meers, P., Sedgwick, J. and Worsley, M. 1995. *The Microbiology and Epidemiology of Infection for Health Science Students.* London: Chapman and Hall.

Medical Devices Agency 1995. *Penile Sheaths: An Evaluation No. A15.* Norwich: HMSO.

Medical Devices Agency 1998. *Disposable, Shaped Bodyworn Pads with Pants for Heavy Incontinence: An evaluation*. London: Medical Devices Agency.

Mohammed, T.A. 2000. Urine testing and catheterization. In Huband, S. and Trigg, E. (eds) *Practices in Children's Nursing: Guidelines for hospital and community*. Edinburgh: Churchill Livingstone, 303–9.

Moore, K.N., Murray, S., Malone-Lee, J. and Wagg, A. 2001. Rapid urinalysis assays for the diagnosis of urinary tract infection. *British Journal of Nursing* **10**, 995–1001.

Mousseau, J. 2001. Contamination of urine specimens from women with acute dysuria did not differ with collection technique *Evidence Based Nursing* **4**(2), 46.

Nazarko, L. 1995. The therapeutic uses of cranberry juice. *Nursing Standard* **9**(34), 33–5.

Nazarko, L. 1997. Continence. The whole story. *Nursing Times* **93**(43), 63–4, 66, 68.

Nazarko, L. 1999. Assess all areas. *Nursing Times* 95(6), 68, 71, 72.

NICE (National Institute for Clinical Excellence) 2003. *Infection Control. Prevention of healthcare-associated infection in primary and community care*. London: NICE. Available from http://www.nice.org.uk. Accessed 2 January 2004.

Noble, J.G., Menzies, D., Cox, P.J. and Edwards, L. 1990. Midnight removal: an improved approach to removal of catheters. *British Journal of Urology* **65**, 615–17.

Norton, C. 1996. Faecal incontinence in adults 1: prevalence and causes. *British Journal of Nursing* **5**, 1367–74.

Norton, C. 1997. Faecal incontinence in adults 2: treatment and management. *British Journal of Nursing* **6**, 23–6.

Norton, C. and Kamm, M.A. 1999. Outcome of biofeedback for faecal incontinence. *British Journal of Surgery* **86**, 1159–63.

Nursing and Midwifery Council 2002. *Code of Professional Conduct*. London: NMC.

O'Meara, B. 1999. Hidden dangers. *Nursing Times* **95**(31), 70–1.

Pomfret, I.J. 2000. Urinary incontinence management – urinary sheaths. *Journal of Community Nursing* **14**(4), www.jcn.co.uk.

Pratt, R.J., Pellowe, C., Loveday, H.P. *et al.* 2001. Department of Health Guidelines for preventing infections associated with the insertion and maintenance of short-term indwelling urethral catheters in acute care. *Journal of Hospital Infection* **47** (Suppl), S39–46.

Pritchard, V. and Hathaway, C. 1988. Patient handwashing practice. *Nursing Times* **84**(36), 68, 70, 72.

Reilly, P., Mills, L. Bessner, D. *et al.* 2002. Using the urine dipstick to screen out unnecessary urine cultures: implementation at one facility. *Clinical Laboratory Science* **15**(1), 9–12.

Robinson, J.P. 2000. Managing urinary incontinence in the nursing home: residents' perspectives. *Journal of Advanced Nursing* **31**, 68–77.

Robinson, J. 2001. Urethral catheter selection. *Nursing Standard* **15**(25), 39–42.

Roe, B. and Williams, K. 1994. *Clinical Handbook for Continence Care*. London: Scutari.

Roe, B., Williams, K. and Palmer, M. 2003. Bladder training for urinary incontinence in adults (Cochrane Review). In *The Cochrane Library*, Issue 3. Oxford: Update Software.

Rogers, J. 1998. RCN continuing education. Promoting continence: the child with special needs. *Nursing Standard* **12**(34), 47–55.

Rowell, D.M. 1998. Evaluation of a urine chemistry analyser. *Professional Nurse* **13**, 553–4.

Royal College of Nursing 2003a. *Digital Rectal Examination: Guidance for nurses working with children and young people*. London: RCN.

Royal College of Nursing 2003b. *Digital Rectal Examination and Manual Removal of Faeces: Guidance for nurses*. London: RCN.

Schmelzer, M. and Wright, K.B. 1996. Enema administration techniques used by experienced registered nurses. *Gastroenterology Nursing* **19**, 171–5.

Schnozzle, J.F., Cruise, P.A., Alessi, C.A. *et al.* 1998. Individualising night time incontinence care in nursing home residents. *Nursing Research* **47**, 197–204.

Shaw, F. 1998. It's never too late. *Nursing Times* **94**(6), 68, 70, 72.

Shirran, E. and Brazzelli, M. 2003. Absorbent products for the containment of urinary and/or faecal incontinence in adults (Cochrane Review). In *The Cochrane Library*, Issue 3. Oxford: Update Software.

Smith, D.B. 1998. A continence care approach for long-term care facilities. *Geriatric Nursing* **19**(2), 81–6.

Smith, P. and Smith, L. 2003. Continence training in intellectual disability. In Getliffe, K. and Dolman, M. (eds) *Promoting Continence: A clinical research resource*, second edition. London: Baillière Tindall, 303–36.

Spiller, J. 1992. For whose sake: the patient or the nurse? Ritual practices in patient washing. *Professional Nurse* **7**, 432–4.

Stanley, R. 1996. Treatment of continence in people with learning disabilities: 2. *British Journal of Nursing* **5**, 492–8.

Stanley, R. 1997. Treatment of continence in people with learning disabilities: 3. *British Journal of Nursing* **6**, 12, 14, 16, 18, 19, 22.

Steeman, E. and Defever, M. 1998. Urinary incontinence among elderly persons who live at home: a literature review. *Geriatric Nursing* **33**, 441–55.

Tarling, C. 1997: Toileting and clothing. In *The Guide to Handling of Patients: Introducing a safer handling policy*, fourth edition. London: National Back Pain Association, 163–71.

Thompson, D.L. and Smith, D.A. 1998. Continence restoration in the cognitively impaired adult. *Geriatric Nursing* **19**(2), 87–90.

Trounce, J. 2000. *Clinical Pharmacology for Nurses*, sixteenth edition. Edinburgh: Churchill Livingstone.

Vernon, S. 1995. Urine collection from infants: a reliable method. *Paediatric Nursing* **7**(6), 26–7.

Vernon, S., Redfearn, A., Pedler, S.J. *et al.* 1994. Urine collection on sanitary towels. *The Lancet* 344, August 27, 612.

Vickerman, J. 2003. The benefits of a lending library for female urinals. *Nursing Times* **99**(44), 56–7.

Vinson, J. and Proch, J. 1998. Inhibition of moisture penetration to the skin by a novel incontinence barrier product. *Journal of Wound, Ostomy and Continence Nursing* **25**, 256–60.

Walsh, K. and Kowanko, I. 2002. Nurses' and patients' perceptions of dignity. *International Journal of Nursing Practice* **8**, 143–51.

Whittingham, K. and May, S. 1998. Cleansing regimens for continence care. *Professional Nurse* **14**, 167–71.

Williams, C. 1998. 3M Cavilon No Sting Barrier Film in the protection of vulnerable skin. *British Journal of Nursing* **10**, 613–15.

Willis, J. 2000. Bowel management and consent. *Nursing Times NT Plus Continence* **96**(6), 7–8.

Wilson, J. 1997. Control and prevention of infection in catheter care. *Nurse Prescriber/Community Nurse* **3**(5), 39–40.

Wilson, J. 2001. *Infection Control in Clinical Practice*, second edition. London: Baillière Tindall.

Winn, C. 1996. Basing catheter care on research principles. *Nursing Standard* **10**(18), 38–40.

Woodward, S. 1996. Impact of neurological problems on urinary continence. *British Journal of Nursing* **5**, 906–13.

Woodward, S. 1997. Complications of allergies to latex urinary catheters. *British Journal of Nursing* **6**, 786, 788, 790, 792–3.

www.bnf.org

USEFUL ORGANISATIONS

The Continence Foundation This company produces a wide range of publications on all aspects of continence, and they have information in ten different languages. They also produce a continence products directory listing main product types and full details about different products available in the UK. The web address is: www.continence-foundation.org.uk. Tel. 0845 345 0165

Incontact is an organisation which supports the development of local self-help groups to support people with incontinence and carers. It is based at United House, North Road, London N7 9DP, UK. The web address is: www.incontact.org. Tel. 0870 770 3246

Assessing and meeting nutritional needs

Kay Child and Sue Higham

Good food in a balanced diet is important in everyone's life, and sound nutrition is an essential prerequisite for health and well-being. Nutrition is a concern to nurses working in any setting and should be regarded as integral and central to patient/client care: 'The provision of food and fluids is a nursing role' (Florence Nightingale 1859, cited in 1980 edition). In care settings people's nutritional demands may be increased due to their impaired health, but hospital meals have been found to be nutritionally inadequate (Fettes and Murray 1999). Up to 40 per cent of patients in acute hospitals are malnourished at any one time (McWhirter and Pennington 1994). The Chief Nurse made a clear statement to all nurses in 1997 that 'it is ultimately the responsibility of nurses to ensure that the nutritional needs of the patients are met' (cited by Bond 1997, p. 1). However nutrition can be seen as basic and taken for granted, and it is sometimes even neglected. A report by the Health Advisory Service 2000 (1998) reported a relative saying: 'nurses did not seem to know about eating/drinking and did not seem to care' (p. 16).

Good nutrition for all people in health care settings is increasingly influenced by initiatives and recommendations by the Department of Health. *The Essence of Care* (Department of Health 2001a) includes a section on nutrition with benchmarking statements for good practice, some of which will be referred to later in this chapter. The provision of food and drink to patients/clients in care environments is a complex process and it involves a range of staff. Nurses are well placed to promote healthy eating because within the caring team they spend most time with the people who require this support. Thus nurses need to recognise the importance of nutrition in their caring role, and prioritise assessment and appropriate interventions.

This chapter includes:
- Recognising the contribution of nutrition to health
- Promoting healthy eating in care settings
- Assessing nutritional status and developing a plan of action
- Preparing and presenting food hygienically
- Assisting people with oral intake of food and drink

- Bottle-feeding infants
- Supporting breast-feeding mothers
- Identifying additional nursing strategies to improve clients' nutritional status.

Recommended biology reading:

The following questions will help you to focus on the biology underpinning the skills in this chapter. Use your recommended text book to find out:

- What are nutrients? Where do nutrients come from?
- What is a balanced diet?
- What is the difference between macronutrients and micronutrients?
- Why do we need these nutrients? What are their roles?
- How are macronutrients digested? Once digested, where do they go?
- What factors may affect the absorption of digested nutrients?
- How does nutrition affect health?
- What are the consequences of under-nutrition and over-nutrition?
- How do nutritional requirements alter across the lifespan?
- What aspects of different age groups (e.g. neonates, infants, children, teenagers, adults and the elderly) may impinge upon nutritional status?
- How does a 'health need' alter our nutritional demands (or supply)?

PRACTICE SCENARIOS

As already stated, nutrition is relevant for everybody. The following practice scenarios highlight situations where nutritional issues would be particularly important, and they will be referred to throughout this chapter.

Adult

Cerebrovascular accident
Cerebral damage caused either by decreased blood flow or haemorrhage. Effects vary but often causes paralysis down one side of the body (hemiplegia), and speech and swallowing difficulty. Commonly termed a stroke.

Miss Alice West is 84 years old and has been transferred from a medical ward to a rehabilitation unit following a **cerebrovascular accident** (CVA) which has caused right-sided weakness. The medical ward staff who transferred her handed over that although she initially had swallowing problems she has since been assessed as being able to swallow. However her appetite is very poor and she often eats only a few small mouthfuls, refusing any more. The staff have been keeping a food chart and a fluid chart which confirm her poor intake. She has dentures but they appear loose. Her niece is concerned that she is 'looking thin' and seems depressed. Miss West is often uncommunicative but on occasions expresses herself clearly. She is also registered partially sighted.

Child

Saba Khan is a 4-week-old full-term infant. She has been admitted to the ward with breathlessness and difficulty in feeding. Saba is fully breast-fed. Until now she has been thriving, having regained her birth weight (3.1 kg) plus 350 g. Her admission weight is 3.32 kg. Saba's mother is resident with her, and her father visits every day. Saba's grandmother is helping to look after her brothers aged 2 and 5 years.

Learning disability

Phillip Picton is a 31-year-old man with a learning disability who lives in a supported living scheme with three other clients. Recently he has become increasingly overweight. His obesity is beginning to interfere with his day-to-day activities. He has expressed concern about two issues: bending over to put his socks on and getting out of breath walking to the local shops. His carers took him to see his GP who referred him to the community team for people with learning disabilities. The community nurse for learning disabilities and the occupational therapist, who is Phillip's **health facilitator**, are going to visit him to carry out an assessment. Phillip does his own food shopping with support.

Health facilitator

A member of the community learning disabilities team (often a nurse) who supports a person with learning disabilities to access the health care they need. See *Valuing People* (Department of Health 2001b).

Mental health

Mr Charles Cooper is an 88-year-old widower (his wife died 15 years ago). He lives alone in a bungalow in a small village. The village has very poor public transport services. The local shop has recently closed. Mr Cooper has a diagnosis of **dementia** for which he is prescribed medication. He is prompted to take this by a home carer who calls twice a day. Recently the community psychiatric nurse (CPN) noticed that Mr Cooper had lost weight. When questioned about his dietary intake Mr Cooper stated that he has a 'good appetite' and manages to prepare all his own meals. On checking the kitchen the CPN observed little evidence of recent food preparation or cooking. The refrigerator contained some dairy products, and these had all expired and were beginning to smell.

Dementia

Dementia is chronic and progressive in nature, has many causes and commonly presents with memory and language impairment, decline in self-care ability, and behavioural and personality changes (Jacques and Jackson 2000).

RECOGNISING THE CONTRIBUTION OF NUTRITION TO HEALTH

Health promotion is considered an essential activity of a registered nurse and student nurses are expected to be able to contribute to health promotion activities (Nursing and Midwifery Council 2002). As sound nutrition plays an essential role in health it is therefore important to understand the key components of a nutritious diet, and be able to identify the factors that might prevent good nutrition.

LEARNING OUTCOMES

By the end of this section you will be able to:

1. Recognise the major nutrients and their contribution to health.
2. Discuss factors that might influence healthy individuals' nutritional needs.
3. Identify situations in which an individual's nutritional status might be impaired.

Learning outcome 1: Recognise the major nutrients and their contribution to health

An adequate supply of essential nutrients is required in the diet to maintain health. Note that the term 'diet' usually refers to the total food eaten, while 'nutrients' refers to components of foodstuffs which have a role in body functioning. For example, bread is composed of the nutrients carbohydrate, protein, fat and some vitamins. The following exercise is designed to help you to check your fundamental knowledge of nutrition. It should be easy if you have worked through the biology questions!

Activity

List all the groups of nutrients you can remember. Can you identify what each of these is used for within the body?

Check your answers against Table 9.1. Note that most foods contain combinations of nutrients.

Activity

Here is a list of the recorded food and fluid intake of Miss West for the day before her transfer to the rehabilitation unit. Note one cup = 200 mL. Miss West takes milk in her tea and coffee but no sugar.

08.15   Small bowl of porridge with milk and sugar, ½ cup of tea
09.00   ½ glass of water
10.30   ½ cup of coffee. Declined snack
12.30   Small amount of mince, mashed potato and peas, one portion of ice cream, ½ glass of water, ½ cup of tea
15.15   ½ cup of tea, declined snack
17.30   ½ bowl of chicken soup, ½ white bread roll with butter, one portion of ice cream, ½ cup of water. ½ cup of tea
20.00   ½ cup of tea, declined snack
22.00   ½ cup of water

Now consider which of the nutrients listed in Table 9.1 does Miss West's diet include, and which nutrients are missing?

Miss West's diet does contain some of the important nutrients listed (e.g. fibre and carbohydrate in her porridge, protein in her mince, fat in the butter, ice cream and milk, and vitamin C in the peas) but her portions are so small that her calorific intake and intake of most nutrients is likely to be inadequate. Healthy people can cope with inadequate nutrition occasionally but up to 40 per cent of people admitted to hospital are already underweight and many more lose further weight in hospital (Meikle 2003). Because Miss West's energy and protein intake are insufficient her body will break down fat and muscle to meet its needs, leading to weight loss. Miss West's diet contains minimal iron and she is at risk of iron deficiency anaemia if her nutritional intake does not improve. Vitamin C helps absorption of iron from non-animal sources (e.g. grains) (Wardlow 1999), but

Table 9.1 Nutrients and their role within the body

Nutrient	Function
Proteins	Used for building, growth or replacement of cells and tissues, or energy source of last resort (Gobbi and Torrance 2000) Major constituent of hormones, enzymes and antibodies (Edwards 1998)
Fats	Source of energy Component of cell membranes (Edwards 1998) Insulation (Gobbi and Torrance 2000)
Carbohydrates	Source of energy and fibre to aid digestion and bowel function (Gobbi and Torrance 2000)
Vitamins	Essential in small quantities for the normal growth and functioning of the body (Gobbi and Torrance 2000)
Minerals	Important building substances (e.g. calcium in bone) and as components of enzymes (Gobbi and Torrance 2000)
Water	Used for building tissues, as a solvent for carrying nutrients and waste, involved in temperature regulation (Tortora and Grabowski 2003)
Fibre	Dietary fibre is not, strictly speaking, a nutrient, but its presence in the diet is necessary for the movement of food through the gastrointestinal tract (Marieb 2001)

her vitamin C intake is small too. Her fluid intake is about 1100 mL which is barely sufficient to maintain her hydration. Recording a food chart, as the nurses have done for Miss West, is a good way of seeing what someone is actually eating and it becomes very clear if their diet is inadequate.

Learning outcome 2: Discuss factors that might influence healthy individuals' nutritional needs

The amounts of various nutrients required for health vary from individual to individual and throughout life.

 Activity — What factors might influence a healthy individual's nutritional needs?

You may have thought of the following:

■ **Age**: Children have higher metabolic rates than adults, and therefore require relatively more energy; they also need to consume sufficient food to support growth (Livingstone 1997). Periods of rapid growth such as infancy and adolescence in particular result in increased energy and nutrient requirements (Kanneh and Ellis 1999). In adulthood, as age increases, the energy requirement decreases because older people have a lower metabolic rate than younger adults (Pender 1994).

- **Gender**: Men require more energy because their relatively greater muscle mass results in a higher metabolic rate than that in women (Pender 1994).
- **Height and build**: The bigger the body the greater the amount of nutrients required to maintain cells (Piper 1996).
- **Amount of physical activity**: As energy is used as fuel, the greater the physical activity the more energy is used up (Pender 1994).
- **Pregnancy**: During the second and third trimesters of pregnancy, rapid growth of the fetus alters the woman's nutritional needs, although the exact demands made on the mother by the fetus vary from individual to individual. In particular the need for energy, protein, and vitamins A, B, C and D are likely to increase (Wardley *et al.* 1997). 'Eating for two' is not necessary, however. The increased energy required by the fetus is often compensated for in part by decreased maternal activity towards the end of pregnancy, and the average British diet generally contains sufficient protein to meet the increased demands (Wardley *et al.* 1997).
- **Lactation**: A breast-feeding woman requires increased energy (as much as 500 calories/day more), increased calcium and increased vitamin A, C and D intake (Wardley *et al.* 1997).

Being aware of factors affecting nutritional demands in the healthy individual is important prior to considering factors that can compromise nutritional status.

Learning outcome 3: Identify situations in which an individual's nutritional status might be impaired

Bond (1997) believes that malnourishment is an overall term that encompasses:

- Undernourishment due to inadequate food intake
- Overnourishment due to excess food consumption, leading to obesity
- Deficiency of specific nutrients, and/or
- Dietary imbalance due to disproportionate intake.

| ■ *Activity* | What do you think might prevent Saba, Miss West, Phillip and Mr Cooper from meeting their nutritional needs? |

Some of the points that you might have considered are:

- Miss West may not be physically able to feed herself as her weak right arm will cause difficulty manipulating eating utensils. Her dentures do not fit properly and this will affect her eating. It also appears that although she can swallow she has lost interest in food. There could be many factors causing this, for example depression or dislike of hospital food. As she is partially sighted she may not be able to see her food or utensils well. When she is discharged, all aspects of food handling could be difficult.

■ In order to feed, infants need to co-ordinate sucking, swallowing and breathing with split second timing (Kanneh and Ellis 1999). Saba's breathlessness may be interfering with her ability to do this, resulting in decreased intake of milk. Nurses caring for Saba should also be aware of her mother's nutritional needs while she is breast-feeding as her food intake could be affected by the hospital environment and its lack of familiar food, and her anxiety about Saba. This might affect her milk production.

■ Phillip is able to feed himself and can also shop with help. As he is obese it might appear that his nutritional intake is more than adequate. However he may not be eating enough of the right foods while eating too many of foods which might lead to obesity, such as a high fat diet or an excess of sugar. He might be unaware of the different nutrients he needs to stay healthy.

■ Mr Cooper has dementia and this could affect his appetite and his ability to shop and prepare food thus leading to an inadequate and inappropriate intake. His access to shops to buy food is very limited.

These examples illustrate that people may be unable to meet their nutritional needs, leading to malnutrition, as a result of inadequate intake, inappropriate intake, increased nutritional demands or any combination of these factors.

Inadequate intake

Activity

What might predispose to an inadequate nutritional intake? The scenarios will give you some clues. Remember to think about psychological and socio-economic factors as well as physical factors.

There are numerous factors that may lead to an inadequate intake.

Appetite
This is the psychological stimulus to eat; it may be connected with and triggered by emotional stimuli (Pender 1994).

■ **Loss of appetite**: **Appetite** loss may be caused by the pain, stress, anxiety, reduced physical activity and fatigue which often accompany illness (Pender 1994). In addition some medicines may suppress the appetite (Holmes 2003).

■ **Stress**: Some people may have an inadequate intake as a result of busy, stressful lives (Edwards 1998).

■ **Lack of knowledge and skills for feeding**: People may not understand the importance of eating, and may be unable to buy suitable food and prepare it.

■ **Dementia**: People with dementia may not be able to physically feed themselves. They may not co-operate with attempts to encourage them to eat and drink, and in very severe cognitive impairment they may no longer recognise food (Manthorpe and Watson 2003).

- **Paranoia**: Some people may not eat because of fear of being poisoned.
- **Nausea and vomiting**: These symptoms can be caused by various illnesses or be side effects of some medicines, and will prevent people from eating even if they feel hungry (Holmes 2003).
- **Nil by mouth**: Some people may be unable to eat for prolonged periods due to their condition (e.g. if they are unconscious) or treatment (e.g. following some types of surgery).
- **Physical factors**: One example of a physical factor is dysphagia (difficulty in swallowing) which results from delayed or absent swallow reflex (Crawley 2003). Initially Miss West had this problem. Chewing difficulty and mouth pain caused by decayed teeth or ill-fitting dentures or mouth ulcers are other physical causes of inadequate intake. Limited dexterity causing difficulty in manipulating cutlery may make feeding oneself slow and difficult (e.g. people with cerebral palsy, stroke or rheumatoid arthritis). The physical effort of eating may be too great for some people with chronic diseases such as heart failure or **emphysema** (Holmes 2003), or children with congenital heart disease.
- **Dependency**: People who are dependent on others and unable to express their needs are at risk of inadequate intake. Examples would be very young children and people unable to communicate as a result of intellectual or neurological impairment, or dementia.
- **Lack of finance**: People who are living on a low income often have many demands on their limited funds, and nutrition may not be the top priority.

Emphysema
Lung disease characterised by over-inflation and destructive changes leading to a lack of elasticity in the alveolar walls.

Inappropriate intake

- **Over-eating**: Some people turn to food as a source of comfort during periods of insecurity, depression or loneliness (Edwards 1998). With Phillip it would be important to consider whether these social and psychological factors are relevant. For example, are there sufficient activities for him to be involved in?
- **Incorrectly made-up feeds**: Lack of knowledge may result in inappropriate intake; for example errors in making up bottle feeds for infants can result in over-concentrated feeds which may cause harm, or weak feeds, resulting in a failure to gain weight.
- **Restricted diets**: Fad diets and erroneous health beliefs may lead people to follow diets that are too restricted to meet their needs. For example, the low-fat, high-fibre diet recommended as healthy eating for adults is inappropriate for very young children who need a diet that is relatively dense in calories because of the smaller volumes consumed (Willis 1997). Recently the 'Atkins diet' has caused much debate as it encourages a high fat and low carbohydrate intake, a combination which many people

believe is unhealthy. Recently published evidence appears to suggest that this diet is safe (Hartley 2003) but debates about it continue.

Increased demands

Basal metabolic rate
The amount of energy needed by the body for essential processes when at complete rest but awake (Brooker 1998).

Holmes (2003) describes how the body's reaction to injury, infection and surgery raises the **basal metabolic rate** and hence increases nutritional demands. Healing of wounds and fractures requires additional nutrients. Some neurological conditions, such as some types of cerebral palsy, can cause excessive body movements using up energy and thus increasing nutritional demands.

Summary

- An adequate intake of the correct balance of nutrients is essential to maintain health, and prevent malnutrition.
- Many people encountered by nurses have increased nutritional demands but their ability to meet these demands is compromised due to an inadequate, and sometimes inappropriate, dietary intake.

PROMOTING HEALTHY EATING IN CARE SETTINGS

An important part of promoting good nutrition is the encouragement of healthy eating. *The Essence of Care* states that best practice is: 'All opportunities are used to encourage the patient/client to eat to promote their health' (Department of Health 2001a, p. 76). A balanced diet contains a particular selection of foods, in the correct proportions to meet the requirements of the body's cells and is essential for maintaining a healthy body that functions efficiently. We have already considered the nutrients necessary for a healthy diet and factors that can affect nutritional status but in care settings, achieving a healthy diet poses particular challenges.

LEARNING OUTCOMES

By the end of this section you will be able to:

1. Identify the factors that influence the food we eat.
2. Discuss the difficulties in maintaining a healthy diet in a care setting.
3. Assist patients/clients to select a healthy diet from a menu in a care setting.

Learning outcome 1: Identify the factors that influence the food we eat

Activity

Make a list of the food you ate yesterday, and think about what led you to eat what you did.

Reasons for eating particular foods might include:

- Hunger
- Personal likes/dislikes
- Knowledge about nutritional value of particular foods
- Time of day, e.g. meal times
- Your environment
- Financial situation
- Your emotional state
- How you were feeling physically
- Culture and religion
- Boredom
- Lifestyle, including work pattern, social events.

Many of the above are linked to personal choice but such choices may be restricted within care settings. How many of the foods you ate were selected for their nutritional value? For example the Department of Health's 'Five a day' campaign (www.dh.gov.uk) to encourage people to increase their fruit and vegetable consumption has received a lot of publicity but has it impacted on your food intake? Among fruit and vegetables most people have their personal favourites but these may not be easily available in hospital. These issues are discussed next.

Learning outcome 2: Discuss the difficulties in maintaining a healthy diet in a care setting

Activity

What difficulties can care settings present for people trying to eat a healthy diet and nurses trying to encourage this? Think about this in relation to an acute hospital setting (as in Miss West's case) or in a setting such as a mental health unit.

Generally, nurses in care settings may not have access to sufficient information regarding clients' nutritional preferences and needs, but even if they do, actually catering for them within an institutional setting can be difficult (Perry 1997). There may be limited availability of appropriate equipment to help people with eating. In hospital settings nurses have restricted access to food due to the food hygiene regulations. Cook chill facilities in many hospitals lead to inflexible meal times so that people have to eat at that time or go without. Staffing levels at meal times are often at their lowest because of staff breaks, and there are frequently other activities going on at the same time, for example medication administration, ward rounds (Edwards 1998; Kowanko *et al.* 1999). Recognising this problem government advisors are recommending that there should be an 'all hands on deck' approach to meal times with staff breaks denied during this period (Meikle 2003).

People's likes and dislikes, and cultural and religious factors can be difficult to cater for in hospital settings. An audit of patient meals found that a third of the hospital vegetarian meals failed to provide the recommended amount of protein (Fettes and Murray 1999). A study of South Asian older people's care experiences found dissatisfaction with their hospital food and a perceived lack of understanding from staff of the food's religious significance (Clegg 2003). One study participant said: 'I am not satisfied with the food, and would prefer Asian food like chapattis and rice made in the traditional way. Sometimes I stay hungry because I do not like the food and I am unable to say. I go to bed and thank Allah that I am getting better and pray that the food will be better tomorrow.'

In mental health units there may be more flexibility over meal times and food provision, but being an institutional setting, this will still be limited. The mental health charity MIND reported that 45 per cent of respondents did not have access to snacks outside of meal times and almost a third of people in in-patient units said they did not have enough access to hot and cold drinks (Baker 2001). There might be facilities for families to bring food in, and to heat food in a microwave. All food brought in should be labelled and dated and staff will need to be informed in case it interacts with medication being taken, any other special diet or the person is to be nil by mouth prior to a treatment. Some mental health units have canteen facilities and these usually provide more choice for service users.

Best practice statements in *The Essence of Care* include:

- 'Food that is provided by the service meets the needs of individual patients/clients', and
- 'Patients/clients have set meal times, are offered a replacement meal if a meal is missed and can access snacks at any time' (Department of Health 2001a, p. 76).

The guidelines also advise that there should be adapted utensils available and inappropriate activity should be curtailed during meal times. They also emphasise throughout that food provided must be in accordance with people's cultural/religious preferences (Department of Health 2001a). Care settings should be working towards these benchmarks of good practice and as you read in Miss West's scenario, she is being offered snacks to encourage her to eat more, so clearly this service is available at her hospital. The Better Hospital Food initiative aims to address the known problems with hospital food and is promoting new NHS menus.

Learning outcome 3: Assist patients/clients to select a healthy diet from a menu in a care setting

■ *Activity*

The menu in Box 9.1 was taken from the Better Hospital Food website (www.betterhospitalfood.com). It is described as a typical NHS hospital menu for lunch and dinner choices. Think about how you might assist a patient in a hospital setting to choose from the menu.

Lunch

- Orange juice or cream of tomato soup with roll
- Moussaka or Pastrami and red onion sandwich
- Peach flan or apple.

Dinner

- Beef braised with button mushrooms in a rich sauce or seafood pasta with fresh dill and parmesan (made with plaice, salmon or prawns) or Gala pie salad
- New potatoes or Parmentier potatoes (diced and fried potatoes), buttered cabbage and green beans
- Baked jam sponge and custard or chocolate mousse or seedless grapes or cheese and biscuits.

Box 9.1 A menu from the Better Hospital Food website (www.betterhospitalfood. com) (Reproduced with kind permission from http://patientexperience.nhsestates. gov.uk/bhf (accessed 15 November 2003))

You might first spend time with the person finding out about their likes and dislikes. As discussed earlier you should consider their religion and culture as some people's food preferences are related to religious beliefs. Thus the menu in Box 9.1 may not provide a choice of food acceptable to your patient. Menus for vegetarians, children and halal meals are also included on the Better Hospital Food website and these choices and others should be available in your care setting. It is important not to make assumptions about what people might eat according to their culture/religion and find out from the individual or family concerned. For example a person who follows Sikhism may refrain from eating beef, eggs or fish or may be a vegetarian (Gill 2002). A person following Judaism is required to eat kosher food (food fit to be eaten in accordance with Jewish law) but there any many diverse practices about this (Collins 2002). Religion apart, people's beliefs and values may lead them to require a vegetarian or vegan diet. Be prepared to explain foods on the menu, as some choices may be unfamiliar to people. For example Miss West may never have eaten moussaka and may not know what pastrami is.

You may need to read out menus and complete them for people. This would be necessary for Miss West who is partially sighted. When going through the menu you can guide your patient towards appropriate foods, ensuring there is a balance of the important food groups discussed earlier in this chapter, while taking preferences into account. Miss West requires food that is not only nourishing but also weight-inducing, so you might encourage her to eat more carbohydrates and dairy products. Many hospitals would allow Saba's mother to eat from the hospital menu. Good nutrition is vital for breast-feeding women and it is unlikely that she would leave her sick baby to eat away from the ward. As well as food intake ensure that your patient consumes sufficient fluid on a daily basis. Two to three litres of fluid daily is considered adequate for an adult; you might remember from an earlier activity that Miss West's intake falls far short of this at present.

Summary

- There are a wide range of factors that affect people's food choices.
- When promoting healthy eating, nurses need to try to find out food preferences.
- Within care settings, choice relating to what is eaten and when can be limited by a number of factors, but hospitals should be working towards the benchmarks of good practice laid down in *The Essence of Care* (Department of Health 2001a). Nurses should be able to guide patients/clients regarding appropriate food choices, with respect for individual preferences, culture, values and beliefs.

ASSESSING NUTRITIONAL STATUS AND DEVELOPING A PLAN OF ACTION

Assessment is the collection of information about a patient/client, and includes obtaining a nutritional history and taking physical measurements. Nurses are in a unique position to assess people's nutritional status, identify people at risk of malnourishment, and then take appropriate action. As recognised already in this chapter, there are many factors that can interfere with nutritional status. If nurses do not carry out nutritional screening carefully, they can put people at unnecessary risk of suffering from the effects of malnourishment. A range of nutritional screening tools is available. The Department of Health defines screening as 'The process of identifying patients who are already malnourished or who are at risk of becoming so' (Department of Health 2001a, p. 78). The benchmark of best practice is 'Nutritional screening progresses to further assessment for all patients/clients identified as "at risk".' (Department of Health 2001a, p. 76).

LEARNING OUTCOMES

By the end of this section you will be able to:

1. Discuss key nursing skills required for successful assessment.
2. Understand the purpose and use of nutritional screening tools.
3. Carry out nutritional screening and recognise if people are at risk of malnutrition.
4. Identify measures to assist people who are at risk of malnutrition.

Learning outcome 1: Discuss key nursing skills required for successful assessment

Assessment comprises measuring, observing and questioning. Each of these are looked at in this section.

Measuring

What measurements do you know of which will help in assessing nutritional status?

Measuring weight is an obvious answer but you might also have heard of the body mass index, for which height measurement is also needed. You might also have seen or heard of growth charts been used for infants and children.

Weighing

All the people in the scenarios could be weighed, using appropriate weighing scales. This may help Miss West, Mr Cooper and Phillip to recognise whether they have lost or gained any significant weight, assuming that they are aware of their previous weights. Parents are often aware of their infant's most recent weight to the last gram. The weights can act as a baseline for future weight measurements, as weekly weighing may be indicated if there is cause for concern.

Height

This measurement is most often used with children but in adults it is necessary for calculating the body mass index (Perry 2003) and so would be measured for all the adults in the scenarios if possible.

Body mass index (BMI)

The BMI is determined by considering a person's weight in relation to height, and it indicates healthy ranges for body weight. It does not distinguish fat from muscle protein. This calculation is not suitable for use with babies and children and therefore would not be relevant to Saba. To calculate the BMI, you need to use the formula:

$$\frac{\text{Weight (kg)}}{\text{Height (m)}^2}$$

Thus if Phillip's weight is 92 kg and his height is 1.68 m you would calculate his BMI by the following calculation:

$$\frac{92}{(1.68 \times 1.68)}$$

However most health care staff use charts as in Fig. 9.1, or in some cases entering the weight and height into an electronic patient record will automatically generate the BMI measurement.

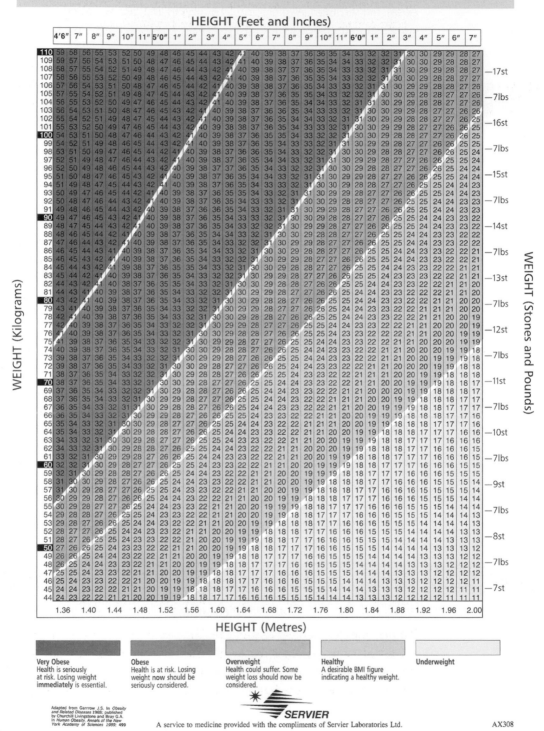

Figure 9.1 The Body Mass Index. (Reproduced with kind permission of Servier Laboratories Limited 1991.)

Activity

Use Fig. 9.1 to calculate:

a) Phillip's BMI, using the measurements above.

b) Mr Cooper's BMI if his height is 1.9 m and his weight is 64 kg.

What category of weight do these BMIs come in to?

(a) You will see that Phillip's BMI according to Fig. 9.1 is 33. The chart classifies this as 'Obese' and advises 'Health is at risk. Losing weight now should be seriously considered'. (b) Mr Cooper's BMI is 18. The chart classifies this as 'Underweight'.

Growth charts

Growth charts are commonly used to assess and monitor the growth of children, which is an indicator of their nutritional status. Growth charts are widely available for boys and girls of different ages. The chart consists of a graph with age on the horizontal axis, and either height, weight or head circumference on the vertical axis. A series of lines are marked on the graph, representing 'centiles'. The value given to a centile represents the percentage of children who are below this height or weight at a given age. This means that 90 per cent of children weigh less than the weight indicated by the ninetieth centile, whereas 97 per cent of children weigh more than that represented by the third centile. Therefore, a child whose weight falls near, for example, the ninetieth centile may be considered 'big' for his age, as only 10 per cent of his peers will be heavier than him.

Children are expected to demonstrate steady weight gain, and broadly, to follow the pattern of the centiles marked on the chart. The growth of children whose weight is plotted below the third centile or above the ninetieth centile is considered outside normal parameters (Moules and Ramsay 1998). It can therefore be seen that weight, height and other measurements must be accurate. It is common practice for weights of infants and children to be checked by two nurses. As explained in Chapter 4, medicines are calculated for infants/children on the basis of their weight so accuracy in weighing is crucial for this purpose too, as well as for monitoring nutrition. Wardley *et al.* (1997) provide a more detailed discussion of the use of growth charts.

Activity

If possible obtain an appropriate growth chart from your practice area and plot Saba's birth weight, last recorded weight and admission weight. What conclusions would you draw as a result?

Plotting Saba's weight reveals that her birth weight was between the twenty-fifth and fiftieth centile and that her weight gain had been within normal expectations. Very recently she has lost 120 g. Whilst this is only a small amount, it could be a significant change as she has previously been growing according to expectations.

Observing

Depending on Miss West's mobility, and the equipment available, it may be difficult to obtain her weight and height measurements. However assessment can be carried out using a range of observations to gain insight into nutritional status.

Activity

> With reference to the scenarios, what observations could be carried out to assist nutritional assessment?

Most senses can be used: eyes to see the physical condition of the client, sense of smell will identify unusual odours, and hands to touch the skin. You may have identified many of the aspects listed below; most would be useful in assessing the patients/clients in the scenarios.

- Observe if clothing, rings and dentures are fitting comfortably. If not, this could suggest an alteration in weight. These could be very useful indicators as to whether Mr Cooper is losing weight and you will remember that Miss West's dentures are loose. Miss West's niece might know whether her aunt's loose dentures are a new problem.
- Look at the skin and check for excessive dryness, scaling and its temperature.
- Check the eyes for brightness and whether they are sunken into their sockets, which could indicate dehydration. These would be important observations with both Mr Cooper (who may not be drinking enough) and Miss West, whose fluid intake we know is poor.
- Note the smell of the breath. Halitosis can indicate poor dental health or dehydration. This could lead you to review the state of the mouth, and to identify a problem with the teeth or gums. A sore mouth can indicate a poor diet. Chapter 7 'Meeting hygiene needs' considers assessment of the condition of the mouth in detail.
- Observe the level of mobility, for example, whether the person can move their arms adequately to feed themselves, or can walk or manoeuvre to get access to food. This is particularly relevant to Miss West but the CPN should also consider Mr Cooper's mobility in relation to obtaining and preparing food.
- Observe for drooling which could be a sign of poor swallowing, as well as poor lip seal. Although Miss West has been assessed as able to swallow now, these are signs which nurses should be aware of due to her previous history.
- While the person is eating and drinking, observe their sequence of breathing and swallowing.
- Observe for non-verbal signals, gestures or signs which the person may use to communicate their wishes, e.g. pushing the dish away. It is important to respect people's wishes.
- In people's own homes, community nurses can observe what food there is around and whether it is within the sell-by date. Out of date food could indicate that food is being bought but not actually eaten. These were

important observations for Mr Cooper's CPN to make. In relation to Phillip the community nurse for learning disability and occupational therapist could observe what food he is buying and storing.

- Observe food intake, which will indicate the amount of food that is actually being consumed. Such details recorded over several days allow for any day-to-day fluctuations. It was good practice that the staff on the medical ward from which Miss West was transferred were recording her food and fluid intake on a food chart. *The Essence of Care*'s benchmark for good practice is 'The amount of food patients actually eat is monitored, recorded and leads to further action when cause for concern' (Department of Health 2001a, p. 76). The nurses on the rehabilitation unit should check back over charts from previous days. Recording Saba's feeding pattern over 24 hours on a fluid balance chart would contribute to her assessment and monitoring. She may also be weighed on a daily basis. If her mother agrees, it would be helpful for a nurse to observe Saba while she is breast-feeding. See Bines *et al.* (2000) for details of technique, positioning and maternal/infant behaviour to be noted during feeding.

Questioning

Nurses can use a range of questioning techniques to acquire information from clients, including closed, open and probing questions (see Chapter 2).

Activity

If you were the CPN visiting Mr Cooper think about the questions you might ask him in relation to assessing his nutritional status. Identify a suitable:

- Closed question
- Open question
- Probing question.

An example of a closed question might be 'Are you hungry?' Closed questions are useful for controlling the interview and for collecting factual information from people. Other examples for Mr Cooper could be 'Did you eat breakfast this morning?' or 'Do you eat fruit?' Closed questions are appropriate to use for people who have speech or breathing difficulties and could be helpful for the rehabilitation unit nurses assessing Miss West. However, replies may not always be accurate, particularly if the person is confused. An example of an open question the CPN might ask Mr Cooper is 'How do you feel about your food intake?' This invites him to choose his response, which can provide a detailed reply. Questioners can ask probing questions to follow up previous questions to gain specific information. If Mr Cooper had said that he had eaten breakfast the CPN could ask 'What did you eat for breakfast this morning?' The CPN should try to avoid leading questions, for example 'You did have breakfast this morning didn't you?' which encourages him to reply 'Yes' whether he did so or not.

Questioning techniques involve key principles but the actual questions asked will be individualised to the person concerned. With an infant the nurse would ask parents questions about the type, amount and frequency of feeds. Parents of older infants who are being weaned onto solid food would be asked for information about weaning practices.

Read Ellis and Kanneh (2000) for a comprehensive overview of formula feeding and weaning, including regulation of baby milks and discussion of the responsibilities of health professionals.

Learning outcome 2: Understand the purpose and use of nutritional screening tools

Nutritional screening is the process of identifying people at risk of malnourishment. Screening should be carried out routinely the first time a nurse meets a client, ideally within 24 hours of admission into the caring setting (Perry 2003), and then at regular intervals afterwards. The nutritional screening tool should be tailored to the patient/client group and be designed to prompt questions about nutritional intake and status. It should be simple and easy to use by the carer and acceptable to the client (Jones 2002). Nutritional status is defined using a simple scoring system which, when totalled, identifies risk categories (Bond 1997). Nurses and dieticians have developed a number of screening tools. Although they vary in content, depending on the client group they are intended for, they all have core themes, for example, body mass changes (weight), evidence of dietary consumption, mobility and capability, physical symptoms, and psychological state. Dieticians may use more comprehensive assessment tools to carry out a more detailed nutritional assessment. Klein (1997), cited by McClaren (1998), suggests that the goals of nutritional assessment are:

- To identify clients who are at risk of protein-energy malnutrition, or specific nutrient deficiencies.
- To quantify clients at risk of developing malnutrition-related complications.
- To monitor accuracy of nutritional therapy.

| ■ *Activity* | Within your own practice area seek out what nutritional screening tools nurses use to determine nutritional status. |

Figure 9.2 shows the Adult Nutritional Screening Tool, which was adapted from the Derby Nutritional Score, by the Bucks Nutrition Project. A score of 0–10 = low risk, 10–12 = moderate risk, 12+ = high risk of malnutrition. Compare this with any that you accessed in practice. You should find that the key features are the same. Note that this tool was developed for adults; similar tools for children are not widely available. The Malnutrition Advisory Group, part of the British Association for Parenteral and Enteral Nutrition (BAPEN), has developed the Malnutrition Universal Screening Tool (MUST) for use with adults at risk of malnutrition (Malnutrition Advisory Group 2003). This is downloadable from www.bapen.org.uk along with screening guidelines.

Name -			Hosp. No. -		
DoB -			Consultant -		

✎ Calculate nutritional risk score on admission
✎ Please complete all sections
✎ Please enter a score for each section – even if it is zero

A. Body weight for height (max score 4)			B. Mobility/capability (max score 4)		
Acceptable		0	Fully independent		0
Over-weight		3	Ill-fitting dentures		3
Under-weight and severly under-nourished		4	Needs help with feeding		4
	Section score:	☐		Section score:	☐

C. Skin type (max score 5)			D. Symptoms (max score 6)		
Healthy		0	Nausea		2
Oedematous and/or discoloured		3	Vomiting		2
Pressure sore/ulceration		5	Constipation and/or diarrhoea		2
			None of the above		0
	Section score:	☐		Section score:	☐

E. Appetite and dietary intake (max score 5)			F. Psychological state (max score 2)		
Normal		0	Fully orientated		0
NBM (pre-operatively)		2	Mildly confused and/or depressed		2
Reduced (no appetite)		5			
	Section score:	☐		Section score:	☐
			Age – If over 65 years score 2		☐
			Total score (maximum total score 28)		

Recent weight loss?   Kg (approx)   Over how long?

Date	Nutritional score							Patient weight	Dietetic referral ✔ or ✕	Nurse signature
	A	B	C	D	E	F	Total			

Figure 9.2 The Adult Nutritional Screening Tool (adapted from the Derby Nutritional Score). (Reproduced with permission of the Bucks Nutrition Project and the Nutritional dietetics department, Derby General Hospital.)

Learning outcome 3: Carry out nutritional screening and recognise if people are at risk of malnutrition

Nutritional screening tools have been designed to enable nurses to make an accurate and quick assessment of patients/clients.

Activity

Using the information provided about Miss West, and the screening tool in Fig. 9.2, work out her risk of malnutrition.

Your assessment should have clearly identified Miss West as being at high risk. Compare your scoring to that below:

■ **Bodyweight for height**: Although you are not given Miss West's BMI, from the information it appears she is underweight so she scores 4.

■ **Mobility/capability**: She has ill-fitting dentures and needs help with feeding so she scores the maximum: 4.

■ **Skin type**: The scenario does not mention any skin problems so for this section we will assume her skin is healthy, scoring 0.

■ **Symptoms**: None of these are mentioned, so she scores 0.

■ **Appetite and dietary intake**: This is reduced, so she scores 5.

■ **Psychological state**: Miss West appears depressed so she scores 2.

As she is over 65 years she scores a further two points, giving her a total score of 17, which is in the high risk category for malnutrition.

There is a scoring system incorporated into all nutritional screening tools and this helps nurses to categorise people's risk status.

■ Activity

Practise using the tool with some other people:

☐ Find a willing colleague and assess his/her nutritional status by working through the screening tool in Fig. 9.2. Hopefully the result will fall into the low risk category.
☐ Think back to a person you have been caring for recently and work through the tool. Are you surprised at the score you obtained?

You have now practised using the screening tool with several individuals. If you accessed a different screening tool, you might like to try using this too, or the one from the BAPEN website.

When people have been identified as being at risk of malnutrition, nurses must then act upon these findings.

Learning outcome 4: Identify measures to assist people who are at risk of malnutrition

Once you have established that a person is at risk of malnutrition you need to develop a plan of action. If the person is at high risk, like Miss West, she will need referral to a dietician for a more in-depth nutritional assessment, and additional nutritional support may be needed. However there are many ways in which nurses can help people to meet their nutritional needs and based on their individual assessment you should identify appropriate helping strategies.

■ Activity

What measures might nurses include in an action plan to help Miss West to eat and drink?

Examples of how you can help are:

■ **Positioning**: Miss West should be positioned so that she can eat comfortably. The most appropriate position is upright, as this lessens the risk of food passing into the respiratory tract, causing choking. Sitting out of bed in a comfortable chair is preferable to sitting up in bed. Ideally the person should sit upright with their feet on the ground, their body well supported and their head tipped slightly forward (Crawley 2003). There may be circumstances when it is not possible for people to be positioned upright, and then a side-lying position can be substituted. It is advisable to use a pillow or similar support placed behind the back to prevent accidental rolling onto the back (Shanley and Starrs 1993).

- **Giving food choices**: Tell the patient what the choices of food are, and ensure that an appropriate size meal is served.
- **Positioning of food**: Ensure that the food is within Miss West's reach and inform her that the food is in front of her. This is particularly important as she is partially sighted. The Health Advisory Service 2000 (1998) reported a relative saying 'Dad often missed breakfast (he is blind and deaf) and it would be taken away uneaten – he did not know it was there and he got very distressed about it' (p. 16).
- **The clock method**: As Miss West has a visual impairment make her aware of the position of the food on the plate using the clock method to explain (see Fig. 9.3). Ensure that the plate is not the same colour as the table, as this helps people who have a visual impairment to identify the plate.
- **Providing the correct equipment**: e.g. appropriately handled cutlery, lipped plates. You may need to liaise with the occupational therapist here. Non-slip mats prevent the plate from moving around and are useful for people, like Miss West, who can only use one hand. Lipped plates are high-rimmed plates and bowls that prevent the food from being pushed off or over the side. This allows people with erratic hand and arm movements to manage with a degree of independence. Plate guards work in a similar way.

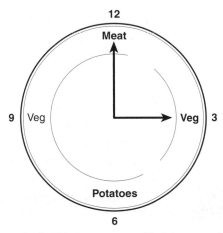

Figure 9.3 The clock method. This is a means of helping people with visual impairment to find their food. Place the food on the plate roughly at the quarter hours. Explain to the person that the meat is at the 12'o clock position on the plate and the vegetables are at quarter past and quarter to the hour, and the potatoes are at the half past position. Ensure that you keep the foods separate.

Cups with two handles or even padded handles can improve an older person's independence (Eberhardie 2003).

■ **Correct consistency**: Many people with eating difficulties, like Miss West, need texture-modified food and fluids, for example pureed/liquidised, or thickened. The speech and language therapist may recommend thickened fluids to help to prevent the choking that can occur with liquid. Nurses need to be aware that such foods may lead to lower energy density meals (Crawley 2003).

■ **Assisting people to eat**: You need to assess exactly how capable Miss West is of feeding herself. This might range from cutting up food, and giving verbal encouragement and reinforcement, to total assistance if she is unable to feed herself at all. The technique for this will be discussed in detail later in this chapter. With some people it is a matter of giving time and not hurrying. Do open cartons, remove lids, cut up food and spread butter on bread, because for some people this is all that is needed to eat independently. Someone who has cerebral palsy might take up to three times as long to eat. They would also need some assistance to ensure that they can safely regulate the flow of liquid. You should observe for signs of fatigue and offer to help when necessary.

For people who are in non-hospital settings other approaches may be employed. For example in some mental health units nurses eat with clients so they can encourage and prompt them to eat. For paranoid clients, it may dispel fear of poisoning if the nurse is eating the same meal from the same source. In some settings facilities to make snacks, for example sandwiches, are available and for a person with paranoia it may be less frightening to make their own food from raw materials than to eat pre-cooked food, which they may fear has been poisoned. Alternatively, they may accept food brought in by their own family.

Summary

- An effective and accurate assessment of nutritional status is essential in order to identify people at risk of nutrition, and their level of risk.
- To assess systematically and comprehensively requires skills in measurement, questioning and observation.
- A nutritional screening tool can provide a more consistent method of assessing nutritional status, and help to identify at risk individuals.
- Once the nutritional assessment is completed, this must be followed up by an appropriate action plan.

PREPARING AND PRESENTING FOOD HYGIENICALLY

Chapter 3 focused on 'Preventing cross-infection', and when involved with food, nurses' adherence to the principles discussed is paramount. This is important when caring for all people of all age groups but babies are particularly vulnerable to cross-infection, as are people who are immunocompromised and older people.

LEARNING OUTCOMES

By the end of this section you will be able to:

1. Identify the need for sterilisation of infant feeding equipment.
2. Clean and sterilise infant feeding equipment using the chemical method.
3. Identify good hygiene practice when serving food.

Learning outcome 1: Identify the need for sterilisation of infant feeding equipment

Activity Can you think of some reasons why hygiene is particularly important for infant feeding equipment?

You may be aware of these important points:

■ Milk and food residues can provide good growth mediums for bacteria (Dare and O'Donovan 1998).

■ Babies are vulnerable to infection, as their immune systems are not fully functional at birth. Bottle-fed infants do not receive protection against infection in the form of antibodies in breast milk (Ellis and Kanneh 2000). Therefore it is recommended that all infant feeding equipment is sterilised, ideally until babies are at least 9 months old (Dare and O'Donovan 1998).

How, then, can we ensure that infant feeding equipment is sterile?

Learning outcome 2: Clean and sterilise infant feeding equipment using the chemical method

Activity Find out what sterilisation methods are available to sterilise infant feeding equipment, in hospital or community.

You may have identified that sterilisation tanks containing either a dilute sodium hypochlorite solution or dissolvable tablets are widely used. In the home, however, many families use either the microwave or steam sterilisation method. In hospital, single-use disposable teats and bottles are often used.

Remember that nothing made of metal should be placed in sterilisation tanks, as the chemicals may react with the metal.

Now note the following important points:

■ All utensils, including cups, bowls and spoons, must be thoroughly cleansed and rinsed to remove all food and milk residues before submersion.

■ Utensils must be carefully placed in the tank to ensure that no air bubbles are trapped and everything is totally submerged. This ensures that the entire surface is in contact with the solution. Utensils will be fully sterilised after the time stated by the manufacturer of the sterilising agent. The tank should be thoroughly washed and the solution renewed daily (Dare and O'Donovan 1998).

Learning outcome 3: Identify good hygiene practice when serving food

■ **Activity**   When next in the practice setting, actively observe what precautions nurses take when handling food.

There is a big drive to ensure good food hygiene practices in all areas. Food poisoning outbreaks in caring areas are not uncommon and in an effort to eradicate this risk the Department of Health (1992) made some suggestions that nurses should adopt.

When serving food nurses should always:

■ Wash hands before touching food and after helping people with personal needs.
■ Wear a clean apron.
■ Keep foods clean and covered.
■ Keep food the correct temperature.
■ Keep utensils clean.

Referring back to Chapter 3 'Preventing cross-infection' will be useful in considering the rationale behind these recommendations.

Summary

■ Food hygiene must be scrupulously adhered to within practice settings, to prevent contamination and cross-infection, particularly amongst vulnerable client groups.
■ Babies are especially vulnerable to infection, so infant feeding equipment must be sterilised effectively, and nurses should be able to advise parents as appropriate.

ASSISTING PEOPLE WITH ORAL INTAKE OF FOOD AND DRINK

To gain the most from this section you need the opportunity to feed and be fed, so you might like to work through the section with a colleague, or another willing volunteer. You will also need a variety of foods: hot, cold, chewy and soft.

Most people eat without assistance. However physical or mental impairment, debilitating illness or generalised weakness may make people physically unable to feed themselves without assistance. Having to be fed can threaten dignity so nurses should make every effort to minimise any negative aspects.

LEARNING OUTCOMES

By the end of this section you will be able to:

1. Appreciate the qualities required by nurses to feed people with care and compassion.
2. Assist a person with oral intake of food and drink.

Learning outcome 1: Appreciate the qualities required by nurses to feed people with care and compassion

Activity

Brainstorm with a colleague what qualities you feel would be important for nurses who are feeding people.

Understanding, patience and knowledge are all important qualities, which your answers might relate to.

Understanding

Nurses need to appreciate how people may feel about not being able to feed themselves, particularly when they were previously independent in this activity. Being fed might engender feelings of helplessness and loss of self-esteem and dignity, and nurses should be alert to signs of such feelings. Nurses also need to appreciate that meal times are social occasions and that to fully enjoy and appreciate food, people need to be allowed time to chew and swallow the food and drink provided. Drawing up a chair close to the person indicates that the nurse is going to spend time with them and values them. Standing up while feeding people gives the impression that the nurse is in a hurry and people are likely to feel rushed at a time when they should be enjoying their food.

Patience

Nurses require patience, especially when feeding a person who is slow at chewing and/or swallowing. The nurse must demonstrate a caring attitude towards the person who may feel vulnerable and if they perceive annoyance or impatience, they may be further inhibited from eating, thus increasing the risk of malnourishment.

Knowledge

As discussed earlier, knowledge of individual preferences regarding food is essential as well as relevant assessment information, and special instructions from other members of the multidisciplinary team. Nurses also require knowledge about all aspects of how to assist someone with eating, including the correct technique and how best to prepare the environment. These aspects are considered next.

Learning outcome 2: Assist a person with oral intake of food and drink

Your assistance should be based on the information collected during assessment. When assisting a person with eating and drinking the following aspects are essential:

- Preparation for eating and drinking
- Food presentation
- Technique
- Reporting/evaluating/documenting.

Preparation for eating and drinking

Preparation relates to both preparing the person for eating and preparing the environment.

- **The person**: You must ensure that the patient is comfortable before you begin, for example, that they have been to the toilet, washed their hands, that their mouths are clean and that dentures have been washed. Many people will leave dentures in soak over night so prior to feeding breakfast ensure that they have been cleaned, rinsed and reinserted. For people with swallowing problems the nurse must think about their position to prevent aspiration or choking. Correct anatomical alignment will help the passage of food through the pharynx and oesophagus. People who can be out of bed should be supported in a chair with their head and trunk flexed slightly forward (Davies 1999).
- The environment

In *The Essence of Care* the best practice benchmark states 'The environment is conducive to enabling the individual patients/clients to eat' (Department of Health 2001a, p. 76).

 Activity   What do you think nurses can do to make the environment in a care setting conducive for eating in?

You might have considered removing any unpleasant odours and sights and making sure that the table is cleaned. Some care settings have a separate dining area, so if possible assist people to leave the bedside and sit at a dining table to eat. The table should be set properly. Ward cleaning must never be carried out during meal times and patients should not be disturbed by other health care professionals carrying out ward rounds.

Food presentation

The Essence of Care's benchmark for best practice is that 'Food is presented to patients/clients in a way that takes into account what appeals to them as individuals' (Department of Health 2001a, p. 76). To make meal time a pleasant experience, food presentation is important. For a person with a poor appetite, particularly if depressed, presentation might influence whether the food will be eaten. The food should be prepared on a tray that is clean with an appropriate drink, a napkin and cutlery. Try to set the meal out so that it tempts the appetite and is enticing to eat. Where food needs to be liquidised, each item should be liquidised separately to preserve distinctive flavours. If appetite is poor, a large meal could be overwhelming, so a small portion is better.

Technique

When people are unable to feed themselves it becomes the nurse's duty, and privilege, to assist with this essential activity of living. The nurse should draw up a chair or stool and sit at eye level with the client because, as discussed earlier, this conveys a relaxed approach.

With the food prepared to the person's liking the nurse should:

- Protect clothing with a napkin. Avoid using plastic bibs or paper towels because this will reduce self-esteem and dignity.
- Ask the person in what order they would like the food. They may communicate this through non-verbal rather than verbal communication, and it is important to observe reactions closely. Food should be cut into bite-sized proportions. If a soft diet is being given, adjust the portion according to the size of the mouth.
- Use normal cutlery/crockery appropriate to the food, as in a fork for the main course, a spoon for the pudding.
- Allow time for the person to chew and swallow the food and drink, before offering the next mouthful. Do not hurry the person.
- Talk to the person during the meal but avoid asking questions.
- Observe for any signs of choking, for example coughing or poor colour, and stop feeding if this is suspected. Be especially vigilant if you know that the person has a history of swallowing problems. This may accompany neurological impairment.
- When the person indicates that they have finished, remove the equipment and offer further drink and the opportunity to clean their mouth and teeth. Particles of food left in the mouth may cause dental decay, or sores can develop around the gums.

Activity

With a willing colleague, feed each other using a variety of food and drink, e.g. cold, hot, soft and chewy. When you have experienced being fed, try some of the following positions:

- Sitting in a scrunched up position.
- Sitting on your hands with a blind-fold covering your eyes.
- Lying fairly flat on your side and pretending that you cannot move. Note: as discussed above, this is not the recommended position for eating. It should only be used for a person who, for medical reasons, has to lie flat.

Now ask your colleague about your technique: what did they feel you did well? What do they feel you could do better?

Then reflect on the experience:

- How did it feel to feed/be fed?
- What would have made the experience better?
- What have you learned from this activity?

Reporting/evaluating/documenting

After assisting a person with eating and drinking you should complete any relevant documentation, for example fill in the food chart and/or fluid balance chart. Remember to report any unusual occurrence to the nurse in charge.

Summary

- When assisting with oral intake of food and drink the nurse should prepare the person, the environment and the food carefully, and try to promote meal time as an enjoyable and relaxed event.
- The nurse's approach should ensure that the person feels valued and does not feel rushed.
- Good hygiene should be maintained, including handwashing and oral care for the patient.
- Monitoring and recording food intake is also important, especially when a patient has been assessed as at high risk of malnutrition.

BOTTLE-FEEDING INFANTS

Parents are encouraged to be active partners in the care of their children in hospital and therefore frequently continue to feed their children as at home. However it is important for nurses to know how to bottle-feed babies so that they can step in if parents are unable to, and also so as to be in a position to offer advice if needed. It may be necessary for a nurse in a mental health setting to supervise a mother caring for her own baby, or to give direct care if the mother is temporarily unable to do so. A nurse working with people with learning disabilities may instruct and supervise a woman in caring for her baby. A baby's usual feeding regime should be maintained wherever possible, that is, the same formula, quantity and frequency. The baby may also have preferences as to whether the feed is given tepid, warm or cold, so it is useful to obtain this information from the parents.

LEARNING OUTCOMES

At the end of this section you will be able to:

1. Make up a formula feed.
2. Feed a baby in a safe manner.

Learning outcome 1: Make up a formula feed

Activity

Find out about the variety of infant feeding formulae by either looking in the unit feed kitchen or looking on the shelves of a local supermarket or chemists. Write down the names of the formulae that you find.

There is a wide range of formulae available. Some are suitable for use from birth, while others, called follow-on milks, are designed to meet the different nutritional needs of babies over 6 months. You may also have identified soya-based formulae. Ready-to-use cartons of some milks are available, and all come in tins of powder for reconstitution with water. In hospital, pre-packed individual bottles of many formulae are readily available.

It is important for nurses to be able to make up feeds, as it may be necessary to instruct parents. In their study of a deprived inner city area, Daly *et al.* (1998) found frequent parental errors were: adding powder before liquid; adding an extra scoop to help the baby sleep; warming feeds in a microwave oven.

Feeds may be made up one bottle at a time or sufficient can be made for 24 hours, providing the formula is then cooled immediately and refrigerated until use (Moules and Ramsay 1998). Equipment that is needed for preparing a formula feed can be seen in Box 9.2. Note that some items must be sterile, while others should be clean. Box 9.3 outlines the key points in preparing a formula feed.

Clean equipment

- Tin of formula
- Measuring scoop for that tin of formula
- Dry knife
- Freshly boiled water that has been allowed to cool slightly.

Sterilised equipment

- Infant feeding bottle with marked measurements (or measuring jug)
- Teat and attachment ring (or attachment ring and disk if feed is to be stored)
- Teat cover
- Large spoon for mixing if using jug.

Box 9.2 Equipment required for preparing a formula feed

To make one bottle of formula:

1. Wash hands.
2. Ensure that you have a clean surface to work on, and wear a plastic apron.
3. Collect equipment (see Box 9.2).
4. Wash hands again.
5. Measure desired volume of boiled water into bottle or jug. Water is always measured first and the appropriate quantity of milk powder added to this volume.
6. Add correct number of scoops of feed for the volume. Check manufacturer's instructions on tin or packet. The scoops should be level and not packed full. Use the back of the knife to level the powder in the scoop before adding to the liquid. Remember to keep count!
7. If using a jug, stir with the sterile spoon to ensure the powder is fully dissolved. Cover, cool and store.
8. If using a bottle, attach teat or disk to bottle using ring. Ensure the connection is not loose. Cover teat with the teat cover. Shake bottle to ensure powder is fully dissolved.

Box 9.3 Preparing a formula feed: key points

Look now at Box 9.3 and note that throughout steps 1–8, touching of the sterilised equipment which will come into contact with the feed should be avoided whenever possible, to reduce the risks of contamination. In hospital, use of a sterile disposable teat, cover and attachment ring units ensures that nurses do not need to touch the teat at all, as once the paper seal is removed, the unit can be securely attached to the bottle without removing the cover.

The feed may now be cooled further before feeding to the baby or cooled and completely and refrigerated until required. In hospital, infant feeds should be stored in a refrigerator used solely for infant feeds. When ready to feed the baby, the feed may be re-heated.

Learning outcome 2: Feed a baby in a safe manner

The baby should be clean and comfortable before commencing the feed. It is common for babies to be fed on demand. This means that they are fed when they are hungry and allowed to take as much as they want. Note that babies should never be left unsupervised with a bottle propped in their mouths, as this represents a choking hazard. It also denies the baby pleasurable intimate physical contact. Box 9.4 outlines the steps in bottle-feeding, and Fig. 9.4 shows the position of the teat in the baby's mouth. Any milk remaining when the baby has completed a feed must always be discarded, not saved and reheated later.

The procedure is as follows:

1. The feed should be prepared as in Box 9.3 or a pre-packed bottle used.
2. Wash hands, and wear apron.
3. Collect the correct feed and teat.
4. Warm the feed to the baby's preference, by immersion in a jug of hot water. **Note the need for safety precautions when carrying the jug of hot water.** Baby feeds should never be microwaved, as the heat distribution within the feed is uneven, so the baby is at risk of being severely burnt by the milk (Moules and Ramsay 1998). Check the temperature of the milk. It should feel comfortably warm when sprinkled on the inside of your wrist.
5. Position the baby comfortably and securely on the nurse's lap, in a semi-upright position.
6. Touch the corner of the baby's mouth with the teat and allow the baby to find the teat and open his or her mouth.
7. Position the teat in the mouth as illustrated in Fig. 9.4. Allow the baby to feed until satisfied. The baby may need to be winded periodically by removing teat and either sitting upright or resting baby against nurse's shoulder and gently massaging his or her back.
8. Ensure that the baby is clean and comfortable on completion of the feed.
9. Record the volume taken and any special comments.
10. Tidy away all equipment.

Box 9.4 Steps in bottle-feeding a baby

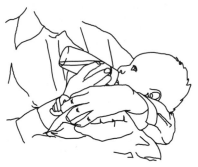

Figure 9.4 Bottle-feeding infants. Note the fluid level: The bottle is held so that the teat remains full of milk, to prevent the baby swallowing air.

Summary

- All nurses should be able to prepare a formula feed and bottle-feed a baby.
- Key principles to adhere to include:
  - scrupulous attention to hygiene
  - following manufacturer's instructions carefully

    – ensuring that the feed is at the correct temperature
    – holding the baby comfortably, and the bottle carefully, to minimise intake of air
    – observing and recording intake.

SUPPORTING BREAST-FEEDING MOTHERS

It is possible for nurses from all branches to care for either women who are breast-feeding, infants who are breast-fed, or both. A community mental health nurse may visit a woman who has post-natal depression. A nurse working with people with learning disabilities may visit a family where there is a newborn child with a congenital condition, or may be supporting a mother with learning disabilities learning to care for her child. An adult branch nurse may care for a woman in hospital with an acute condition who has brought a breast-feeding infant with her.

A world-wide campaign – the Baby Friendly Initiative – has been organised by the World Health Organization and the United Nations Children's Fund to improve hospital practices so that health care professionals are able to support mothers who choose to breast-feed (Radford 1997). It is therefore important that all nurses are aware of current recommendations with regards to breast-feeding.

In the UK, 69 per cent of women breast-feed initially, falling to 28 per cent still fully breast-feeding at four months (Department of Health 2002). It is outside the scope of this book to consider breast-feeding and the socio-political, cultural and other influences on breast-feeding practices in detail.

LEARNING OUTCOMES

At the end of this section you will be able to:

1. Identify the health benefits of breast-feeding for babies.
2. Provide an appropriate and supportive environment for a breast-feeding woman in a care setting.

Learning outcome 1: Identify the health benefits of breast-feeding for babies

Activity What do you think might be the benefits of breast-feeding for babies?

The health benefits to both mother and child are widely known (Royal College of Nursing 1998). Infants who are breast-fed are less likely to develop gastro-intestinal disorders and allergic reactions; breast milk also contains antibodies to protect against infections (Kanneh and Ellis 1999). The constituents of breast milk match closely the infant's nutritional needs, changing over time as the infant's needs change (Kanneh and Ellis 1999).

Learning outcome 2: Provide an appropriate and supportive environment for a breast-feeding woman in a care setting

Activity — Lactation is the production of milk during breast-feeding. From your biology book find out about the physiology of lactation and identify factors that might support breast-feeding in a care setting.

You will have found that breast-feeding is a complex process. Earlier in this chapter, the increased nutritional needs of lactating women were discussed, and these should be borne in mind. A crucial element in successful breast-feeding is the 'let-down' reflex, resulting from the release of oxytocin from the posterior pituitary gland in response initially to the physical stimulus of the baby's contact with the breast (Henshel and Inch 1996).

Over time this reflex becomes conditioned so that even thinking about her baby can cause a woman's breasts to leak (Henshel and Inch 1996). Once conditioned, the reflex can be affected by physical stress (for example caused by painful nipples), emotional stress (e.g. embarrassment), lack of confidence, worry and shock (Henshel and Inch 1996). Whilst breast-feeding is evidently natural, it is not entirely instinctive and is at least in part, a skill which has to be learned by both mother and baby. About a third of women experience difficulties breast-feeding while in hospital after the birth and in the first few weeks of the baby's life (Department of Health 2002). It is also important to acknowledge the emotional element of breast-feeding. Women may see breast-feeding as an essential part of good mothering (Hauck and Irurita 2002). Saba's mother might feel guilt and a sense of failure about Saba's weight loss. She would therefore need sensitive, knowledgeable and consistent information and support from health professionals.

A number of factors contribute to successful breast-feeding:

- In order for lactation to become established, the baby must attach properly to the breast. Correct positioning is vital. The mother should be in a comfortable well-supported position and the baby should face the mother's breast (see Fig. 9.5).

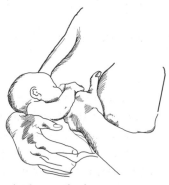

Figure 9.5 Correct position for breast-feeding.

■ It is important to ensure that the baby opens the mouth wide and grasps the whole of the nipple, including the areola, into their mouth. Correct positioning in this way reduces the risk of sore or cracked nipples (Huband and Trigg 2000).

■ The mother should be encouraged to respond to the baby's needs and offer the breast frequently. Many babies are fed 'on demand' rather than at pre-determined intervals, therefore mother and child should be together at all times.

■ A suitably comfortable and private environment should be provided, and respected by all members of the health care team.

■ Breast-feeding women should have access to a balanced diet and regular fluids, and nurses caring for Saba must be aware of this.

■ Breast-fed infants should not be given dummies, pacifiers or liquids via a bottle and teat as the sucking technique for these is different from the technique of sucking at the breast (Huband and Trigg 2000).

■ If unable to feed the baby for a short time (e.g. because of surgery to mother or child), the mother should be encouraged to express milk, and comfortable, private facilities made available for her to do so. The milk may be stored safely and given to the baby by cup or spoon in her absence. In this instance, nurses should seek advice about the correct procedure for the storage of human milk. If the baby is unable to breast-feed for any reason, encouraging the mother to express milk will help maintain milk production until the baby is able to feed again. If the mother is expressing to maintain milk supply over several days, she should express 6–8 times a day, including at night (Huband and Trigg 2000). Note that if a mother is on some medications, these may either interfere with breast-feeding or contraindicate breast-feeding. The British National Formulary (www.bnf.org) carries details of these drugs in an appendix.

Activity

Find out what provision is made in your clinical area for breast-feeding. Is there an identified breast-feeding support nurse/midwife? Consider the wider environment, such as out-patients departments, reception areas or A&E departments. How might the recommendations outlined above be achieved in these areas?

If you are working on a paediatric unit, you might like to carry out the audit suggested in the Royal College of Nursing's *Guidance for Good Practice* (1998).

If difficulties with breast-feeding arise, staff should know who to refer to. A hospital may have a designated person to provide support and advice across departments to breast-feeding women. In the community, midwives and health visitors may be available for advice. There are also support groups whose volunteers may be available (see Box 9.5).

- **National Childbirth Trust Breast-feeding Promotion Group**, Alexandra House, Oldham Terrace, Acton, London W3 6NH. Enquiry line: 0870 4448707. Breast-feeding line: 0870 4448708.
- **La Leche League (Great Britain)**, PO Box 29, West Bridgeford, Nottingham NG2 27NB. Breast-feeding help and information. Tel: 020 7242 1278.

Box 9.5 Breast-feeding support groups

Summary

■ Breast-feeding has clear health benefits for babies, and thus all health care professionals should understand how they can support breast-feeding mothers and know where to access advice.

■ All care settings should provide facilities for breast-feeding mothers, including a conducive environment and access to food and drink.

IDENTIFYING ADDITIONAL NURSING STRATEGIES TO IMPROVE CLIENTS' NUTRITIONAL STATUS

Nurses have a responsibility to assess systematically their patients'/clients' nutritional status and needs, and to assist and support them in meeting nutritional needs. This section considers the nurse's role when a client is unable to meet her nutritional needs fully from a normal oral dietary intake.

LEARNING OUTCOMES

At the end of this section you will be able to:

1. Identify other health care professionals who may be involved in the nutritional care of clients.
2. Discuss strategies to enhance the nutritional value of a person's oral intake.
3. Show understanding of appropriate interventions if a client is unable to meet their nutritional needs orally.

Learning outcome 1: Identify other health care professionals who may be involved in the nutritional care of clients

Activity

List other health care professionals who you think might be able to help people with meeting their nutritional needs. Some have already been mentioned in this chapter. Think back to the patients/clients in the scenarios and identify health care professionals who might be appropriate for referrals.

Your list may include the following:

- **Dieticians**: Dieticians are experts in nutrition, able to perform comprehensive assessments of people's nutritional status and needs. They are able to offer general healthy eating advice, guidance for the use of dietary supplements and specific advice for dietary management in relation to medical disorders, e.g. diabetes mellitus. Some dieticians specialise in certain age groups, for example children or older people. As Miss West has been assessed as being at high risk of malnutrition she must be referred to the dietician. If Mr Cooper is found to be high risk when nutritional screening is carried out, referral to a dietician would be appropriate for him too. A dietician can educate Phillip about eating healthily but also his carers so they can support Phillip in making healthy food choices, and also make Phillip and his carers aware of the implications of not making dietary changes.

- **Speech and language therapists (SLT)**: SLTs are able to assist people of all ages and abilities with chewing and swallowing problems, for example, an older person, like Miss West, who had dysphagia following a stroke, or an infant with a **cleft palate**. It could be worthwhile asking an SLT to reassess Miss West's swallowing as she is still having problems eating. SLTs will advise on whether it is possible for people to take food orally and if so whether special precautions are necessary, for example using thickening agents.

- **Physicians**: Dietary supplements may need to be prescribed by a doctor. For some people there may be an underlying medical problem affecting their nutrition, which needs to be treated. Saba may need some investigations to find out if there is a physical cause for her weight loss. In some instances weight gain, as experienced by Phillip, can be caused by an underlying medical condition, for example an underactive thyroid gland (hypothyroidism).

- **Pharmacists**: Pharmacists may have a role in advising physicians and may also be involved in aspects of enteral and parenteral nutrition (see Learning outcome 3).

- **Dentists**: Dentists may assist people with dental or denture problems. If Miss West's dentures fitted properly, this could help considerably with her eating. The CPN should check whether referral to a dentist would be appropriate for Mr Cooper too.

- **Health visitors**: Helath visitors are able to offer general advice on healthy eating, particularly for the under-fives. The health visitor will be an important source of support for Saba's mother, and will help with monitoring Saba's growth and weight gain. Some health centres have health advisors for the elderly too, and this could be relevant to Miss West when she is discharged, and for providing additional support for Mr Cooper.

- **Psychologists**: A referral to a psychologist would be appropriate if a person has an eating disorder, for example but could also be relevant to Miss West in relation to her possible depression.

Cleft palate

A congenital defect characterised by a fissure on the midline of the palate. This may cause difficulty in sucking, as there may be a connection between the nasal passages and the mouth.

- **Physiotherapists**: Physiotherapists can assist people with motor problems, for example following a stroke, and help with their positioning. This is likely to be helpful for Miss West.
- **Occupational therapists** (OT): An OT may be able to identify suitable aids to assist with eating and drinking and positioning, thus promoting independence. Miss West would be likely to benefit from this help. The OT could assist Phillip in improving his skills in food preparation.
- **Social workers**: A social worker would be involved in arranging home care packages, including home-carers to serve meals and shop, and meals on wheels. This may well be essential to enable Miss West to maintain her nutrition after discharge from hospital. The CPN visiting Mr Cooper will belong to a Community Mental Health Team for the over 65s, which is a multidisciplinary team and includes social workers. The different members of the team will appear on his Care Programme Approach plan, with their input identified. His plan may well need reviewing and additional support planned.

An additional source of help for Phillip could be to attend a 'Healthy lifestyles' course, aimed at his age group and covering a range of issues such as nutrition and exercise, which will be run by a group of professionals including the dietician, occupational therapist and community nurse for learning disabilities.

Learning outcome 2: Discuss strategies to enhance the nutritional value of a person's oral intake

Sometimes if appetite is poor or a person is very unwell, food intake may be insufficient to meet nutritional needs. Other people might have increased nutritional needs as a result of a higher metabolic rate caused by chronic illness (Moules and Ramsay 1998). A wide range of supplements are available, some of which are designed to be added to the normal diet (e.g. powdered glucose polymers such as Maxijul and Polycal), or to be taken as a drink between normal meals (e.g. Fresubin, Fortisip and Enlive) (Holden and MacDonald 1997). The purpose of these is to increase the nutritional value of oral intake; some provide just calories while others provide proteins, vitamins and minerals in addition to calories. A dietician can advise which is most appropriate for an individual person following a comprehensive nutritional assessment. There are a wide variety of flavours available, and for both Miss West and Mr Cooper it may be possible to find some acceptable. These supplements can be a very good way of increasing nutritional intake.

Learning outcome 3: Show understanding of appropriate interventions if a client is unable to meet their nutritional needs orally

Even with the use of supplements, it may not be possible for some people to fully meet their nutritional needs with oral intake. Other people may not be able to take food and drink orally at all due to an inability to swallow. This may be for a temporary period (e.g. if a person is unconscious for a few days) but for some people it can be permanent.

Activity

| If you were unable to eat, how might you be helped to meet your nutritional needs? Have you seen any methods used in practice to provide nutrition for people unable to eat and drink? |

You might have seen people fed by tube (enteral feeding) or through an intra-venous infusion (parenteral feeding).

Enteral feeding

This may be used to supplement or completely replace oral intake. Examples might be to maintain adequate nutrition for a person with severe neurological impairment as a result of cerebral palsy or stroke where swallowing is extremely difficult or hazardous, or for people whose nutritional needs exceed their oral intake, due to a health problem. Enteral feeding may be achieved via a naso-gastric tube (a tube passed via the nose down the oesophagus and into the stomach) or via percutaneous endoscopic gastrostomy (PEG) which is an opening in the abdominal wall, through which a tube is passed to allow feeds to enter the stomach directly. Both these procedures are invasive and consent must be gained from the patient/client. For insertion of a PEG, which is a surgical procedure, written consent would be gained. Both these methods have benefits and hazards associated with them (Davies 1999).

Naso-gastric tubes can be used for short-term problems, for example a baby with a respiratory infection who is temporarily too breathless to feed normally. Nurses can insert naso-gastric tubes for feeding if they have been given training. Employers may have a policy about who can insert naso-gastric tubes for feeding and what training is required. The tube must be placed correctly, and not introduced into the respiratory tract in error. The fine-bore tubes that are often used have a guide wire and the position of the tube must be checked by X-ray prior to the wire being removed and feeding commencing. A PEG tube is used when the problem is longer term or permanent (Arrowsmith 1996).

Most enteral feeds come prepared from the manufacturers. Feeds may be given continuously, overnight, or by bolus at regular intervals, and nurses in collaboration with dieticians will decide on the most appropriate feed regime. The feeds are often administered by an enteral feed pump so the rate can be set accurately. It is increasingly common for people to administer their own enteral feeds at home, with training and support from community nurses. The procedures to follow when administering enteral feeds via naso-gastric tube or gastrostomy are described in detail in Nicol *et al.* (2003). The correct position for feeding described earlier in this chapter is equally necessary for people being fed by tube.

Activity | If a person is unable to take food or fluids orally and is being fed enterally, what special care do you think they would need?

You might have included the following:

- Observation of fluid intake and output
- Ensuring the prescribed feeding regime is adhered to
- Observing for and reporting any untoward effects (like vomiting, diarrhoea or constipation)
- Maintaining mouth care (see Chapter 7)
- Ensuring that the position of the tube is maintained, for example that a naso-gastric tube is secured adequately
- Taking measures to prevent cross-infection (e.g. hand hygiene, changing the administration set)
- Ensuring that the tube remains patent
- Being aware of, and trying to minimise, the psycho-social effects of enteral feeding for example, effects on body image (see Chapter 2) and the loss associated with inability to enjoy eating and join in with the associated social aspects.

Parenteral feeding

Parenteral feeding (often referred to as total parenteral nutrition – TPN) may be used when a person is unable to use the gastrointestinal tract for nutrition, either temporarily or long term. An example would be a person who has had major surgery to the gastrointestinal tract. Parenteral nutrition involves the administration of all nutrients and micronutrients directly into the circulation intravenously via a device in the vein (Moules and Ramsay 1998), and therefore only qualified nurses can administer TPN.

Summary

- A multidisciplinary approach to promoting nutrition will optimise specialist skills and knowledge, giving patients and clients the best chance of having their individual nutritional needs met in full.
- If nutritional needs cannot be met through a person's usual oral diet, other alternatives must be found. These could be oral supplements, enteral feeding or parenteral feeding. The dietician's input and advice is essential in these situations.

CHAPTER SUMMARY

This chapter has highlighted throughout the importance of nutrition for the maintenance of health. As has been suggested, nurses are in an excellent position to screen patients/clients for nutritional risk as part of their assessment, and should work collaboratively with other health care professionals to identify and implement strategies to meet the differing nutritional needs of individuals. This chapter has included general principles that apply across a range of ages and settings. Nutrition is, however, a vast subject, and readers are encouraged to undertake further reading if wishing to enquire into specialist areas in more depth. To conclude, all nurses should recognise the importance of nutrition, and be able to promote nutrition in their everyday practice.

REFERENCES

Arrowsmith, H. 1996. Nursing management of a patient receiving gastrostomy feeding. *British Journal of Nursing* **5**, 268–73.

Baker, S. 2001. *Environmentally Friendly: Patients' views of conditions on psychiatric wards*. London: MIND.

Bond, S. 1997. *Eating Matters*. Newcastle: Centre for Health Services Research, University of Newcastle upon Tyne.

Bines, J., Gibbons, K., Meehan, M. *et al.* 2000. Infant nutrition. In Smart, J. (ed.) *Paediatric Handbook*, sixth edition. Oxford: Blackwell Science.

Brooker, C. 1998. *Human Structure and Function*, second edition. London: Mosby.

Clegg, A. 2003. Older Asian patient and carer perceptions of culturally sensitive care in a community hospital setting. *Journal of Clinical Nursing* **12**, 283–90.

Collins, A. 2002. Nursing with dignity Part 1: Judaism. *Nursing Times* **98**(9), 34–5.

Crawley 2003. Neurological eating disorders. In Shuttleworth, A. (ed.) *Nutrition: A practical guide*. London: EMAP Healthcare, 14–15.

Daly, A., MacDonald, A. and Booth, I.W. 1998. Diet and disadvantage: observations on infant feeding from an inner city. *Journal of Human Nutrition and Dietetics* **11**, 381–9.

Dare, A. and O'Donovan, M. 1998. *A Practical Guide to Working with Babies*, second edition. Cheltenham: Stanley Thornes.

Davies, S. 1999. Dysphagia in acute strokes. *Nursing Standard* **13**(30), 49–55.

Department of Health 1992. *The Nutrition of Elderly People. Report 43 on Health and Social Subjects*. London: HMSO.

Department of Health 2001a. *The Essence of Care: Patient focused benchmarking for health care practitioners*. London: DH.

Department of Health 2001b. *Valuing People: A new strategy for learning disability for the 21st century*. London: DH.

Department of Health 2002. *Infant Feeding 2000*. London: HMSO.

Eberhardie, C. 2003. Nutrition in older people. In Shuttleworth, A. (ed.) *Nutrition: A practical guide*. London: EMAP Healthcare, 16–17.

Edwards, S. 1998. Malnutrition in hospital patients: where does it come from? *British Journal of Nursing* **7**, 954, 956–8, 971–4.

Ellis, M. and Kanneh, A. 2000. Infant nutrition: Part two. *Paediatric Nursing* **12**(1), 38–43.

Fettes, S.B. and Murray, M. 1999. Audit of the nutritional content of patient meals in Ayrshire and Arran. *Health Bulletin* **57**, 374–83.

Gill, B.K. 2002. Nursing with dignity Part 6: Sikhism. *Nursing Times* **98**(14), 39–41.

Gobbi, M. and Torrance, C. 2000. Nutrition. In Alexander, M., Fawcett, J. and Runciman, P. (eds) *Nursing Practice Hospital and Home: The adult,* second edition. Edinburgh: Churchill Livingstone, 697–718.

Hartley, J. 2003. Studies show Atkins diet is safe. *Nursing Times* **99**(36), 7.

Hauck, Y.L. and Irurita, V.F. 2002. Constructing compatibility: managing breast-feeding and weaning from the mother's perspective. *Qualitative Health Research* **12**, 897–911.

Health Advisory Service 2000 1998. *"Not because they are old": An independent inquiry into the care of older people on acute wards in general hospitals.* London: Health Advisory Service 2000.

Henshel, D. and Inch, S. 1996. *Breastfeeding: A guide for midwives.* Cheshire: Books for Midwives Press.

Holden, C. and MacDonald, A. 1997. Nutritional care: the nurse's role. *Paediatric Nursing* **9**(4), 29–34.

Holmes, S. 2003. Undernutrition in hospital patients. *Nursing Standard* **17**(19), 45–52.

Huband, S. and Trigg, E. 2000. *Practices in Children's Nursing: Guidelines for hospital and community.* London: Churchill Livingstone.

Jacques, A. and Jackson, G.A. 2000. *Understanding Dementia,* third edition. Edinburgh: Churchill Livingstone.

Jones, J.M. 2002. The methodology of nutritional screening and assessment tools. *Journal of Human Nutrition and Dietetics* **15**(1), 59–71, 73–5.

Kanneh, A. and Ellis, M. 1999. Infant feeding: Part One. *Paediatric Nursing* **11**(10), 36–43.

Kowanko, I., Simon, S. and Wood, J. 1999. Nutritional care of the patient: nurses' knowledge and attitude in the acute care setting. *Journal of Clinical Nursing* **8**, 217–24.

Livingstone, B. 1997. Healthy eating in infancy. *Professional Care of the Mother and Child* **7**(1), 9–11.

Malnutrition Advisory Group 2003. A consistent and reliable tool for malnutrition screening. *Nursing Times* **99**(46), 26–7.

Manthorpe, J. and Watson, R. 2003. Poorly served? Eating and dementia. *Journal of Advanced Nursing* **41**, 162–9.

Marieb, E. 2001. *Human Anatomy and Physiology,* fifth edition. San Francisco: Benjamin Cummins.

McClaren, S. 1998. Nutritional assessment and screening. *Professional Nursing Studies Supplement* **13**(6), S9–15.

McWhirter, J.P. and Pennington, C.R. 1994. Incidence and recognition of malnutrition in hospital. *British Medical Journal* **308**, 495–8.

Meikle, J. 2003. Hospital visitors may be locked out at mealtimes. *The Guardian* 12 November, 10.

Moules, T. and Ramsay, J. 1998. *The Textbook of Children's Nursing*. Cheltenham: Stanley Thornes.

Nicol, M., Bavin, C., Bedford-Turner, S. *et al.* 2003. *Essential nursing skills*. Edinburgh: Mosby.

Nightingale, F. 1980. *Notes on Nursing: What It Is and What It Is Not*. Edinburgh: Churchill Livingstone.

Nursing and Midwifery Council 2002. *Requirements for Pre-registration Nursing Programmes*. London: NMC.

Pender, F. 1994. *Nutrition and Dietetics*. Edinburgh: Campion Press.

Perry, L. 1997. Nutrition: a hard nut to crack. An exploration of knowledge, attitudes and activities of qualified nurses in relation to nutritional nursing care. *Journal of Clinical Nursing* **6**, 315–24.

Perry, L. 2003. Nutritional screening tools. In Shuttleworth, A. (ed.) *Nutrition: A practical guide*. London: EMAP Healthcare, 6–8.

Piper, B. 1996. *Diet and Nutrition: A guide for students and practitioners*. London: Chapman and Hall.

Radford, A. 1997. The baby friendly initiative – supporting a mother's choice. *Paediatric Nursing* **9**(2), 9–10.

Royal College of Nursing 1998. *Breastfeeding in Paediatric Units: Guidance for good practice*. London: Royal College of Nursing.

Shanley, E. and Starrs, T. 1993. *Learning Disabilities: A handbook of care*, second edition. Edinburgh: Churchill Livingstone.

Tortora, G. and Grabowski, S. 2003. *Principles of Anatomy and Physiology*, tenth edition. New York: John Wiley and Sons.

Wardley, B., Puntis, J. and Taitz, S. 1997. *Handbook of Child Nutrition*. Oxford: Oxford University Press.

Wardlow, G.M. 1999. *Perspectives in Nutrition*, fourth edition. Boston: McGraw-Hill.

Willis, J. 1997. Food fads and scares: the nutritional health of the nation's children. *Health Visitor* **70**(9), 354–55.

www.betterhospitalfood.com (accessed 15th November 2003)

www.dh.gov.uk (accessed 10th July 2004)

10

Monitoring vital signs

Sue Higham and Sue Maddex

Millions of nurse hours each year are spent measuring vital signs (Salvage 2000). These observations contribute to the overall assessment of people by nurses, establish a baseline for future comparison, and identify abnormalities that might indicate disease or injury. The Nursing and Midwifery Council (2002) requires student nurses to be able to contribute to patient assessments by the end of the Common Foundation Programme, and to carry out physiological measurements. This chapter aims to prepare nurses to undertake these measurements skillfully, based on best evidence, and with the knowledge to begin to interpret findings.

When carrying out nursing observations, effective non-verbal and verbal communication skills are essential. Chapter 2 will assist you in considering your approach to people while carrying out practical skills. It is important to promote patients/clients' confidence and trust in your ability to perform these techniques accurately. Uncertainty of your skills may produce fear and anxiety in people, thus altering measurements of their vital signs. Documenting and reporting observations is also crucial to ensure that any abnormalities or potential problems with people's vital signs are identified and addressed.

This chapter includes:
- Measuring and recording temperature
- Measuring and recording the pulse
- Measuring and recording blood pressure
- Neurological assessment

Note that Chapter 11 'Respiratory care: assessment and interventions' discusses the measurement and recording of respiratory rate, and oxygen saturations via pulse oximetry, and these are other important vital signs. Pain assessment is sometimes referred to as a vital sign too and this is addressed in Chapter 12.

> **Recommended biology reading:**
> The following questions will help you to focus on the biology underpinning this chapter's skills. Use your recommended text book to find out:
>
> - Which body systems are involved in thermoregulation?
> - How is heat generated within the body?
> - How is heat lost from the body?
> - What effect does temperature have on cellular function?
> - What happens if the body starts to get too hot or too cold?
> - Why do we appear flushed when too warm?
> - What are the components of the cardiovascular system?
> - Which vessels usually carry oxygenated blood?
> - Why does blood travel in one direction?
> - What are the names for the four chambers of the heart, the great vessels and valves? Draw a diagram of the heart and label these structures. Indicate the direction in which oxygenated and deoxygenated blood flows through the heart.
> - What are the layers of the heart wall and what types of tissue are they composed of?
> - How does the heart contract in such a co-ordinated way? Explore the route taken by impulses through the myocardium.
> - Myocardial tissue works very hard and needs its own blood supply. Where are the coronary vessels located and what would be the consequence of their blockage?
> - Compare the structure of arteries, capillaries and veins. Which vessels permit gaseous exchange and why? Which vessels contain valves?
> - When tissues are damaged, an inflammatory process is initiated to repair the damage. What are the clinical signs of inflammation? What role does histamine play in inflammation? Why is inflammation of brain tissue potentially life-threatening?
> - What role does blood play in maintaining cellular homeostasis?
> - What are the components of blood and what specific roles do they play?
> - Where are blood cells produced?
> - What is haemostasis? Why is it important?

PRACTICE SCENARIOS

Observation and recording of a person's vital signs are carried out for a variety of reasons. The following scenarios are used to assist you to relate your learning of these skills to patients/clients you might encounter in the practice setting.

Adult

Mrs Anne Parkinson is a 56-year-old woman who has been taken to the Accident and Emergency (A&E) unit by ambulance following a head injury after falling from her bicycle. She cannot remember the accident but was apparently unresponsive for 2–3 minutes afterwards. She is alert but appears disorientated. Her husband is present.

Child

Max Skinner is 18 months old. He has been admitted to the children's ward following a brief febrile convultion. He has been found to have an ear infection. A short while ago, Max had a further convulsion lasting 7 minutes. His parents are both with him.

Learning disability

Health facilitator

A member of the community learning disabilities team (often a nurse) who supports a person with learning disabilities to access the health care they need. See *Valuing People* (Department of Health 2001).

Emma Campbell is a 25-year-old woman with a severe learning disability. She lives in a group home. This morning the community nurse for learning disability, her **health facilitator**, is visiting to advise on her hydration and nutrition. When the nurse arrives, her carers report that a short while ago Emma slumped forward in her wheelchair and seemed unable to hold herself up. When a staff member spoke to her she was initially unable to respond but is now responsive though 'not her usual self'. Her GP has been contacted and is on her way. The nurse checks Emma's blood pressure and finds the reading is low. Her pulse is weak and rapid.

Mental health

Natalie Turney is 21 years old. She has been admitted as a voluntary patient to an acute mental health ward with severe depression. After going home for a day she returns, appearing unsteady on her feet and she has a strong smell of alcohol. Her speech is very slurred and she is quite uncommunicative. When the staff ask her if she has taken any tablets she mentions some 'little yellow pills' and paracetamol. However, she won't give details about the quantity or when she took them.

EQUIPMENT REQUIRED FOR THIS CHAPTER

Before embarking upon this chapter, find out what equipment is available locally within the skills laboratory or your practice area, for recording vital signs. Look for:

- **Thermometers**: may be mercury in glass, tympanic, electronic probes and/or chemical disposable.
- **Sphygmomanometers**: electronic and/or manual.

Some of this equipment may be available for you to practise with, in the skills laboratory. You also need a watch with a second hand, a pen torch, and observation charts, for temperature, pulse and blood pressure, and for neurological assessment. You may wish to work through the sections with a colleague so that you can practise this chapter's skills.

MEASURING AND RECORDING TEMPERATURE

Nurses frequently measure temperature as it is often important to assess whether body temperature is within the normal range. A person's body temperature is measured by a thermometer in degrees Celsius (°C). Body temperature results from a balance between heat production within the body and heat loss from the body (Marieb 2001). In health, various physiological and behavioural mechanisms operate to maintain the core body temperature (the temperature of the organs within the cranial, thoracic and abdominal cavities) within a range of 36–37.6°C (Brooker 1998). This process is called thermoregulation, and is controlled by the hypothalamus, which acts as a thermostat (Tortora and Grabowski 2003). There may be times when this process is ineffective for a variety of reasons. Body temperature which is higher than 37°C (usually 37.2–41°C) is known as pyrexia, and if a person's body temperature is lower than 35°C, this is termed hypothermia (Brooker 1998).

LEARNING OUTCOMES

By the end of this section you will be able to:

1. Explain the rationale for monitoring temperature.
2. Identify the sites and equipment used for measuring temperature.
3. Accurately measure a person's temperature.

Learning outcome 1: Explain the rationale for monitoring temperature

Temperature readings can be used to help identify disease or dysfunction.

Activity

What factors can you think of that might influence a person's body temperature?

You may have identified the following factors:

- **Age**: The newborn's ability to regulate temperature is not fully developed due to a number of factors. A relatively thin subcutaneous fat layer, providing little insulation, and a higher ratio of surface area to body weight, combine to increase the potential for heat loss. The inability to shiver of the newborn reduces their capacity to generate heat (Mohammed 2000). This explains why some pre-term babies need to be nursed in a highly regulated environment such as an incubator. Young children grow rapidly, producing heat through metabolic processes involved in growth, resulting in a slightly higher body temperature in this age group (Childs 2000). Older people often have a lower body temperature as metabolic rate falls after the age of 50 years (Childs 2000).
- **Environment**: Heat loss is influenced by environmental temperature and humidity. The ability of the body to thermoregulate cannot accommodate

extremes of heat and cold for long periods. Hence hypothermia may result from prolonged exposure to cold, and heat exhaustion from a very hot environment. If thermoregulation is impaired, people become susceptible to overheating or cooling. Older people are less able to respond metabolically to falling body temperature and may have decreased perception of cold (Tortora and Grabowski 2003), increasing the risk of hypothermia. People with impaired cognitive function, confusion or perceptual disturbance may be unable to recognise and respond appropriately to changes in environmental temperature. They may, for example, go out inadequately dressed in cold weather.

■ **Level of physical activity**: Muscular activity produces heat energy that contributes to maintaining body temperature, and changes to muscle activity are an important part of thermoregulation (Marieb 2001). Intense muscular contraction, such as shivering, produces a large amount of heat (Brooker 1998), and is a physiological response to cold, an attempt by the body to raise its temperature. Strenuous exercise may lead to a higher core body temperature for several hours afterwards as a result of heat production by muscles (Childs 2000). People with diminished mobility as a result of conditions such as cerebral palsy or arthritis may thus be susceptible to cold, and they may be unable to respond behaviourally by, for example, adding another layer of clothing, without assistance from others.

■ **Metabolic rate**: The body's metabolic processes are a source of heat production. People with an excessive metabolic rate, for example those with an overactive thyroid gland, may have a higher than normal body temperature (Edwards 1997). Underactivity of the thyroid gland, results in a condition termed myxoedema and a low metabolic rate. Low metabolic rates may cause low body temperatures.

■ **Time of day**: Body temperatures normally fall during sleep, so tend to be lowest at night, and rise during the day, peaking in the early evening (Edwards 1997).

■ **Drugs**: Alcohol diminishes perception of cold, impairs shivering and causes vasodilation, thus predisposing to a lowering of body temperature. Sedative and narcotic drugs may reduce the perception of cold, and thus the likelihood of appropriate behavioural responses (Fritsch 1995).

■ **Infection**: One of the body's responses to infection is to raise body temperature; in effect the thermostat of the hypothalamus is reset resulting in increased heat production and inhibition of heat loss (Marieb 2001).

■ **Menstrual cycle**: Many women have higher oral body temperatures around ovulation (Childs 2000).

■ **Eating**: The process of digesting and metabolising food can produce enough heat to raise body temperature slightly (Childs 2000).

Nurses must take all these factors into account when interpreting the results of temperature measurement.

Bearing in mind the above points, identify the reasons why you might record the person's temperature in each of the scenarios.

Compare your answers with the points below:

- You would take Anne's temperature as part of her initial patient assessment and as a baseline for future recordings. Also she may have become hypothermic if she was lying on the ground outside in very cold weather.
- Max will have his temperature recorded hourly initially, as he is pyrexial.
- Emma's temperature might be recorded as part of her general assessment, particularly if she feels hot or cold to touch.
- Natalie's temperature would have been recorded on admission as part of her assessment. This measurement acts as a baseline against which any future measurements can be compared. Her body temperature may be lower at present as a result of alcohol consumption.

Body temperature is routinely recorded when a person is admitted to hospital, pre- and post-operatively, following invasive procedures and during various treatments. In each of these instances, temperature measurement is part of the overall assessment and monitoring of the person's condition. For people with learning disabilities, recording body temperature can help identify whether changes in behaviour are due to a physical health problem. Also recording temperature regularly for people with learning disabilities, perhaps during routine health check-ups at the local surgery, promotes familiarity with the equipment and procedure so if temperature needs to be recorded when they are unwell, this should not cause undue distress. Frequency of measurements may range from just one recording on admission, to hourly in a child with a high temperature, like Max.

Learning outcome 2: Identify the sites and equipment used for measuring temperature

Ideally the same site and method should be used each time a person's temperature is measured (Edwards 1997), as this promotes greater consistency. Different sites and methods are appropriate in different circumstances.

From your experience in practice, as well as personal experience of having your temperature taken, list the equipment and sites that you have seen used to record body temperature.

There are advantages and disadvantages to using the different sites and equipment and these are discussed below. All temperature recordings should be accurate, safe and suitable for each person's needs, so choice of equipment and site varies according to the individual.

Sites

You are likely to have seen the following sites used:

- The mouth
- The axilla
- The tympanic membrane.

You may be aware that the rectum can also be used to measure temperature but this site is rarely used in children or adults, except in a few special circumstances. Taking temperatures rectally is an invasive procedure that can cause people embarrassment. It may be unacceptable to a child or family (Craig *et al.* 2000) and there is a potential risk of bowel perforation (Casey 2000).

The oral site is not used for temperature recording in children, unless the child is old enough to understand and co-operate with holding the thermometer in the mouth and not biting it. Oral measurements are also unsuitable for people who are confused, unconscious or breathless. A breathless person tends to mouth breathe so oral temperature measurement would then be both distressing and inaccurate.

To record a temperature in the axilla requires good contact between the two skin surfaces. This site will probably be inaccurate if used for a very thin person, and it does require the person to keep the arm still by the side of the chest. A very young child or a confused person may be unable to co-operate with this. The axillary temperature is not an accurate indicator of core body temperature if the person is vasoconstricted or chilled (Casey 2000), as Anne may be if she has been outside for a prolonged period. The tympanic membrane is a convenient site for temperature recording, and can be used with most people if the equipment is available.

Activity — When you are next in the practice setting, observe which routes are being used for temperature measurement for different people, and try to identify the rationale for their choice.

Equipment

You may have seen mercury in glass, chemical disposable, electronic and infrared light reflectance thermometers.

Mercury in glass thermometers

These may be used in the mouth, the axilla and the rectum; they are familiar to nurses and patients, relatively inexpensive and widely available. However, there have been concerns about the potential risks to nurses and clients of mercury spillage from broken glass thermometers, and Salvage (2000) suggests that nurses have little awareness of these hazards. Mercury vaporises rapidly and can be inhaled and absorbed into the bloodstream, causing skin irritation, organ damage and reproductive problems (Salvage 2000). The Medicines and Healthcare products Regulatory Agency (MHRA) (2003a) advises that these devices can still be

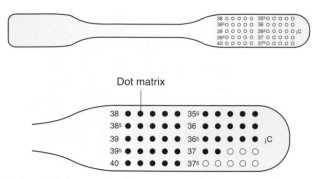

Figure 10.1 A chemical dot matrix thermometer, showing 37.1°C.

used if there is no available substitute. However staff must be trained in safe handling of them and what to do if there is mercury spillage, and there should be local procedures for mercury spillage and disposal (MHRA 2003a). There have also been reports of people being injured by broken glass from thermometers (O'Toole 1998).

The thermometer must be disinfected after use; if this is ineffective, cross-infection could occur. Sometimes a disposable plastic sleeve is used over the thermometer, but these can easily perforate so the thermometer still needs to be cleaned. Carroll's audit (2000) on one ward found no glass thermometer was cleaned between patients when disposable sheaths were used.

Disinfection and the costs associated with the correct disposal of mercury following breakage thus add to the overall cost of using this traditional equipment. Accuracy is dependent upon correct technique, for example leaving the thermometer in place for long enough. Carroll (2000) found the majority of axilla and oral thermometers were left in place for an insufficient time to obtain accurate readings. The use of mercury in glass thermometers has declined recently due to the availability of newer methods that are seen as less hazardous.

Chemical disposable thermometers (Fig. 10.1)

These may be used in the mouth or axilla. They are thin plastic strips that have 50 small dots of thermosensitive chemicals that change colour with increasing temperature (Torrance and Semple 1998a). As these are disposed of after use there is no risk of cross-infection. Accuracy depends on correct technique in relation to timing and positioning. Research suggests this method is as reliable as mercury in glass and tympanic thermometers (Molton *et al.* 2001). They must be stored at under 30°C.

Electronic thermometers

These consist of a probe, which is placed in the mouth, the axilla or the rectum, usually connected to a power supply and display unit. The purchase cost is significant, as are the ongoing costs of probe covers needed for each use. Most produce an auditory signal after a preset time or when maximum temperature is reached (Carroll 2000), so the user does not determine the timing.

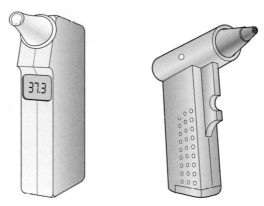

Figure 10.2 An infra-red tympanic thermometer.

Infrared light reflectance thermometers (Fig. 10.2)

These detect heat radiated as infrared energy from the tympanic membrane. The temperature registers within a few seconds, causing very little inconvenience or discomfort (Edwards 1997). There is ongoing debate about the accuracy of these infrared devices in some circumstances. Inaccurate readings mainly result from incorrect placement of the thermometer probe (Casey 2000). The thermometers are designed to detect heat from the tympanic membrane but will also detect heat from the ear canal (which may be 2°C lower) if not correctly placed to provide a snug fit (MHRA 2003b). In a study on a neonatal unit, Leick-Rude and Bloom (1998) found that tympanic thermometers were excessively influenced by environmental factors, such as overhead heaters. However, Schmitz *et al.* (1995) suggest that their use is effective in pyrexial people, and they highlight their accuracy in measuring temperatures of 38°C and above. One concern is that the size of the probe makes the method unsuitable for babies and very young children (Molton *et al.* 2001). The use of disposable probe covers prevents cross-infection but adds to the ongoing costs in use.

 Activity | Which method and site do you think is most appropriate for each of the people in the scenarios, and why?

Compare your answers with the points below:

■ **Adult**: For Anne, a tympanic thermometer would probably be used at this stage. The oral route is not appropriate as she is disorientated, and she may be in pain, anxious about being in A&E, and receiving oxygen via a mask. A tympanic thermometer would record her temperature without being invasive to her or affecting her other treatments and observations. Alternatively a thermometer (either disposable or mercury in glass) could be used in her axilla.

■ **Child**: A child of Max's age is very unlikely to tolerate the restriction of being held still for an axilla temperature to be taken. It is likely that a tympanic thermometer would be used in the ear without an infection. Although the recording time is very short, this may still cause him some distress because he may anticipate pain, like when his infected ear was examined with an auroscope.

■ **Learning disability**: Emma's temperature could be measured in the axilla using either a chemical disposable or electronic thermometer. A mercury in glass thermometer would need to be used with great care, as there is a potential risk of the glass thermometer being broken if Emma moves suddenly. The oral route is inappropriate as Emma has had a recent episode of unconsciousness. An infrared tympanic thermometer could be used and some community nurses for learning disabilities will carry this equipment.

■ **Mental health**: Natalie's temperature could be recorded tympanically if an infrared thermometer is available. The oral route is not suitable as it sounds as though she is not fully conscious. The axilla route could be used, preferably using a chemical disposable thermometer. The nurse would need to help her keep her arm by her side for the required length of time.

Learning outcome 3: Accurately measure a person's temperature

Oral measurements

■ *Activity*	Find a willing volunteer with whom to practise this activity. You will need a clean mercury in glass thermometer and a chemical disposable thermometer from the skills laboratory. Carefully work through the instructions in Box 10.1.

When recording an oral temperature there are a number of other considerations too. You might have thought of the following:

■ *Activity*	List the factors that you think might affect the accuracy of oral temperature measurements.

■ Eating or drinking hot or cold substances shortly before the procedure.
■ Smoking.
■ Talking.
■ Breathing through the mouth.
■ Incorrect positioning of the thermometer.
■ Thermometer in the mouth for too short a time.

It is suggested that an oral temperature should not be recorded within 15 minutes of the patient eating, drinking or smoking (Torrance and Semple 1998b). The time that a mercury in glass thermometer should be left in place is controversial. Torrance and Semple (1998b) recommend a minimum of 2 minutes, whereas Edwards (1997) cites studies recommending times ranging from no more than 3 minutes (Pugh-Davies *et al.* 1986) to 8–9 minutes (Nichols and Kucha 1972).

Explain the procedure to the person, including the need to keep lips closed whilst the thermometer is in position.

Using a mercury in glass thermometer

- Holding the thermometer horizontally at eye level, rotate it slightly between thumb and forefinger so that the silver column of mercury can be seen clearly.
- Check that the mercury is below the level at which the numbers start. If not, shake the thermometer in a downward direction, and check again.
- Position the thermometer (bulb first) under the person's tongue to the side; see diagram below for correct positioning.
- Ask the person to hold the thermometer in place with lips closed.
- Keep the thermometer in position for a minimum of 2 minutes (Torrance and Semple 1998b). This should be timed with a watch, not guessed.
- Remove the thermometer and, holding it at eye level, read at the level to which the mercury has risen.
- Record the measurement on an observation chart, as per example below, of a temperature of 36.8°C. Report abnormal temperatures. Clean the thermometer thoroughly according to the local infection control policy in your practice area.

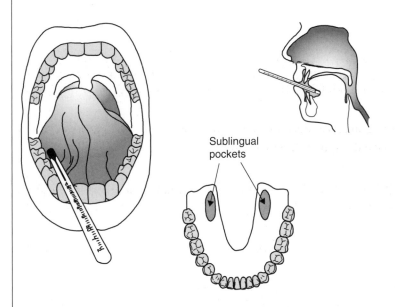

Sublingual pockets

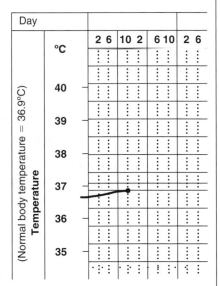

Using a disposable thermometer

- Position the plastic strip in the person's mouth (as for the glass thermometer), with the face with the dots on (dot matrix) either way up for 1 minute (Torrance and Semple 1998b).
- Remove the thermometer and read the measurement by counting the number of dots that have changed colour. Dispose of the plastic strip.
- Record the measurement on an observation chart as above.

Box 10.1 Oral temperature measurement

■ Activity

Try taking your temperature with a mercury in glass thermometer at 1-minute intervals, from 2 to 7 minutes. You won't need to shake the thermometer down in between each recording, just read it and put it back in your mouth for a further minute. Does it actually make a difference to the reading? A further exercise to try is to take your temperature just after a hot or cold drink, and see for yourself how this affects oral temperature recording.

Axilla measurements

■ Activity

Now try using a chemical disposable or mercury in glass thermometer to measure someone's temperature in the axilla, using the instructions in Box 10.2. Compare this reading with the previous oral measurement.

- Explain the procedure to the person, including the need to remain still while the thermometer is in position.
- Prepare glass thermometer as for oral temperature measurement (see Box 10.1).
- Raise the person's arm. Place the thermometer in the centre of the person's axilla (see diagram). If using a disposable thermometer, position it with the dot matrix against the torso (Torrance and Semple 1998b).
- Check to ensure that there is good contact with the skin when the arm is lowered.
- Rest the person's arm across the chest and maintain the thermometer in position for a minimum of 3 minutes for a chemical strip and 5 minutes for a mercury in glass thermometer (Torrance and Semple 1998b).
- Remove the thermometer, read and record the result as in Box 10.1.
- Report any abnormal readings.
- Dispose of the chemical thermometer, or clean and disinfect the glass thermometer according to local policy.

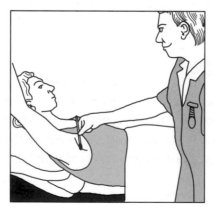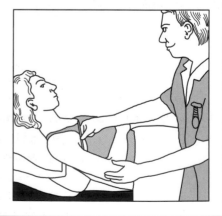

Box 10.2 Measurement of a temperature in the axilla, using a mercury in glass or a disposable thermometer

Electronic devices

For instructions for using electronic thermometers see Box 10.3. You may be able to practise these if the equipment is available. Note that the tympanic temperature should not be taken with a hearing aid in place, in an ear that is infected nor following ear surgery (Molton *et al.* 2001).

Using an electronic thermometer to record oral or axilla temperature

- The positioning of electronic probes in the mouth or the axilla is the same as for mercury in glass or chemical disposable thermometers.
- A new probe cover should be used for each person.
- Devices have either an auditory (e.g. bleeping sound) or visual (e.g. flashing) indicator when maximum temperature is reached; the probe should remain in place until this is noted.

Using an infrared tympanic membrane thermometer

- The speculum is covered with a disposable cover.
- The ear is pulled gently but firmly to straighten the ear canal. To achieve this for adults over one year pull the ear up and back, and for children under one year pull the ear straight back (MHRA 2003b).
- The speculum is inserted gently into the ear canal, ensuring a snug fit.
- The start button is pressed.
- The reading is obtained within 1–2 seconds, indicated by a bleeping sound.

Box 10.3 Temperature measurement using the electronic thermometer and the tympanic thermometer

Activity

Using a thermometer will give you an accurate measurement of temperature but can you think of other observations which could help you to assess body temperature?

You could observe the person's colour, whether they are pale or flushed in appearance. You can feel whether the person has cold extremities or is hot to touch. You can look for whether the person is shivering or sweating, and ask them how they feel. It is particularly important to use these observations if people are unable to communicate verbally about whether they feel cold or hot. Your observations may prompt you to record their temperature.

Summary
■ Choice of route and equipment for measuring temperature should take into account individual factors such as age, and

physical and mental condition, as well as the devices available in the particular practice setting.

■ For each route and device used, the measurement should be carried out and recorded carefully and accurately.

■ Abnormal measurements should be reported as action, for example administration of anti-pyretic medication (e.g. paracetamol), may be needed.

■ As temperature can vary between body sites the site of measurement should be recorded and the same site used for subsequent recordings whenever possible.

MEASURING AND RECORDING THE PULSE

When the left ventricle of the heart pumps blood into the already full aorta and out into the arterial system, this causes a wave of expansion throughout the arteries. Where arteries are near the surface of the body, this expansion – the pulse – can be felt when lightly pressing (palpating) the artery against bone. The pulse thus represents each ventricular contraction of the heart and in the healthy heart, one heart beat corresponds to one pulse beat. However, disease can affect the cardiac cycle, leading to a difference between the heart rate and the pulse rate. The pulse rate is the number of beats of the heart in a 60-second period.

LEARNING OUTCOMES

By the end of this section you will be able to:

1. Explain the rationale for monitoring pulse rate.
2. Identify the normal values of the pulse for different age groups.
3. Locate pulses in different areas of the body, and identify which might be used in specific situations.
4. Accurately measure a person's pulse rate.

Learning outcome 1: Explain the rationale for monitoring pulse rate

■ **Activity**   Look again at the definition of a pulse above, and then identify what a person's pulse might actually tell you about their body.

The pulse is measured to identify the rate and strength of the ventricular contraction, and to gain information regarding a person's health. For example, in the case of trauma and severe bleeding, the pulse rate might be weak and fast.

When measuring a pulse, the following should be considered:

- **The frequency of the pulse**: This indicates the rate of contraction of the left ventricle. It is affected by numerous factors such as age, exercise, stress, injury and disease. Emma has a fast pulse rate and there could be many reasons for this. For example, a fever, an over-active thyroid gland and certain drugs speed up the pulse, while an under-active thyroid gland, hypothermia and some drugs will slow the pulse. As Max has an infection and is pyrexial his pulse will be faster than usual.

- **The volume**: This indicates the strength of the ventricular contraction. For example, a weak contraction produces a pulse that feels weak, or it may not be strong enough to produce a pulse at the periphery, such as the wrist, at all. A weak pulse may also be present when there is a lack of blood volume.

- **The rhythm**: This helps to establish if the heart is beating regularly. An irregular pulse indicates a possible abnormality in the heart's conduction system.

Note that the thickness and tension of a patient's arteriole walls will also influence the pulse. Atherosclerosis is present in many people over the age of 40 years, and this degenerative process can lead to structural changes in the arteries. Brooker (1996) identifies how this common disease affects the elasticity of the arteries, thus altering the pulse rate.

Measuring the pulse can provide very useful information about health status. As with temperature, it will be recorded on admission to hospital as a baseline and subsequent measurements may be performed for monitoring purposes.

Learning outcome 2: Identify the normal values of the pulse for different age groups

Activity

Discuss with a colleague what might be the normal range of pulse rates for the following age groups:

- Less than 3 months
- 3–24 months
- 2–10 years
- Child over 10 years
- Adulthood.

The normal adult heart rate ranges from 60 to 100 beats per minute, but at rest is usually between 60 and 80 (Waugh and Grant 2001). For children's values, see Table 10.1. You may have known that the younger the person, the faster the pulse rate. It is important to be aware of these expected ranges when assessing an individual's pulse rate. Note also that the heart rate diminishes by 10–20 beats per minute during sleep (Herbert and Alison 1996).

Table 10.1 Normal heart rate ranges for different age groups (Rudolph and Levene 1999, p. 33)

Age group	Beats per minute
Less than 3 months	100–180
3–24 months	80–150
2–10 years	70–110
Child over 10 years	55–90

Useful terms

- The term used for a pulse which is considered abnormally slow is **bradycardia**. In an adult this would usually be a pulse rate below 60 beats per minute.
- The term used for an abnormally fast pulse is **tachycardia**. This would usually be a pulse rate above 100 beats per minute in an adult.

Learning outcome 3: Locate pulses in different areas of the body, and identify which might be used in specific situations

It is important to know the sites where a pulse can be found.

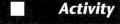

Activity

Here is a list of pulses that can be palpated (Fig. 10.3). How many can you find on yourself?

- Temporal artery – on the side of the forehead
- Facial artery – on the side of the face
- Carotid artery – at the neck
- Brachial artery – in the antecubital fossa of the arm
- Radial artery – at the wrist
- Femoral artery – in the groin
- Popliteal artery – behind the knee
- Posterior tibial artery – at the inner side of each ankle

Note that the apex beat can be listened to with a stethoscope, and is located to the left side of the sternum over the heart.

You will have found that some of these pulses are easier to palpate and more accessible than others. Choice of site for taking a pulse depends on the individual and the situation. For adults in a non-emergency situation, the radial pulse is usually recorded because this site is non-invasive and easily accessible. Anne, Emma and Natalie could all have their radial pulses taken. However Moules and Ramsay (1998) highlight that a child's pulse can be difficult to feel. Also young children are often reluctant to be held still for the 60 seconds required for an accurate pulse measurement. So with a young child like Max, nurses would probably record the apex by listening through a stethoscope. The radial pulse or brachial pulse is used for children over 2 years. In an emergency

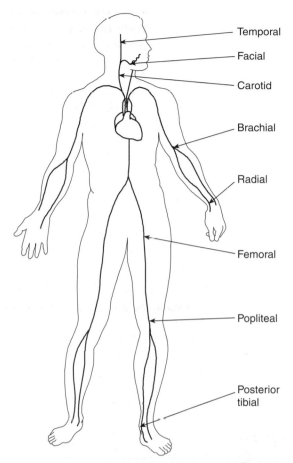

Figure 10.3 Location of pulses within the body.

situation, for example a collapsed person where there could be respiratory or cardiac arrest, it is often difficult to locate the peripheral pulses (e.g. the radial pulse). The carotid or femoral pulse may then used. The basic life support guidelines for adults and children (Resuscitation Council Guidelines 2000) discuss in detail how circulation can be checked in an emergency.

With all individuals, psychological state needs to be considered, and co-operation sought, prior to measuring the pulse. This involves explaining why the pulse needs to be measured. It may be difficult to palpate some pulse sites in people with contractures. Pulses in the lower legs are usually only palpated when assessing the presence of circulation to the limbs. This might be after trauma or surgery.

Learning outcome 4: Accurately measure a person's pulse rate

Activity

You need a willing volunteer, a watch with a second hand or a digital watch, and an observation chart from your skills laboratory. Now follow the steps in Box 10.4 (overleaf) to measure and record the radial pulse.

- Identify the radial artery. This is found with the palm of the hand facing upwards and gently pressing at the wrist region at the thumb side. See the diagram to assist you.
- Press the artery gently against the bone with your fingers (not your thumb, which itself has a pulse) and feel the pulse bounding.
- Using your watch, count the beats of the pulse for 1 minute. The number of beats corresponds to the pulse rate. For example, 70 beats indicates the person's pulse rate is 70.
- Using the example, which shows a pulse rate of 70 beats per minute (bpm), record the pulse on the observation chart.

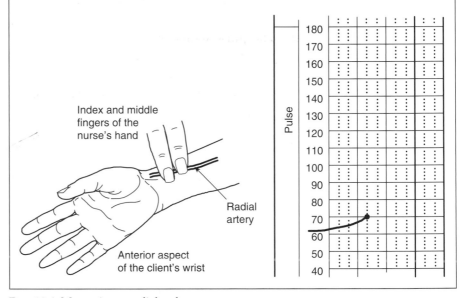

Box 10.4 Measuring a radial pulse

When measuring the pulse rate, nurses often count the pulse for 15 seconds and multiply by four, or for 30 seconds and multiply by two. With a regular pulse this will give a reasonably accurate measurement, but an irregular pulse should always be counted for a full minute. An irregular pulse rate is usually caused by an abnormality in the conduction system of the heart, and the word 'irregular' should be written by the rate. In children too, it is recommended that the pulse is always counted for a whole minute (Moules and Ramsay 1998).

Activity

Now ask your volunteer to jog on the spot for 1 minute and then record the pulse rate again. You will probably find that their pulse rate has risen, which is due to the extra oxygen demands caused by exercise. Can you remember any other reasons why the pulse may be faster in a healthy person?

Anxiety or stress also raises the pulse rate. Thus Anne's pulse rate could be raised due to the stress of being brought into hospital and the anxiety about what is happening to her. Max would not understand what is happening to him and may be frightened of all the new people, and this would increase his pulse too. As discussed at the start of this chapter, you need to put people at ease when recording vital signs, thus relieving anxiety and gaining an accurate measurement.

Electronic measurement of the pulse rate

A range of devices are available to electronically record the pulse rate, including the following:

■ **The electronic sphygmomanometer** (discussed in the next section): As well as giving a blood pressure reading, the pulse rate is usually displayed too.
■ **The pulse oximeter** (as discussed in Chapter 11): As well as measuring oxygen saturation, the pulse rate is usually displayed.
■ **The cardiac monitor**: This displays the heart rate which, as we have discussed, will usually reflect the pulse rate.

While all these devices record a pulse rate, they will not indicate either the volume of the pulse or its regularity. With the pulse oximeter and cardiac monitor, movement of the person may cause an artefact, which leads to an inaccurate figure displayed. These devices should be used with caution as errors in recording may occur. Ensure that the pulse rate accurately represents your patient's physical appearance and your own assessment. If you doubt the accuracy of any observation, re-record it and inform a qualified member of the health care team.

Summary
■ Measuring a person's pulse is minimally invasive and uses little equipment but is a useful vital sign as it gives a helpful insight into health status.
■ Nurses must be able to palpate a range of pulses, and be aware of which pulse would be appropriate to measure for different age groups and in different situations.
■ When measuring pulses, it is important to be aware of the normal range and to assess the volume and regularity of the pulse as well as the rate.

MEASURING AND RECORDING BLOOD PRESSURE

Blood pressure is defined as the 'force or pressure which the blood exerts on the walls of the blood vessels' (Waugh and Grant 2001, p. 91). Blood pressure is different in different blood vessels but in everyday clinical practice the term 'blood pressure' is used to mean systemic arterial blood pressure (Thompson and Webster 2000). Blood pressure results from the combination of cardiac output, circulating blood volume and peripheral resistance, which is the opposition to blood flow from friction between blood and blood vessel walls (Marieb 2001). It is regulated by complex neural and hormonal systems, discussed further by Tortora and Grabowski (2003). Currently blood pressure is measured in millimeters of mercury (mmHg) using a sphygmomanometer or electronic device (O'Brien 2001).

LEARNING OUTCOMES

By the end of this section you will be able to:

1. Discuss the equipment used for blood pressure measurements and the meaning of the reading obtained.
2. Identify the normal values for blood pressure and factors affecting blood pressure recordings.
3. Accurately measure a person's blood pressure using manual equipment.

Learning outcome 1: Discuss the equipment used for blood pressure measurements and the meaning of the reading obtained

Activity

What sort of equipment have you seen used to measure blood pressure? If you are not familiar with the sphygmomanometer, try to access one in the skills laboratory or the practice setting and, if possible, look at electronic equipment too.

The two main ways of measuring blood pressure are:

■ Indirectly by use of electronic monitoring, for example, oscillometry. An oscillometer is a machine which is attached to the patient's arm by means of a cuff. The cuff is inflated by the machine, which then reads the pressure within the artery. The result is displayed as two readings: the systolic and the diastolic. Some machines also display mean arterial pressure (MAP), which is the mean blood pressure during the reading.

■ A more conventional method of blood pressure recording is use of a stethoscope and a mercury sphygmomanometer (Fig. 10.4). Blood pressures were traditionally recorded manually this way, but in acute settings they are increasingly recorded electronically. Nevertheless, nurses need to learn how to record a blood pressure manually, as electronic devices are not always available, particularly in community and non-acute settings. Although there are concerns about using mercury devices, as discussed earlier there are no current plans to ban their use. The MHRA advise that they can be used if

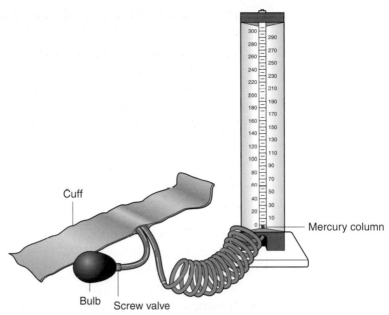

Figure 10.4 A mercury syphygmomanometer.

there are no alternatives and if staff have been trained appropriately, including what to do if mercury spillage occurs (MHRA 2003a).

Note: The use of anaeroid sphygmomanometers – those with a cuff attached to a dial – is discouraged as they are known to become inaccurate over time and result in false measurements (O'Brien 2001).

A blood pressure reading has two values: the systolic and the diastolic. The **systolic** is the maximum pressure of the blood against the wall of the artery, and occurs during ventricular contraction. This is recorded as the top figure when documenting the blood pressure. The **diastolic** is the minimum pressure of the blood against the wall of the artery, which occurs following closure of the aortic valve. This measurement, therefore, assesses the pressure when the ventricles are at rest. It is recorded as the bottom figure when documenting a blood pressure.

Thus a blood pressure recorded as 120/70, means that the systolic pressure is 120 mmHg, and the diastolic pressure is 70 mmHg. The measurements of diastolic and systolic should be judged as one reading. The difference between systolic and diastolic readings is termed the 'pulse pressure' (Thompson and Webster 2000).

Learning outcome 2: Identify the normal values for blood pressure and factors affecting blood pressure recordings

When measuring blood pressure, as with any other vital signs, it is important to be aware of expected normal ranges. However, there is no such thing as a

Table 10.2 Typical childhood blood pressure readings in mmHg (from Hull and Johnstone 1999, p. 357)

Age	Systolic	Diastolic
Neonate	60–85	35–57
Infant (6 months)	75–110	40–70
Toddler (2 years)	75–110	45–80
School age (7-year-old)	75–115	50–80
Adolescent (15-year-old)	100–145	60–95

normal blood pressure as it can vary greatly between one person and another and from moment to moment (Thompson and Webster 2000). Normal adult blood pressure is generally considered to range from 100/60 to 140/90 (Mallet and Dougherty 2000). The term used for high blood pressure is **hypertension** and the term used for low blood pressure is **hypotension**. The physiological changes that occur during hypotension and hypertension are outlined by Marieb (2001). In children the blood pressure varies with the size and age of the child (Table 10.2).

 Activity   Consider the people in the scenarios at the start of this chapter. What factors can you identify that might affect their blood pressure recordings?

Age is a factor that influences blood pressure so Max is likely to have the lowest blood pressure, and Anne may have a higher blood pressure than Natalie and Emma who are younger adults. Disease, injury and drugs all influence blood pressure and these are factors relevant to all four scenarios. As you know, the nurse has found Emma's blood pressure to be low and there could be a variety of reasons for this.

Factors influencing blood pressure include:

- **Blood volume**: The regulatory mechanisms are able to cope with minor fluctuations in circulating blood volume, but losses of 10 per cent or more – as a result of trauma, haemorrhage or severe dehydration – result in a fall in blood pressure (Tortora and Grabowski 2003).
- **Age**: Blood pressure increases from birth and throughout life (Marieb 2001). Therefore a measurement for a 70 year old might be considered normal and healthy, yet in a younger person this same value might be considered to be hypertension.
- **Disease**: Elasticity of the arteries is affected directly by diseases such as atherosclerosis (Thompson and Webster 2000). Many other diseases can raise blood pressure, including heart disease, kidney disease, endocrine

disorders and neurological conditions (Marieb 2001). In these instances high blood pressure is termed secondary hypertension.

- **Gravity**: A change in a person's postural position may affect the blood pressure. For example, if a person is lying down and stands up quickly, the blood pressure may fall. This is termed **orthostatic hypotension** and is more common in older people (Marieb 2001). As a complication of immobility it is considered in Chapter 5.
- **Drug usage**: Certain therapeutic prescribed drugs can affect blood pressure, for example diuretics and tranquillisers (Tortora and Grabowski 2003). If Natalie has taken an overdose of tranquillisers, depending on the quantity, this is likely to lower her blood pressure.
- **Emotional factors**: Stress, fear and anxiety all increase blood pressure. Crying and sucking are known to raise blood pressure in children (O'Brien *et al.* 1999), as are anxiety and excitement (Roy 1997). Relaxation techniques such as yoga and meditation can lower blood pressure (Leefarr 2000).
- **White coat hypertension**: This term is used when a person's blood pressure is consistently higher when recorded in a medical situation, such as a hospital, clinic or GP's surgery, than at home (O'Brien *et al.* 1999). It is a common phenomenon, affecting up to 25 per cent of those who appear to have hypertension (O'Brien 2001).
- **Time of day**: Blood pressure is known to be lowest in the morning and then rises throughout the day, reaching its peak in the afternoon, and then falls in the evening (Thompson and Webster 2000).
- **Weight**: An obese person's heart has to work harder and so the blood pressure may be higher (Marieb 2001).
- **Diet**: High salt and low calcium dietary intakes may lead to a rise in blood pressure (Marieb 2001).

Finally, faulty equipment and poor technique can affect blood pressure measurements. This is discussed in Learning outcome 3.

Learning outcome 3: Accurately measure a person's blood pressure using manual equipment

■ Activity

Look back to the areas where a pulse can be found. Bearing in mind the need to attach a cuff above an artery, which arteries do you think blood pressure could be measured from? Which arteries have you seen used in practice?

Any of the following arteries could be used:

- **The brachial artery**: The pulse is situated in the antecubital fossa on the inside of the elbow joint when the palm of the hand is uppermost. The cuff is placed around the upper arm.

- **The radial artery**: This pulse (as already palpated in the previous section) is found where the wrist meets the palm of the hand on the side of the thumb. The cuff is placed around the lower arm.
- **The popliteal artery**: The pulse is found behind the knee, and the cuff is placed around the thigh.
- **The posterior tibial artery**: The pulse can be palpated where the ankle meets the inside of the foot just at the heel. The cuff is placed around the calf or ankle.

As you have seen, blood pressure can be measured at a number of sites but in the majority of clinical situations the brachial artery is used as it is convenient for patients and easily accessible for nurses, so it is the artery you are most likely to have seen used in practice. Some of the newer electronic devices measure blood pressure at the radial artery. It is advisable to avoid recording the blood pressure on an arm that is affected by disability (e.g. weakness due to a CVA), or where an intravenous infusion is *in situ*. When a person has suffered trauma or surgery affecting both arms, the thigh can be used. In this instance, a larger cuff is needed.

Errors in taking blood pressure

Although blood pressure recordings are frequently carried out in practice, they remain a contentious issue. O'Brien *et al.* (1999) highlight sources of error in blood pressure measurement, including equipment failure and operator error. They note that controversy exists over when to record the diastolic pressure. This relates to the sounds termed **Korotkoff sounds**, which are the sounds heard through the stethoscope when you are manually recording a blood pressure (Table 10.3). They are named after Nikolai Korotkoff who first identified the audible sounds of blood pressure in 1905 (Korotkoff 1905, cited by Roy 1997).

There may be a period between phase 2 and 3 where no sounds are audible, yet they become audible again at a lower pressure. This phenomenon is known as an **auscultatory gap** (O'Brien *et al.* 1999), and is the reason that correct

Table 10.3 Korotkoff sounds (Korotkoff 1905, cited by O'Brien *et al.* 1999)

Phase	Sound	When they are normally heard
1	Clear tapping	Usually above 120 mmHg
2	Blowing or whistling	Around 110 mmHg
3	Soft thud	Around 100 mmHg
4	Low pitched, muffled sound	Around 90 mmHg
5	Disappearance of all sounds	Around 80 mmHg

procedure involves palpation to find systolic blood pressure before using the sphygmomanometer. This technique is explained later.

The main area of debate is whether the diastolic should be recorded at phase 4 or phase 5. Generally guidelines recommend phase 5 as the point of diastolic pressure (O'Brien *et al.* 1999), for children as well as adults (Roy 1997). Phase 4 should only be used to record diastolic blood pressure if sounds are heard to virtually 0 mmHg, which can occur in pregnancy and states of high cardiac output (Armstrong 2002). Accuracy in measurement is important because human or mechanical error in recording blood pressure can affect the person's future management, yet Armstrong's research (2002) suggests that nurses have poor knowledge of some aspects of correct technique. Table 10.4 lists possible problems you may encounter and how to resolve them. Every effort must be made to reduce these errors so that blood pressure monitoring is accurate.

Steps in recording blood pressure

Blood pressure recording is frequently carried out by nurses and is a common experience for most people, but always remember that for some people it will be the first time. Always give adequate explanation, warning about the tightness of the cuff, which some people find quite uncomfortable. For people with learning disabilities it is good practice for their blood pressure to be recorded as part of routine health checks, leading to familiarity with the procedure and the establishment of a sound baseline.

Table 10.4 Common problems with blood pressure measurement, and suggested solutions (O'Brien *et al.* 1999)

Problem	*Solution*
Incorrect blood pressure reading	Ensure that the measurement is made to the nearest 2 mmHg
Incorrect size and position of cuff for the patient	Use the appropriate size of cuff for the individual. The cuff bladder should cover 80 per cent of the arm's circumference. A too large or too small cuff will give a false reading
Confusion about diastolic blood pressure reading	Diastolic measurement taken at cessation of sounds
Poorly maintained equipment causing errors in measurement	Ensure that the manometer mercury is visible at zero and that the machine is calibrated according to the manufacturer's instructions. The tubing and all connections should be carefully checked prior to use

If you can access manual blood pressure recording equipment – a sphygmomanometer and a stethoscope – practise taking and recording a blood pressure with a colleague, using the steps in taking a manual blood pressure given in Box 10.5. Figure 10.5 illustrates how the screw valve and bulb are used to inflate or deflate the cuff bladder.

1. Allow the person to sit down and relax, for 5–15 minutes if possible, prior to the recording.
2. Collect and check equipment – stethoscope and sphygmomanometer. Ensure that the tubing, bladder and cuff are intact.
3. Explain what you are going to do, to allay anxiety, and try to promote comfort and privacy.
4. Position arm on secure surface where it is in line with the person's heart (see diagram).

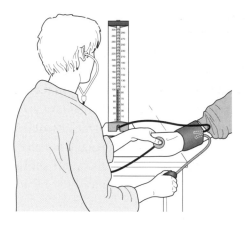

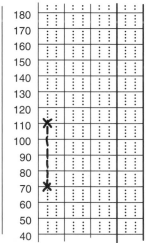

5. Locate the brachial artery with your fingers and palpate to identify the pulse.
6. Place the cuff on the arm 2.5 cm above the brachial artery.
7. Ensure that the cuff fits snugly to the arm and is secured. It is advised that the cuff bladder (the insert of the cuff, made of rubber) should cover 80 per cent of the circumference of the upper arm. The average arm circumference is 30 cm. This needs to be considered when choosing a cuff for your client. The measurement of a cuff should be clearly visible on each cuff you use in practice.

The following sizes are suggested as a guide only:
- A standard bladder 12 by 26 cm is suitable for the majority of adults.
- An obese bladder 12 by 40 cm for obese arms.
- A small bladder measuring 10 by 18 cm for lean adults and older children.

Note: Each person's arm measurements are different and it is important that you seek the advice of a qualified nurse to ensure the correct choice. The sizes indicate the size of the bladder within the velcro fastening or wrap around cuff.

8. See Fig. 10.5 showing how to hold the bulb and screw valve. While palpating the radial pulse, inflate the cuff until the pulse disappears. Note the level at which this occurs, as this equates to the systolic pressure.
9. Deflate the cuff fully and wait 1 minute.
10. Place the stethoscope over the brachial pulse.
11. Inflate the cuff, to 30 mmHg above your estimated systolic measurement, and then open the screw valve so the cuff deflates slowly, listening carefully.
12. When you hear the first sound, note the measurement on the column of mercury in front of you. This is the systolic blood pressure – the top number.
13. Continue listening whilst deflating the cuff slowly and evenly. Note the changing sounds. When the sound disappears completely, this is the diastolic blood pressure – the bottom number.
14. Record the results on your observation chart (as shown) and interpret the results, i.e. consider whether the blood pressure is high (hypertension) or low (hypotension) or within the normal range for the person.

Box 10.5 Steps in recording a blood pressure manually (adapted from O'Brien *et al.* 1999)

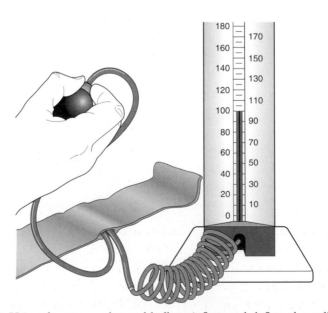

Figure 10.5 Using the screw valve and bulb to inflate and deflate the cuff bladder.

Some people have difficulty in straightening their arms, or may have pulses that are not easy to find. Always ask for supervision when needed.

Recording children's blood pressure

The most important factor in accurate blood pressure recording in children is the cuff size (Moules and Ramsay 1998). When recording a child's blood pressure, a cuff should be used that has an inflatable bladder long enough to encircle 80 per cent of the arm's circumference, with the widest cuff that the arm will accommodate (O'Brien *et al.* 1999). The size of cuff used should be recorded, so that if serial readings are taken the same size cuff is used on each occasion, enabling reliable comparisons to be made. Cuffs with bladders $4 \times 13\,cm$, $10 \times 18\,cm$ and $12 \times 26\,cm$ are available for children aged 0–14 years (O'Brien *et al.* 1999).

The steps for recording blood pressure in Box 10.5 apply equally to children. However, it can be difficult to hear a young child's blood pressure with a stethoscope and this problem is increased by the fact that a young child is unlikely to remain still for long (Fearon 2000a). Electronic oscillometric blood pressure devices are therefore recommended for children under 5 years (O'Brien *et al.* 1999). Movement can adversely affect the recording. It is important to explain to the child what will happen during the procedure. A demonstration on a parent or carer may help toddlers or pre-school children to understand the procedure and what is expected of them. This enhances co-operation and reduces anxiety, thereby increasing the validity of the reading.

Summary

- Blood pressure measurements can be affected by a number of factors, psychological, physical and environmental, but technique and equipment are also important aspects.
- While electronic devices are increasingly used for recording blood pressure, an understanding of how to use manual equipment accurately remains important for nurses.

NEUROLOGICAL ASSESSMENT

Neurological observations are performed in order to assess a person's neurological status and are appropriate whenever there is impaired consciousness, a history of loss of consciousness, or a risk that the level of consciousness might deteriorate. This can be necessary for a variety of reasons and may be performed at the scene of an accident or incident and/or in the hospital setting. Neurological observation consists of an evaluation of the level of consciousness, pupil size and reaction, motor and sensory function and vital signs (pulse, blood pressure, temperature, oxygen saturation and respiration). This assessment will inform the health care professionals' decisions regarding the treatment, diagnosis and prognosis of the people in their care.

LEARNING OUTCOMES

By the end of this section you will be able to:

1. Understand why a neurological assessment would be needed and what instruments are used.
2. Accurately perform and record an assessment of an adult's neurological status.
3. Show awareness of how neurological assessment can be carried out with children, and the special considerations that are necessary.

Learning outcome 1: Understand why a neurological assessment would be needed and what instruments are used

Activity

For which of the people in the scenarios would a neurological assessment be appropriate and why?

Neurological assessment would be appropriate for all four people in the scenarios as all have a history of impaired consciousness. Anne has a head injury and was unconscious briefly. Natalie is not fully alert and she has ingested an unknown quantity and variety of drugs that may affect her neurological function. Emma was briefly unresponsive and her carers report that she is not her usual self. Max has had a prolonged fit which will have caused unresponsiveness.

A head injury (as in Anne's case) is a particularly important reason for performing neurological assessment. In 2003 the National Institute for Clinical Excellence (NICE) published guidelines for all aspects of managing people who have head injuries and these include recommendations for assessment. These guidelines can be downloaded from the NICE website (www.nice.org.uk) and are referred to throughout this section. Because of the importance of neurological observations being recorded accurately for people with a head injury it is recommended that they are only conducted by professionals competent in assessment of head injury (NICE 2003). The Glasgow Coma Scale (GCS) score, which forms part of this assessment, directly affects subsequent investigations and management for such patients.

Assessment can help to identify a neurological problem, establish what impact a neurological condition has on a person's independence or activities, assist in establishing a baseline assessment of neurological function, identify changes in neurological status, and detect life-threatening situations (Aucken and Crawford 1998, van Carrapiett 2003). This is particularly important where there is a concern about the development of raised intracranial pressure (Box 10.6). Being a rigid vault, the skull (cranium) cannot accommodate any swelling without the function of the brain being impaired. In disease or injury, the brain tissue, blood or cerebral spinal fluid (CSF) can increase in volume or

- Level of consciousness: decrease in arousal and awareness. This is the most sensitive indicator of neurological function.
- Increasing headache.
- Pupils: enlargement, asymmetry, oval shape, decreased reaction. A new unilateral, dilated fixed pupil is a medical emergency.
- Slowing of the pulse rate: this is a late sign.
- Respirations: abnormal or irregular pattern.
- Raised systolic blood pressure.
- Limb movements: variable responses.

If any of the above changes occur it is extremely important that you report these immediately to a qualified nurse or doctor.

Box 10.6 Signs of raised intracranial pressure (Winkelman 1995)

Extra-dural haematoma

This is an accumulation of blood between the dura and the skull. The meningeal artery passes through the extra-dural space, and can become torn after a head injury, resulting in an arterial bleed into the extra-dural space. The brain then becomes compressed and displaced. This is a serious life-threatening condition, requiring urgent treatment.

Sub-dural haematoma

Here, blood accumulates in the sub-dural space and gradually builds up to produce a haematoma. This can lead to compression of the brain, which in turn can result in loss of brain function.

size, causing a rise in intracranial pressure. This adversely affects cerebral blood flow (Winkelman 1995).

In some situations, particularly head injury where an **extra-dural or sub-dural haematoma** can develop, detection of deteriorating consciousness level is paramount, as life-saving treatment could be needed. Neurological observations should be carried out under supervision of a registered nurse, and any concerns reported immediately.

Instruments used to assess neurological status

The Glasgow Coma Scale (GCS) was developed by Jennet and Teasdale (1974) and is one of several neurological assessment tools available. It is widely used and recognised, and is often incorporated into the trauma assessment chart (see Skinner et al. 2000). There are other scales available; for example, Lowry (1998) describes an alternative instrument for observation of people with actual or suspected neurological dysfunction. However, Hickey (2003) reports that the Glasgow Coma Scale is the most commonly used neurological assessment tool and it is recommended for use with people with head injuries in the NICE guidelines (NICE 2003). See later section on 'Neurological assessment of children' for details of the coma scales used with children.

Activity

Access a neurological observation scale from your local practice setting. Look at the sections and how they are laid out. They should include the GCS, pupil reactions and limb movements and a section for charting vital signs.

As the GCS is currently the most widely used neurological assessment tool, the following text focuses on it. The GCS is used to assist nurses in providing a consistent and standard measurement of people's neurological status (NICE 2003). Scoring using the GCS is done in three sections: eye opening, verbal response and motor response. Different versions of the GCS exist, but Box 10.7 contains

Best eye response (4)

1. No eye opening
2. Eye opening to pain
3. Eye opening to verbal command
4. Eyes open spontaneously

Best verbal response (5)

1. No verbal response
2. Incomprehensible sounds
3. Inappropriate words
4. Confused
5. Orientated

Best motor response (6)

1. No motor response
2. Extension to pain
3. Flexion to pain
4. Withdrawal from pain
5. Localising pain
6. Obeys commands

Box 10.7 The Glasgow Coma Scale for adults. Source: National Institute for Clinical Excellence (2003) Head injury – triage, assessment, investigation and early management of head injury in infants, children and adults, June 2003; London: National Institute for Clinical Excellence. Available from: www.nice.org.uk. Reproduced with kind permission from the National Institute for Clinical Excellence

the scale as detailed in the NICE guidelines (NICE 2003). Each section is given a score and these are totalled to give a score ranging from 15 (best) to 3 (worst). As a person's neurological condition improves, so their GCS score should improve.

The severity of a head injury can be indicated by the score attained (Jennet and Teasdale 1974). A score of 8 or less indicates a severe head injury and the person will be in a coma. A score of more than 8 indicates that the person is conscious. People with a minor head injury might have a score of 13–15. Use of the GCS for people with head injuries is well documented but it can be used for anyone who requires a neurological assessment, regardless of the underlying cause, so it would be relevant for Emma, Max and Natalie as well as for Anne.

Learning outcome 2: Accurately perform and record an assessment of an adult's neurological status

When assessing any person in your care the first priorities are to check responsiveness, ensure the patient has an open airway, check breathing and maintain an adequate circulation following the adult and paediatric basic life support algorithms (Resuscitation Council Guidelines 2000). It is important to establish quickly if the person lost consciousness at any stage and appears to be deteriorating, particularly following an accident (NICE 2003). Find out what the person and any bystanders recall about the incident; the value of using bystanders to assist with collecting information regarding a person's head injury, fit or collapse is well recognised (Dolan and Holt 2000; Walsh *et al.* 1999). Thus gaining a detailed history from Emma's carers, Anne's husband and Max's parents about exactly what they observed, is essential. The onset and duration of signs and symptoms, previous medical history and any recent illnesses (e.g. flu-like symptoms or a sore throat) are all useful to note. After taking a history, the person's neurological status can be assessed using the Glasgow Coma Scale (GCS). This assessment provides a quantitative score for assessing eye opening, verbal response and motor response.

Activity

Find a willing adult volunteer to help you to work through the GCS. Look at the scale in Box 10.7 and consider how you might assess whether your volunteer's GCS score was 15/15 – the best response.

A person with a GCS score of 15/15 will have airway, breathing and circulation that is present and normal, and will speak to you and answer questions appropriately. In brief, a talking, breathing, alert, coherent and orientated person will have a score of 15. Hopefully this applies to your volunteer!

NICE (2003) recommends that the scores for each of the three sections (eye opening, verbal response and motor response) should be documented separately to explain exactly what score has been awarded in each category. You may therefore see the score documented as $E = 4$, $V = 5$, $M = 6$, to indicate a person's GCS score is 15. If a person's score is 14 then you may see the score recorded as $E = 4$, $V = 4$ (instead of 5), $M = 6$, indicating that the deficit lies in the patient's verbal response.

Each section of the scale, and how people can be assessed in relation to it, will now be explained in more detail. This will be linked to how you might assess Anne, who has fallen from her bicycle and sustained a head injury.

Eye opening

Assessment of Anne's eye opening response indicates the arousal mechanisms found within her brainstem. When observing her eye opening response, gently touch her arm when you ask a question. Touch is a very important way of communicating non-verbally and is particularly important for people with hearing and visual deficits. Anne's husband could inform you if these apply to Anne. Remember that some people with a head injury might have difficulty opening their eyes due to swelling of the eyelids, particularly if there is an accompanying facial injury.

■ **Eyes open spontaneously** (Scores 4): Anne will score 4 if she opens her eyes or already has her eyes open when you approach her.

- **Eye opening to verbal command** (Score 3): It is important to differentiate between a person sleeping and being unresponsive. This can be done by asking a simple question, such as 'Can you open your eyes?'
- **Eye opening to pain** (Score 2): If Anne does not open her eyes to speech, you would need to assess whether she responds to pain. How pain should be inflicted remains controversial. You may only use appropriate touch and must take care not to cause damage such as bruising. One way is to squeeze the trapezius muscle. Use your thumb and two fingers and place them where the neck meets the shoulder and gently squeeze this muscle. Alternatively, you can apply supra-orbital pressure by pressing the skin just below the eyebrow, or apply the sternal rub by using the knuckles of a clenched fist to apply pressure to Anne's sternum. Underlying injuries must be taken into account when applying these techniques to avoid causing more pain or injury to people and only the minimum stimulus to elicit a response should be used. For example, do not press over the sternum if you know the person has fractured ribs and do not apply supra-orbital pressure if there is an injury in this area. You should discuss the accepted practice within your area with your supervising practitioner.
- **No eye opening** (Score 1): This score is recorded where applying pain causes no eye opening response.

■ **Activity**   It your volunteer agrees you could try out the different techniques for applying painful stimuli on them, or even try them on yourself!

Causing pain in children is also controversial. Ferguson-Clark and Williams (1998) suggest the same sites used in adults are appropriate for children. However, Fearon (2000b) advises against supra-orbital pressure, and cites Frawley (1990)'s suggested alternative, which is to hold a pen at right angles to the child's extended finger and gently press the pen against the side of the finger. However, this is then peripheral rather than central stimulation (van Carrapiett 2003).

Best verbal response

The verbal response should be assessed in relation to a person's usual communication so you need to be aware of how they would communicate normally. Anne's neurological status is being assessed by staff who do not know her and how she communicates so her husband's input would be particularly helpful.

- **Orientated** (Score 5): If Anne is fully orientated she should be able to answer your questions appropriately. She will tell you her name, where she is and the date.
- **Confused** (Score 4): In this case, Anne can discuss something with you but may not give accurate information. For example, when asked 'Where are you?' she may respond: 'I'm in the town'.

- **Inappropriate words** (Score 3): Here Anne will use words which do not make sense. She may appear agitated and at times aggressive when you ask questions.
- **Incomprehensible sounds** (Score 2): Anne will not use any understandable words but will make verbal noises such as mumbling, moaning or groaning.
- **No verbal response** (Score 1): The person will not respond verbally at all. Note that if a person is intubated, they will be unable to talk, and this should be recorded as: 'I'.

Best motor response

When assessing motor response you need to take into account pre-existing disabilities and also any new injuries, which in Anne's case could have been sustained in her fall. The assessment of motor response is done in relation to upper limbs as lower limb responses can reflect spinal function (Aucken and Crawford 1998).

- **Obeys commands** (Score 6): When you are carrying out Anne's other observations you can assess whether she co-ordinates her actions in response to your requests. For example, you might ask Anne to roll up her sleeve to assist you in recording her blood pressure. Alternatives would be to ask her to close/open her eyes or stick out her tongue. If Anne were unable to obey commands, you would next apply painful stimuli (as discussed previously), and note her motor response to this.
- **Localising pain** (Score 5): In this instance, when you apply painful stimuli Anne would move her hand towards the pain to attempt to move you away. For example if you apply supra-orbital pressure she would try to push your hand away.
- **Withdrawal from pain** (Score 4): If Anne attempts to move away from the pain, this response is termed withdrawal and scores a 4.
- **Flexion to pain** (Score 3): Flexion is bending the elbow as a response to a painful stimulus.
- **Extension to pain** (Score 2): Extension is straightening the arm as a response to painful stimuli.
- **No motor response** (Score 1): Here no motor response to any painful stimulus is made.

 Activity   When assessing a person's GCS, what factors could affect the accuracy of the assessment and how could you overcome these?

You may have considered the following:

- **Hearing loss**: If the person has impaired hearing it may be difficult to communicate with them verbally, which could affect the accuracy of the result in all three categories. Sign language could be used or a communication board, providing that this is appropriate to the person's level of consciousness, and that their vision is not impaired. The person may lip read and therefore be able to communicate effectively with you, and written responses are also valuable in this situation.

- **Language barrier**: If a person cannot understand or speak English, this could lead to difficulties with obtaining an accurate response, for example assessing orientation or whether commands are obeyed. A communication board may help, or interpretation via a relative or interpreter.
- **Speech difficulties and physical impairment**: A person with learning disabilities, for example, may communicate by a signing system, in which case information from their family or carers would be important.
- **Alcohol**: If a person has ingested alcohol and has a suspected head injury, it is difficult to assess accurately. However, nurses should always err on the side of caution. A person's neurological assessment should never be assumed to be due to alcohol until other causes, for example a head injury, have been ruled out.

A nurse carrying out neurological assessment of any of the people in the scenarios would need to be aware of all the above factors. For example, any of them could have impaired hearing. Involvement by family or significant others who know the person's usual level of response is invaluable.

Pupil reaction

Assessment of pupil reactions usually forms part of neurological observation, as alteration in pupil sizes and reaction could indicate a rise in intracranial pressure. Take note, now, of the pupil sizes shown in Fig. 10.6. You will see that they are shown in varying sizes in millimetres, ranging from 1 to 8 mm. When recording pupil reactions, the person should be examined in dim light as bright light affects pupil reactions to torchlight.

 Activity Ask your willing volunteer to walk into a brightly lit room, and observe what happens to their pupils. Now observe the pupils in a dimly lit room. When did the pupil size appear the greatest?

When recording pupil reactions, the size and reaction of each eye is checked and recorded individually, L denoting the left eye and R denoting the right eye. A light beam (usually from a pen torch) is directed into the eye to assess the reaction to the light and the size of the pupil against the chart.

You need to look at both eyes and ask yourself:

- Are the pupils equal?
- Do they look between 2 and 5 mm?
- Do they look round?

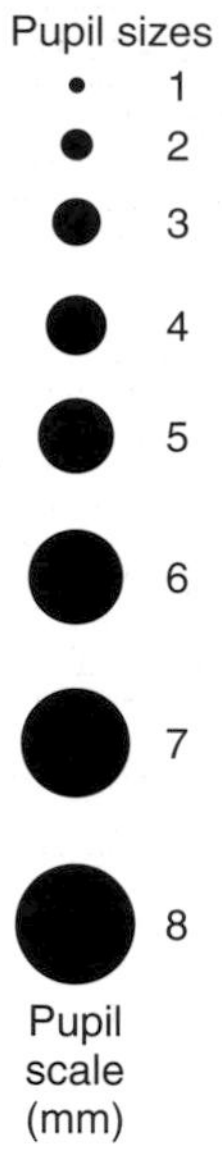

Pupil sizes

Figure 10.6 Pupil sizes and recording reactions.

- What happens when a light is shined into them?
  - Are the reactions brisk? If so, record B.
  - Are they sluggish? If so record SL.
  - Is there no reaction? If so, record – (Aucken and Crawford 1998).

Always note whether a person is wearing contact lenses or has a false eye as these will obviously affect the results. In the chart in Fig. 10.6, you will see that both the left and right pupils have been recorded as 4, B, meaning that the pupils are approximately 4 mm in size and react to light briskly.

| ■ *Activity* | Now assess the size and reaction of your volunteer's pupils. |

Glaucoma

An increase in the intraocular pressure of the eye causing reduced vision in the affected eye.

People with visual impairment and those who have had ocular surgery or disease may have altered pupil reactions, so it is then important to try to establish what is normal for this person. For example a person who has **glaucoma** may use eyedrops that constrict the pupil.

Limb movements

A neurological chart also contains a section for recording limb movements. There are different versions used in practice but Box 10.8 gives one example. Verbal commands are used to examine these movements. For example the nurse may ask the person to push and pull against them with each limb. The responses are recorded for arms and legs separately. If there is a difference between the limbs, they are recorded separately.

				Normal power	R		
L I M B	M O V E M E N T S	A R M S		Mild weakness	L		
				Severe weakness			
				Flexion			
				Extension			
				No response			
		L E G S		Normal power	R/L		
				Mild weakness			
				Severe weakness			
				Flexion			
				Extension			
				No response			

Box 10.8 Recording limb movements

In Box 10.8 the assessment indicates normal power in both legs, a mild weakness in the left arm, and normal power in the right arm. Normal power is recorded when the person responds appropriately to commands and shows normal function and strength of the limb. Mild weakness implies that the limb can be moved but with reduced power. The arm weakness recorded on the chart shown may be due to a CVA or other pre-existing condition, such as cerebral palsy. Severe weakness implies movement is possible but with no real strength. 'Flexion' is recorded when the knee or elbow is bent, and 'extension' is recorded when the arm or leg straightens, when a painful stimulus is applied. 'No response' is recorded when no stimulus (as used in best motor response) obtains any motor response from the person.

Activity

Practise all the skills included in this chapter by recording a full set of neurological observations with your willing volunteer, which will include vital signs as well as level of consciousness, pupil reactions and limb movements.

The complexity and importance of neurological observations

Neurological assessment is complex and requires practice in the clinical setting (NICE 2003). You should first observe a qualified nurse recording a neurological assessment and then take part under supervision, according to local policy. The first set of neurological observations forms the baseline for future assessment. Ingram (1994) warned that people perform neurological observations differently, thus leading to unreliable results. However, Juarez and Lyons (1995) discuss how the GCS score can provide an accurate and reliable assessment of a person's conscious level. To improve reliability it is recommended that before a new nurse takes over the care of the person, the previous nurse should demonstrate a neurological assessment. Neurological observations should be carried out and recorded on a half-hourly basis until GCS score equal to 15 has been achieved. The minimum frequency of observations for patients with GCS score equal to 15 should be half-hourly for 2 hours then hourly for 4 hours and 2 hourly thereafter (NICE 2003).

Learning outcome 3: Show awareness of how neurological assessment can be carried out with children, and the special considerations that are necessary

Activity

It has already been identified that the Glasgow Coma Scale was developed for use with adults but is often used to assess children (Orfanelli 2001). What difficulties might there be in using this scale for children?

You may have identified the following:

- **Motor response**: An infant or young child may not have yet developed the motor control required to co-operate, so even when fully conscious and orientated, they may not understand what they are being asked to do.
- **Verbal response**: A child may not have the language skills required to answer questions. Also it is common for young children in an unfamiliar environment to refuse to speak to strangers, particularly if they are fearful or anxious. A child who has motor, language or developmental delay or impairment may be unable to achieve a maximum score even when fully conscious. Regression (behaving as one would expect a younger child to do) is also a common reaction to hospital and stressful events (Ferguson-Clark and Williams 1998).
- **Vital signs**: Bradycardia and hypertension, seen in response to raised intracranial pressure in adults, are rare in children and a very late sign of deterioration (Orfanelli 2001).

A number of modified versions of the GCS have been published for use with children that take into account these developmental and behavioural factors (Ferguson-Clark and Williams 1998). NICE (2003) have published a modified GCS for children, which can be found in Box 10.9.

Parental involvement

Parents are important allies in the neurological assessment of their children. Irritability and altered behaviour may be significant indicators of deterioration in very young children (NICE 2003). Parents have the knowledge of their child's normal behaviour when well and when under stress, and can therefore help the nurse to identify abnormal behaviour that might be a cause for concern, even if these changes are very subtle. For example, the child's carer may be able to identify that the child's crying sounds different to their usual cry, whereas the nurse

Best eye response (4)

1. No eye opening
2. Eye opening to pain
3. Eye opening to verbal command
4. Eyes open spontaneously

Best verbal response (5)

1. No vocal response
2. Occasionally whimpers and/or moans
3. Cries inappropriately
4. Less than usual ability and/or spontaneous irritable cry
5. Alert, babbles, coos, words or sentences to usual ability

Communication with the infant or child's caregivers is required to establish the best usual verbal response. A 'grimace' alternative to verbal responses should be used in pre-verbal or intubated patients.

Best grimace response (5)

1. No response to pain
2. Mild grimace to pain
3. Vigorous grimace to pain
4. Less than usual spontaneous ability or only response to touch stimuli
5. Spontaneous normal facial/oro-motor activity

Best motor response (6)

1. No motor response to pain
2. Abnormal extension to pain (decerebrate)
3. Abnormal flexion to pain (decorticate)
4. Withdrawal to painful stimuli
5. Localises to painful stimuli or withdraws to touch
6. Obeys commands or performs normal spontaneous movements

Box 10.9 Paediatric version of the Glasgow Coma Scale. Source: National Institute for Clinical Excellence (2003) Head injury – triage, assessment, investigation and early management of head injury in infants, children and adults, June 2003; London: National Institute for Clinical Excellence. Available from: www.nice.org.uk. Reproduced with kind permission from the National Institute for Clinical Excellence

is not in a position to recognise this. Parents or carers might also help with coaxing a child to co-operate with testing pupil reactions. The use of play and toys, for example, shining the light in teddy's eyes first, might also help.

The most important observation of a child following a head injury is level of consciousness and behaviour, as if the child deteriorates, changes to vital signs occur late (Campbell and Glasper 1995). Changes to pupil size and reaction are also late signs of deterioration in children (Orfanelli 2001). However, assessing level of consciousness is complicated by the fact that frequent disturbance to a child (to perform an assessment) may in itself cause fatigue, sleepiness and irritability, which may also be a sign of deterioration (Campbell and Glasper 1995).

Please note

The neurological assessment of children is a complex activity for which nurses need a detailed knowledge of normal child development and behaviour and the ability to work in partnership with parents, in addition to training in the use of the assessment tool being used. NICE (2003) recommends that it should be undertaken only by those with specific training. It is therefore beyond the scope of this chapter to enable nurses to make judgements on the neurological status of children. The reader is advised to pursue further reading (Fearon 2000b; Ferguson-Clark and Williams 1998), and should not undertake the neurological assessment of children unsupervised.

Summary

- Neurological observations are frequently performed by nurses, and are very important when monitoring the condition of a person with actual or potential neurological impairment.
- The Glasgow Coma Scale, and its adapted versions for children, have been developed to promote consistency in assessment. Nevertheless, how the scale is used in practice could differ, so to promote reliability between readings, one nurse should carry out the observations, and demonstrate how they were carried out to any other nurse who is taking over the care.
- The Glasgow Coma Scale score can be highly influential in terms of treatment and further investigation. Therefore students carrying out these observations should be working under supervision, and report immediately any concerns.
- Neurological assessment of children is particularly complex, and a depth of knowledge of child development, and the ability to work with parents, is required to enable an accurate assessment to be made.
- Most head injuries are mild but a small number of patients suffer serious injuries to their brain, resulting in severe disability or death. It is imperative that nurses who observe, measure and record neurological observations are aware that people who have experienced neurological trauma can deteriorate very

quickly. Noticing any changes in neurological function and notifying senior nursing and medical personnel of these changes is imperative so that life-saving procedures can be carried out.

CHAPTER SUMMARY

This chapter aimed to begin to assist you in developing your skills in assessing vital signs within the practice setting. These observations should not be considered in isolation but as part of a person's holistic assessment which will include a range of other observations and gaining information from various sources. Vital signs must be assessed and recorded accurately, using the appropriate equipment in the recommended manner. They must also be reported and guidance sought in their interpretation. Some vital signs can change quickly along with the person's level of consciousness so they must be carried out at the required frequency. It can take considerable practice with a range of people in a variety of settings to become really confident and competent in these skills.

REFERENCES

Armstrong, R. 2002. Nurses' knowledge of error in blood pressure measurement technique. *International Journal of Nursing Practice* **8**, 116–19.

Aucken, S. and Crawford, B. 1998. Neurological assessment. In Guerrero, D. (ed.) *Neuro Oncology for Nurses*. London: Whurr Publishers.

Brooker, C. 1996. *Nursing Applications in Clinical Practice: Human structure and function*, second edition. London: Mosby.

Brooker, C. 1998. *Human Structure and Function*, second edition. London: Mosby.

Campbell, S. and Glasper, E.A. 1995. *Whaley and Wong's Children's Nursing*. London: Mosby.

Carroll, M. 2000. An evaluation of temperature measurement. *Nursing Standard* **14**(4), 1174–8.

Casey, G. 2000. Fever management in children. *Nursing Standard* **14**(40), 36–42.

Childs, C. 2000. Temperature control. In Alexander, M., Fawcett, J. and Runciman, P. (eds) *Nursing Practice in Hospital and Home: The adult*, second edition. Edinburgh: Churchill Livingstone, 719–35.

Craig, J., Lancaster, G., Williamson, P. and Smyth, R. 2000. Temperature measurement at the axilla compared with the rectum in children and young people: a systematic review. *British Medical Journal* **320**(7234), 1174–8.

Department of Health 2001. *Valuing People: A new strategy for learning disability for the 21st century*. London: DH.

Dolan, B. and Holt, L. 2000. *Accident and Emergency Theory into Practice*. London: Baillière Tindall.

Edwards, S. 1997. Measuring temperature. *Professional Nurse* **13**(2), s5–7.

Fearon, J. 2000a. Assessment. In Huband, S. and Trigg, E. (eds) *Practices in Children's Nursing: Guidelines for hospital and community*. Edinburgh: Churchill Livingstone, 45–54.

Fearon, J. 2000b. Neurological observations and coma scales. In Huband, S. and Trigg, E. (eds) *Practices in Children's Nursing: Guidelines for hospital and community*. Edinburgh: Churchill Livingstone, 171–8.

Ferguson-Clark, L. and Williams, C. 1998. Neurological assessment in children. *Paediatric Nursing* **10**(4), 29–33.

Fritsch, D.E. 1995. Hypothermia in the trauma patient. *American Association of Critical Care Nurses Clinical Issues* **6**(2), 196–211.

Herbert, R.A. and Alison, J.A. 1996. Cardiovascular function. In Hinchliff, S.M., Montague, S.E. and Watson, R. (eds) *Physiology for Nursing Practice*, second edition. London: Baillière Tindall, 374–451.

Hickey, J.V. 2003. *The Clinical Practice of Neurological and Neurosurgical Nursing*, fifth edition. New York: Lippincott.

Hull, D. and Johnstone, D.I. 1999. *Essential Paediatrics*, fourth edition. Edinburgh: Churchill Livingstone.

Ingram, N. 1994. Knowledge and level of consciousness: application to nursing practice. *Journal of Advanced Nursing* **20**, 881–4.

Jennet, B. and Teasdale, G. 1974. Assessment of the coma and impaired consciousness. *Lancet* **2**, 81–4.

Juarez, V. and Lyons, M. 1995. Interrater reliability of the Glasgow Coma Score. *Journal of Neuroscience Nursing* **27**(5), 283–86.

Leefarr,V. 2000. Stress. In Alexander, M., Fawcett, J. and Runciman, P. (eds) *Nursing Practice in Hospital and Home: The adult*, second edition. Edinburgh: Churchill Livingstone, 613–33.

Leick-Rude, M. and Bloom, L. 1998. A comparison of temperature taking methods in neonates *Neonatal Network* **17**(5), 21–37.

Lowry, M. 1998. Emergency nursing and the Glasgow Coma Score. *Accident and Emergency Nursing* **6**, 143–8.

Mallet, J. and Dougherty, L. 2000. *Manual of Clinical Nursing Procedures*, fifth edition. Oxford: Blackwell Science.

Marieb, E. 2001. *Human Anatomy and Physiology*, fifth edition. San Francisco: Benjamin Cummings.

MHRA (Medicines and Healthcare products Regulatory Agency) 2003a. Medical devices containing mercury. http//www.medical-devices.gov.uk. Accessed 11 December 2003.

MHRA 2003b. Infra-red thermometers: important advice. http//www. mhra. gov.uk. Accessed 17 November 2003.

Mohammed, T.A. 2000. Incubator care. In Huband, S. and Trigg, E. (eds) *Practices in Children's Nursing: Guidelines for hospital and community*. Edinburgh: Churchill Livingstone, 139–42.

Molton, A., Blacktop, J. and Hall, C. 2001. Temperature taking in children. *Journal of Child Health Care* **5**(1), 5–10.

Moules, T. and Ramsey, J. 1998. *The Textbook of Children's Nursing*. Cheltenham: Stanley Thornes.

NICE (National Institute for Clinical Excellence) 2003. Head injury – triage, assessment, investigation and early management of head injury in infants, children and adults, June 2003. London: National Institue for Clinical Excellence. Available from http://www.nice.org.uk. Accessed 27 July 2003.

Nursing and Midwifery Council 2002. *Requirements for Pre-registration Nursing Programmes*. London: Nursing and Midwifery Council.

O'Brien, E. 2001. Blood pressure measurement is changing! *Heart* **85**(1), 3–5.

O'Brien, E., Petrie, J., Littler, W. *et al.* 1999. *Blood Pressure Measurement Recommendations of the British Hypertension Society*. London: British Medical Journal Publication.

Orfanelli, L. 2001. Neurologic examination of the toddler: how to assess for raised intracranial pressure following head trauma *American Journal of Nursing* **101**(12), 24cc–24ff.

O'Toole, S. 1998. Temperature measurement devices. *Professional Nurse* **13**, 779–86.

Resuscitation Council Guidelines 2000. Basic life support guidelines/algorithm. Available from http://www.resus.org.uk. Accessed 12 August 2003.

Roy, L. 1997. Measurement of blood pressure in children. *Journal of Paediatrics and Child Health* **33**(6), 477–8.

Rudolph, M. and Levene, M. 1999. *Paediatrics and Child Health*. Oxford: Blackwell Science.

Salvage, J. 2000. Go slow on quicksilver. *Nursing Times* **96**(45), 22.

Schmitz, T., Bair, N., Falk, N. and Levine, C. 1995. A comparison of five methods of temperature measurement devices in febrile intensive care patients. *American Journal of Critical Care* **4**, 286–96.

Skinner, D., Driscoll, P. and Earlam, P. 2000. *ABC of Major Trauma*, third edition. London: British Medical Journal Publication.

Thompson, D. and Webster, R. 2000. The cardiovascular system. Alexander, M., Fawcett, J. and Runciman, P. (eds) *Nursing Practice in Hospital and Home: The adult*, second edition. Edinburgh: Churchill Livingstone, 7–58.

Torrance, C. and Semple, M.C. 1998a. Recording temperature. *Nursing Times* **94**(2), Practical Procedures for Nurses Suppl.

Torrance, C. and Semple, M.C. 1998b. Recording temperature. *Nursing Times* **94**(3), Practical Procedures for Nurses Suppl.

Tortora, G. and Grabowski, S. 2003. *Principles of Anatomy and Physiology*, tenth edition. New York: John Wiley and Sons.

Van Carrapiett, D. 2003 Neurological observations – Introduction. Available from http://www.emergency-nurse.com/resource/neuro/intro. Accessed 12 August 2003.

Walsh, M., Crumbie, A. and Reveley, S. 1999. *Nurse Practitioners: Clinical skills and professional issues*. Oxford: Butterworth-Heinemann.

Waugh, A. and Grant, A. 2001. *Ross and Wilson Anatomy and Physiology in Health and Illness*, ninth edition. London: Churchill Livingstone.

Winkelman, C. 1995. Increased intracranial pressure. In Urban, N.A., Greenlee, K.K., Krumberger, J.M. and Winkelman, C. (eds) *Guidelines for Critical Care Nursing*. St Louis: Mosby, 3–11.

Respiratory care:
assessment and interventions

Lesley Baillie, Veronica Corben and Sue Higham

In many settings people being cared for by nurses will require assessment and monitoring of their respiratory status, and interventions to relieve or prevent respiratory symptoms. Problems with breathing are often frightening and require nurses to be supportive and understanding. Nurses need to be able to assess people accurately and know how to deliver some key interventions safely, and sometimes speedily. People with chronic respiratory disease need assistance and support to monitor their own conditions and maintain their health status. The aim of this chapter is to help you to develop practical skills involved in respiratory care, with a sound underpinning knowledge.

This chapter includes:
- ■ Measuring and recording respirations
- ■ Measuring and recording peak expiratory flow rate
- ■ Pulse oximetry
- ■ Observation of sputum and collection of sputum specimens
- ■ Oxygen therapy
- ■ Administering inhaled medication
- ■ Managing nebulised therapy.

Recommended biology reading:
The following questions will help you to focus on the biology underpinning this chapter's skills. Use your recommended text book to find out:

- What are the components of the respiratory system (e.g. airways, respiratory muscles, control mechanisms) and what are their functions?
- How do these functions contribute towards maintaining homeostasis?
- Where does gaseous exchange occur? Which gases are being exchanged?
- Why does this exchange occur? What may affect this exchange?
- How does inspiration occur? What is the stimulus for us to breathe?
- What are the proportions of gases in atmospheric, alveolar and expired air?

- How does the respiratory system respond to respiratory tract infection? What role do cilia play? What symptoms are associated with respiratory tract infection?
- What other situations could cause respiratory distress or respiratory dysfunction?
- Where is bronchial smooth muscle located?
- What is the consequence of bronchoconstriction?
- Where are the pleural membranes? What functions do they have?
- What is surfactant? How does it prevent lung collapse?
- How can lung function be assessed? What factors could affect lung function?
- What factors are required for adequate tissue oxygenation to occur? Consider the role blood plays in this.

PRACTICE SCENARIOS

The following scenarios illustrate when respiratory assessment and care may be needed, and will be referred to throughout this chapter.

Adult

George Phillips is 69 years old. He has had **chronic obstructive pulmonary disease** (COPD) for many years, and has had several hospital admissions. Previously a heavy smoker, George blames himself for his disease and the impact it has had on his wife, Julia, who is now his main carer. They have no children, and he now refuses to go into hospital any more, as he says 'they can't cure me'. He has continuous oxygen via an oxygen concentrator, regular nebulisers, and lives in one room, sleeping in a chair at night.

Child

Samir Hashmi is 7 weeks old and has been admitted to the children's ward with **bronchiolitis**. He is quite pale, with an elevated heart and respiratory rate. He needs to have oxygen. Samir is too breathless to continue his normal breast-feeds. His mother is resident with him.

Learning disability

Anthony Horton is 22 years old and has a moderate learning disability. He lives in a small group home. He is known to have **asthma** for which he uses inhalers. He recently had to be taken to Accident and Emergency (A&E), from where he was admitted overnight, as he became suddenly very wheezy. He has now been asked to attend the practice nurse's asthma clinic and he is accompanied there by his **health facilitator**, the community nurse for learning disability. She aims to liaise between the surgery and the staff at the home, and develop an educational programme with the care staff and Anthony so that his asthma can be managed

---

Chronic obstructive pulmonary disease

This is a chronic respiratory disease, including conditions such as emphysema, chronic bronchitis and chronic asthma. It causes debilitating breathlessness which affects day-to-day living.

Bronchiolitis

Infection of the bronchioles which affects mainly babies.

Asthma

A respiratory disorder characterised by recurrent episodes of difficulty in breathing, wheezing on expiration, coughing and viscous mucoid bronchial secretions.

Health facilitator

A member of the community learning disabilities team (often a nurse) who supports a person with learning disabilities to access the health care they need. See *Valuing People* (Department of Health 2001).

as well as possible. The practice nurse says she is concerned about Anthony's inhaler technique, and would also like Anthony to be able to use a peak flow meter to help to monitor his condition if possible. She also discusses how an asthma attack can be recognised by observing his respiration.

Mental health

Tina Lunn is 58 years old and has a long history of mental illness. She has been admitted to an acute mental health unit due to her deteriorating mental state. She is known to have asthma, has becotide (a **corticosteroid**) and salbutamol (a **bronchodilator**) inhalers, and also takes oral prednisolone (also a **cortico-steroid**). The staff are encouraging her to manage her asthma, to monitor her peak flow and take her inhalers as prescribed, but one morning after a restless night, her respiration is so laboured she has difficulty completing sentences and she is very distressed and wheezy. Her peak flow is found to be around half her normal measurement. A salbutamol nebuliser (prescribed on an as required basis) is administered via oxygen with some effect. The doctor diagnoses a chest infection and asks for a sputum specimen to be collected.

MEASURING AND RECORDING RESPIRATIONS

The major function of the respiratory system is to supply the body with oxygen and remove carbon dioxide. When the respiratory rate is measured, it is the act of ventilation which is observed. One respiration consists of one inspiration (breathing in), and one expiration (breathing out).

Bronchodilator

A drug that relaxes the smooth muscle of the bronchioles to improve ventilation to the lungs. Commonly used examples are salbutamol and terbutaline.

Corticosteroid

Inhaled corticosteroids such as becotide are used for asthma as a preventative treatment. They appear to reduce bronchial mucosal inflammation, and thus decrease oedema and secretion of mucus in the airway. Corticosteriods can be administered via most other routes too. Prednisolone is an oral preparation.

LEARNING OUTCOMES

By the end of this section you will be able to:

1. Discuss when and why observation of respiration is performed.
2. State the normal respiratory rates for different age groups.
3. Discuss what other aspects of breathing nurses observe when measuring respiratory rates.
4. Accurately measure and record the respiratory rate.
5. Define terms commonly used for breathing abnormalities.

Equipment required:

■ A watch with a second hand.
■ An observation chart.

Learning outcome 1: Discuss when and why observation of respiration is performed

| ■ *Activity* | Why would a person's respiration be observed by a nurse? The practice scenarios will give you some clues. List possible reasons. |

You may have thought of the following situations:

- Admission to hospital or pre-operatively, providing a baseline for future comparison.
- When a person (in hospital or in the community) is unwell or injured, for example, loss of consciousness, chest injury, difficulty with breathing, chest pain. Both Anthony and Tina's respiratory rates should be observed when they appear breathless, and Samir's respirations will be observed regularly while he is acutely ill.
- To monitor a patient's condition, for example after surgery, or during treatment, such as a morphine infusion.
- To monitor a patient's response to treatments or medication that affect the respiratory system.

Learning outcome 2: State the normal respiratory rates for different age groups

When assessing respiratory rate you need to know the expected normal rate for the person's age group, and if a baseline reading is available, you can make a comparison with this.

 Activity | What do you think the normal respiratory rate would be for Tina, as an adult, and for a baby of Samir's age? In health, when would respirations be slower or faster, and why?

There is considerable individual variation in respiratory rates (Stocks 1996). The respiratory rate varies according to age, size and gender, and can also fluctuate in well people, for example if metabolic demands change. The normal adult respiratory rate is about 10–15 breaths per minute (Stocks 1996). For children's respiratory rates see Table 11.1. Exercise, stress and fear will all increase the respiratory rate; this is a normal bodily response. Thus if Anthony was running, his respiratory rate would be increased as his body requires more oxygen. If you count people's respiratory rates when they have just arrived for admission to hospital, the anxiety and stress of the situation may lead to a raised respiratory rate, which would not

Table 11.1 Normal range for respiratory rates in children (Hull and Johnstone 1999)

Age (years)	Respiratory rate (breaths per minute)
Under 1 year	25–35
1–5 years	20–30
5–12 years	20–25
Over 12 years	15–25

be an accurate baseline. In deep (stage 4) sleep, respiratory rate drops to its lowest normal level. Knowledge of normal biological functioning will help you to recognise abnormalities, and causes for concern.

An increased respiratory rate is termed **tachypnoea**. Samir is tachypnoeic and Anthony would probably have been tachypnoeic when he went to A&E with his acute asthmatic attack. A decreased respiratory rate is termed **bradypnoea**. This might occur if sedation has been administered. One of the most serious side effects of opioid drugs, like morphine, is a depressed respiratory rate.

In healthy people, the relationship between pulse and respiration is fairly constant, being a ratio of one respiration to every four or five heart beats. Very rapid respirations, such as over forty per minute in an adult (in the absence of exercise) or very slow respirations, such as eight per minute, are cause for alarm and should be reported promptly.

Learning outcome 3: Discuss what other aspects of breathing nurses would observe when measuring respiratory rates

| **Activity** | When you are counting the respiratory rates of the people in the scenarios, what else about their respiration should you be observing? |

You should be observing the difficulty, sound, depth and pattern of breathing, as discussed below.

Difficulty

Respirations are normally effortless, and you should therefore observe whether breathing is difficult or laboured (termed **dyspnoea**). Dyspnoeic patients, like Tina, may use accessory muscles of respiration such as their neck and abdominal muscles. However babies like Samir and, to a lesser extent, children up to 6 years, rely predominantly on diaphragmatic movement to breathe, resulting in greater abdominal movements during normal breathing than adults (Carter 1995). Signs of dyspnoea in babies and younger children include recession (sinking in of the soft tissues during inspiration) below the sternum and under and between the ribs, and flaring of the nostrils (Campbell and Glasper 1995). The nurses caring for Samir should be looking out for these signs of laboured breathing, which can be tiring for babies and young children.

People with dyspnoea often mouth breathe, as there is less resistance to airflow through the mouth than the nose, and this can cause drying of the oral mucosa (Stocks 1996). Oral hygiene (see Chapter 7) is therefore essential. People with dyspnoea need to be sitting up, either in an armchair, or in bed well supported by pillows, to optimise ventilation (Fig. 11.1). A baby, like Samir, or a young child, can be held in this position by a parent. **Orthopnoea** is the term used when people cannot breathe unless they are upright. This will be the reason that George is sleeping in a chair at night. Note that dyspnoea is frightening and psychological support is essential.

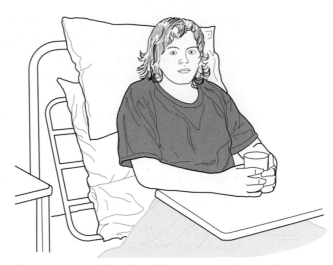

Figure 11.1 Correct position for a breathless person. An upright position, well supported by pillows, optimises ventilation.

Sound

You should also observe the sound of breathing, which is normally quiet. You may hear a variety of abnormal breath sounds, such as a wheeze or a stridor. A **wheeze** is a high-pitched sound which occurs when air is forced through narrowed respiratory passages. This is often heard in people with asthma, like Anthony and Tina. A **stridor** is a harsh, high-pitched sound that is heard during respiration when the larynx is obstructed.

Depth

Depth of breathing should also be observed. This relates to the volume of air moving in and out of the respiratory tract with each breath, and is referred to as tidal volume. The term **hyperventilation** is used to describe prolonged, rapid and deep ventilations which can occur in someone who is having an anxiety attack. This can cause dizziness and fainting as the resulting low carbon dioxide level causes cerebral vasoconstriction. If you encounter someone who is hyperventilating you can help by being calm and asking them to breathe more slowly in and out of a paper bag. This enables rebreathing of expired air, which is rich in carbon dioxide, thus restoring normal levels. **Hypoventilation** is the term used for slow and shallow breathing, which could lead to inadequate gaseous exchange. You should also observe whether the chest expands equally on both sides, particularly if there is a history of chest injury.

Pattern

The pattern of breathing should also be observed. Terms are given to certain abnormalities:

- **Apnoea**: This is a period without breathing. It could occur during hypoventilation, with another breath only taking place when arterial carbon dioxide levels rise and breathing is stimulated.

- **Cheyne–Stokes respirations**: These are when there is a gradual increase in the depth of respirations leading to an episode of hyperventilation, followed by a gradual decrease in the depth of respirations, and then a period of apnoea lasting about 15–20 seconds.

Note that it is common for infants to have an irregular breathing pattern, with alternating short (a few seconds) periods of apnoea and rapid breathing.

Learning outcome 4: Accurately measure and record the respiratory rate

For the following activities you need a willing volunteer. If a colleague is not available, another friend or family member may oblige!

 Activity | Measure your volunteer's respiratory rate, using the instructions in Box 11.1.

1. Observe the rise and fall of the chest. Note that in practice you should do this when people are unaware that they are being observed, as otherwise they may alter their breathing pattern. However in an unresponsive person, or a very small baby, this precaution is not relevant. In an alert individual the respiratory rate may be counted directly after the pulse, while still outwardly counting the pulse.
2. With infants and young children you should observe for abdominal movements. This may be done by placing the hand gently against the lower part of their chest to feel movement while continuing to hold the wrist as if taking the pulse. However if the child resists the wrist being held, this should be discontinued. With an infant, it may be necessary to listen for the sounds of inspiration with a stethoscope placed on the chest in order to record the respiratory rate.
3. Note the placement of the second hand of your watch. Count each rise and fall of the chest.
4. If respirations are regular, even and unlaboured, count the number that occur over half a minute, and multiply by two to obtain the rate for one minute. If the respirations are abnormal in any way, count them for one minute. You should not count for only 10 or 15 seconds as with numbers as small as respiratory rates, there is too much room for error. The irregular breathing pattern of infants means it is essential for accuracy that respirations are counted for a full minute in babies aged less than one year (Wong *et al.* 1999).

Box 11.1 Measuring respiratory rate

Respiratory rates, particularly on admission assessment sheets, may be recorded simply as a number (the number of respirations per minute). However if the person's respiratory rate is to be recorded regularly over a period of time a graph sheet may be used. How often recordings are made varies considerably according to their condition. They may be quarter hourly (for a patient with acute breathing difficulties), hourly, four hourly or daily. For example, it is likely that when Anthony attended A&E his respirations were recorded quarter hourly initially, and then reduced to hourly and then four hourly as he stabilised.

Activity

Ask your volunteer to spend a couple of minutes exercising (e.g. running up and down stairs), and then count their respiratory rate again. Using the example in Fig. 11.2 as a guide, note how you would record the two respiratory rates which you have taken on an observation chart.

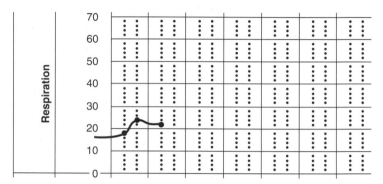

Figure 11.2 Observation chart, showing how respirations could be recorded.

Learning outcome 5: Define terms commonly used for breathing abnormalities

Throughout this section a number of terms have been used which you may commonly hear used in relation to breathing abnormalities. For example Tina is likely to be orthopnoeic and dyspnoeic.

Activity

Can you remember what the following terms mean?

- Dyspnoea
- Hyperventilation
- Tachypnoea
- Orthopnoea
- Hypoventilation
- Bradypnoea
- Apnoea.

All the terms in the list can be found in this section. Check the answers if you are unsure.

Summary

- Measurement of respirations is performed as part of an acutely ill person's assessment, as a baseline for future comparison, and to monitor and evaluate a person's condition and response to treatment.
- It is important to be aware of normal respiratory rates, and of possible abnormalities of respiration that can occur.

MEASURING AND RECORDING PEAK EXPIRATORY FLOW RATE

In brief, a **peak flow meter** measures an individual's ability to exhale. The **peak flow** is a measure, in litres per minute, of the maximum flow rate that an individual can achieve on forced expiration, when starting at full inspiration (Leach 1994). The more accurate term to use is **peak expiratory flow rate** (PEFR). The measurement helps to determine lung volume, and is one of the most accurate clinical measures of a person's current respiratory status.

Peak flow measurement is relatively convenient and inexpensive, and can play a key role in identifying acute exacerbations of asthma (Donohue 1996). It is therefore important that you understand how to measure and record the peak flow rate, and understand its implications.

LEARNING OUTCOMES

On completion of this section you will be able to:

1. Discuss for which individuals peak flow measurement may be useful.
2. Accurately measure and record peak flow rate.
3. Show awareness of how normal peak flow measurements differ for individuals.
4. Show insight into how monitoring peak flow measurements can be used for self-management.

Try to access from the skills laboratory or in the practice setting:

- A peak flow meter and mouthpiece.
- An observation chart.

Learning outcome 1: Discuss for which individuals peak flow measurement may be useful

Activity

Bearing in mind the definition of peak flow, and drawing on the scenarios, for people with which conditions might peak flow measurements be useful?

It is for people who have asthma, like Tina and Anthony, that peak flow measurements are particularly important. This is because asthma is characterised by reduced lung volume and variable obstruction of the airways (Woollons 1995), which thus reduces the amount of air the individual can expel from the lungs in a single blow. Donohue (1996) recommends that peak flow monitoring is indicated in people with moderate to severe asthma. It is particularly useful for people who have difficulty recognising that their asthma control is worsening (McGrath *et al.* 2001).

Peak flow measurements can usually be performed on children from the age of 5 years old (Seymour 1995). Young children can be confused between 'blowing' for peak flow measurements, and 'sucking' for inhaler use. Generally children can distinguish between these two activities by the age of 4–5 years. Peak flows in children should not be measured, therefore, until inhaler technique is established (Wooler 1994).

Learning outcome 2: Accurately measure and record peak flow rate

A peak flow meter is needed with a disposable mouthpiece for each person. Two types of meter that are commonly available are the Wright meter, a robust device which is often seen in hospital wards, and the mini-Wright (Fig. 11.3), which is less robust and cheaper, and is ideal for self-monitoring, being designed for single patient use. You should be aware that as well as the standard meters which measure up to 1000 L per minute, there are low reading or paediatric meters available, which should be used for children and for adults with widespread airways disease. There are also 'child friendly' meters available for self-monitoring, which are easy to hold for small hands, and include windmills or sails which move when the child blows. For step-by-step instructions and diagrams for measuring peak flow, see Fig. 11.3.

Activity

Using the instructions and diagrams in Fig. 11.3, take the measurement on yourself, writing down each recording. Now work through the list below jotting down your thoughts.

1. Try measuring your peak flow while in only a semi-upright position. How does it compare with your original reading? What does that tell you about positioning of patients prior to taking peak flow measurements?
2. What would you do if a measurement seemed rather low?
3. How could the peak flow measurement be recorded?
4. How often might the peak flow rate be measured?

Points which you may have considered:

1. Peak flow readings can be misleading if the person is not in an upright position and does not use the correct technique. This could lead to inappropriate choice of treatment, and be demoralising to the patient (Cartridge 1990).

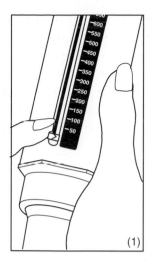
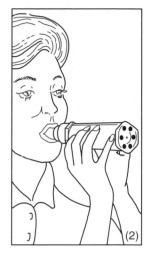
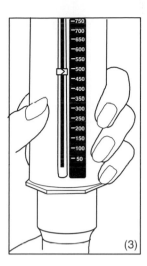

- First the mouthpiece should be slotted into the meter.
- The flow indicator should be at its lowest setting (*see* Diagram 1).
- The meter should be held horizontally without fingers obstructing the scale. (*see* Diagram 2).
- The person should stand or sit upright, take a deep breath, clamp his or her lips around the mouthpiece and blow out as hard as possible, in a short, sharp manner (like blowing out birthday candles).
- The number indicated on the scale should be noted (*see* Diagram 3).
- Two further attempts should be made and then the best of three readings is recorded. The dial should be returned to the lowest setting in between each attempt (as Diagram 1).

Figure 11.3 Procedure for measuring peak flow. (Reproduced with kind permission from Clement Clarke International Ltd.)

2. If a low reading is obtained you first need to check that the person's position and technique are correct. Then, as with any other observation, you would need to report abnormal measurements to the qualified nurse, who is accountable for the patient's care. Little can usually be deduced from a single peak flow reading as a series of readings are required to produce a comprehensive picture. However a single low reading may need a quick response. Obviously the patient's general condition and other observations will be taken into account too.

3. On most adult wards peak flow will be recorded simply as a figure at the bottom of the observation chart. There are special charts available, particularly for when there needs to be ongoing monitoring, and these are often used for children, and for home monitoring of peak flow (Fig. 11.4). This would be a useful record for Anthony to keep.

4. Generally twice daily (morning and early evening) measurements are sufficient, except during acute episodes. Donohue (1996) recommends that measuring a morning pre-bronchodilator peak flow is one of the best ways of monitoring asthma. In mild cases of asthma, once or twice weekly measurements may be enough. Often it is necessary to monitor effects of medication, for example inhaled bronchodilators. Peak flows are then measured before and 30 minutes after medication (when the medication is having the maximum

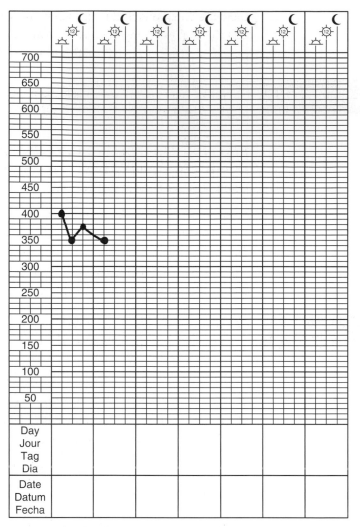

Figure 11.4 Example of a chart to monitor peak flow. (Reproduced with kind permission of Clement Clarke International Ltd.)

effect) (Brewin and Hughes 1995). These pre- and post-medication measurements need to be recorded clearly. Many wards use different coloured pens.

Learning outcome 3: Show awareness of how normal peak flow measurements differ for individuals

The normal peak flow reading varies according to a person's age, height and gender. Generally an adult should achieve 400–600 L per minute, but males achieve a higher figure than females, and greater height increases the peak flow reading. A smaller measurement would obviously be expected of a child, and there are charts available on paediatric wards that can help to calculate the expected peak flow. A child of 9 could be expected to achieve 175 L per minute, but again this varies according to height. Therefore accurate height measurement is essential prior to peak flow measurement in children. Even in individuals without asthma there are variations in the measurement, with the morning figure being lower, and the highest being achieved in early evening. This tendency is likely to be exaggerated in people with asthma, like Anthony and Tina.

Activity Compare your peak flow measurement with the information above. Does it fulfil what would be expected for you?

Learning outcome 4: Show insight into how monitoring peak flow measurements can be used for self-management

Peak flow meters are increasingly used by people with asthma to monitor and manage their condition. They have been available on prescription since 1990. Patients are normally advised about their baseline peak flow rate, according to age, height and gender. The same peak flow meter should be used for a particular individual to ensure consistency.

Activity Why might teaching people who have asthma to measure their peak flow rate be useful in managing their condition?

Points which you may have identified include:

■ To find out how well their asthma is controlled.

■ Doing regular readings may reveal a gradual (and possibly asymptomatic) deterioration, which requires action (e.g. change of medication) to prevent an acute episode. If the reading falls below 80 per cent of an individual's best level, then preventive medicine (usually an inhaled steroid) should be increased (Seymour 1995).

■ Without peak flow monitoring, people can be unaware of worsening symptoms and the peak flow may fall by up to 50 per cent before symptoms are noticed (Bellamy and Bellamy 1990).

■ Circumstances affecting peak flow may be identified, for example contact with a cat. This could enable asthma triggers to be recognised.

■ The measurement may indicate the severity of the asthma at that particular time. The lower the measurement, the narrower the airways. A measurement of below 50 per cent of the baseline requires immediate medical attention (Matthews 1997).

■ To monitor how any change in medication is affecting respiratory status.

Donohue (1996) emphasises that teaching people to monitor their peak flow should be only part of a comprehensive asthma management programme. This should also include: instruction about avoiding asthma triggers, correct use of medication, identification of warning signs of worsening asthma, and what action to take. On-going education and monitoring can be achieved through attendance at asthma clinics like those run by Anthony's practice nurse. This will include checking correct technique in peak flow measurement. The community nurse for learning disabilities will be able to suggest suitable strategies and provide resource materials to help Anthony develop an understanding of his asthma and how to monitor his peak flow and use his inhalers (see later section). Anthony's manual dexterity and co-ordination for using both his peak flow meter and his inhaler needs to be assessed. This could be relevant to other people too.

Despite the potential benefits of peak flow monitoring, studies have indicated that long-term levels of use can be somewhat low, even in motivated patients who have taken part in an educational programme (Cote *et al.* 1998). One study found that 66 per cent of children with asthma who had peak flow meters did not actually use them (Scarfone *et al.* 2001). McCullen *et al.* (2002) also studied the use of peak flow meters in childhood asthma and concluded that families tend to use them when children are symptomatic but daily use is probably an unrealistic expectation as families do not perceive this as useful.

Summary

- Peak flow measurements are important indicators of respiratory function, particularly in people who have asthma.
- They must be recorded accurately and consistently, as treatment may be adjusted according to their values.
- They may be recorded in hospital, during acute episodes, but also at home to enable self-monitoring. Effective education is then essential.

PULSE OXIMETRY

Pulse oximetry enables continuous non-invasive monitoring of the oxygen saturation of haemoglobin in arterial blood which is updated with each pulse wave. It involves the use of a microprocessor with a probe attached to the patient and is used in a range of settings but particularly with people with respiratory problems. Although pulse oximetry is technically complex, it is easy to apply and has therefore gained rapid acceptance (Moyle 1999). However studies have indicated that doctors and nurses do not always understand how pulse oximetry works nor its limitations (Howell 2002; Stoneham *et al.* 1994).

LEARNING OUTCOMES

By the end of this section you will be able to:

1. Explain how pulse oximetry works and what it actually measures.
2. Discuss how a pulse oximeter should be used in practice.
3. Identify when pulse oximetry is used and its advantages.
4. Show understanding of the limitations of pulse oximetry.

You may be able to access a pulse oximeter in the skills laboratory or your practice setting.

Learning outcome 1: Explain how pulse oximetry works and what it actually measures

What do pulse oximeters actually measure?

You may recall that haemoglobin (Hb) is a molecule, present in erythrocytes (red blood cells), which transports gases (especially oxygen) around the body. About 98 per cent of the oxygen in the blood is transported attached to these haemoglobin molecules (then called oxyhaemoglobin – HbO_2) while about 2 per cent is carried dissolved in the plasma. Pulse oximetry measurements of oxygen saturation are used to calculate how saturated with oxygen the haemoglobin molecules are. The result is denoted by the abbreviation SpO_2.

The equipment

There are a number of pulse oximeters available, varying in sophistication from small hand-held devices which simply display the percentage of oxygen saturation and the pulse rate, to more substantial and less portable devices, which also show the pulsatile waveform (Fig. 11.5). Cowan (1997) summarises the key features of a number of different devices. The box always has a wire leading to the sensor or probe. The probe may be in the form of a clip or sleeve which can be placed on a finger, toe or earlobe, or it may be in a form which can be taped to the skin or wrapped round an infant's foot or a palm. Probes can be disposable or re-usable, and are available in different sizes. Figure 11.6 shows a selection of probes.

How the equipment works

On one side of the sensor is the light source, which consists of two light-emitting diodes, one giving red light (of a short wavelength) and one giving infrared light (of a longer wavelength). On the other side of the sensor is a photodetector, which detects the light that passes through the area of the body to which it is attached. As the oxyhaemoglobin (HbO_2) absorbs more of the infrared light, the microprocessor can calculate the oxyhaemoglobin saturation (SpO_2), and this is displayed on the screen, along with the pulse rate. The diagram in Fig. 11.7 shows how the sensor works.

The pulse oximeter works on the premise that anything that pulses and absorbs red and infrared light between the light source and the light detector must be arterial blood (Lowton 1999). Pulse oximeters therefore only monitor light absorption from tissue with a pulsatile flow, so preventing false readings from fat, bone, connective tissue and venous blood. A good arterial blood flow is therefore needed for a reliable reading (Carroll 1997a).

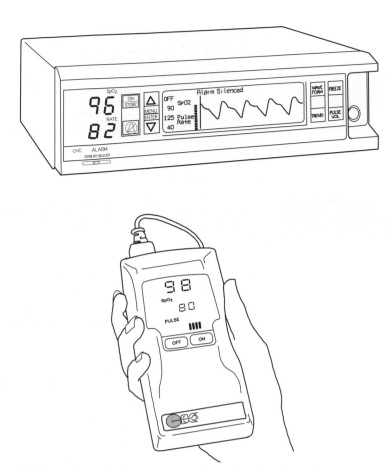

Figure 11.5 Examples of pulse oximeters. (Reproduced with kind permission from Smiths Medical PM, Inc.)

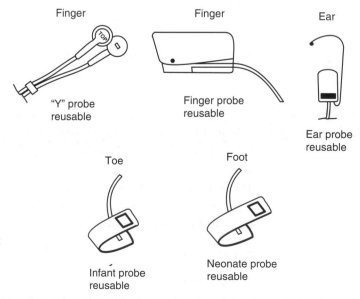

Figure 11.6 Examples of probes. (Reproduced with kind permission from Smiths Medical PM, Inc.)

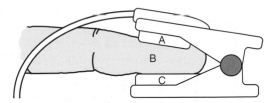

Λ Light omitting diodes

B Finger through which the red and infrared light passes

C Photodetector

Figure 11.7 Diagram showing how a pulse oximeter works.

Normal readings

The normal value of oxygen saturation is 95–100 per cent, so hopefully your reading should have fallen within this range! This figure refers to the percentage of haemoglobin molecules fully saturated with oxygen. **SpO_2 readings below 90 per cent give cause for concern (Place 1998), and must be reported.** Nursing measures such as repositioning the person to a more upright position, if not contraindicated, may provide significant improvement (see Fig. 11.1). Pulse oximeters have alarm systems, which sound if the measurement falls below a normal level. Most manufacturers claim that their devices are accurate to plus or minus 2 per cent, at oxygen saturations of 70–99 per cent. The ability of pulse oximeters to detect **hypoxaemia** (insufficient oxygenation of blood) has been confirmed by a systematic review (Pedersen *et al.* 2003). However as hypoxaemia rises, pulse oximetry does become less accurate, and at 80–85 per cent a more detailed assessment is necessary. If at any stage there is any doubt about the accuracy of pulse oximetry, blood gas analysis, which involves analysis of a sample of blood obtained from an artery, should be performed. This is usually a medical procedure.

Learning outcome 2: Discuss how a pulse oximeter should be used in practice

There are a number of factors that can interfere with obtaining an accurate measurement and these are listed in Box 11.2. Discussion about some of these factors and possible solutions will now follow.

Positioning

The sensor must always be placed correctly, with the diodes and detector positioned directly opposite each other. If inaccurately positioned, the light may pass directly from the light-emitting diode to the photodetector without passing

- Incorrect positioning of probe
- Use of pierced ear for probe
- Probe applied to hand of arm with blood pressure cuff attached
- Incorrect size probe
- Tape applied too tightly
- Dark nail varnish
- Bright light: sunlight or artificial light
- Movement
- Interference from other equipment or cellular telephones
- Poor peripheral perfusion

Box 11.2 Factors that can cause inaccurate pulse oximeter measurements

through the vascular bed (Carroll 1997a). If the earlobe is used, the appropriate sensor will be needed. However, a pierced earlobe should not be used as the light-emitting diodes will reach the photodetector without passing through the vascular bed. Fingers should be fully inserted into the finger probes and flexible sensors should be applied correctly (Cowan 1997). Always ensure that the sensor is not applied to the finger of an arm with a blood pressure cuff attached, which leads to inaccurate or absent readings when the cuff is inflated.

 Activity

If you can access a pulse oximeter, attach the probe to your finger, and rather than removing it as soon as a reading appears, keep it on for 5 minutes. Is it uncomfortable? Can you imagine how you would feel if you had to wear it for several hours? How would a child or a person with confusion respond to this?

Note that the oximeter probe can lead to skin damage due to pressure, particularly if the person has poor peripheral perfusion (as in heart failure), or has sensitive skin (such as with older people or children). The probe site should be checked frequently in people with continuous pulse oximetry (Le Grand and Peters 1999), and the site should be changed every 4–8 hours in pre-term infants (Wong *et al.* 1999). Often it is preferable with babies and children to take frequent readings, removing the probe after each reading, rather than continually monitoring.

Correct size probes and use of tape

With babies and children accuracy and safety is only achieved if the correct size probe for the size of the child is used in the correct manner (Moyle 1999). There are special probes available for neonates, babies and small children, which usually work through the palm, foot or arm; the manufacturer's instructions should be strictly adhered to (Moyle 1999). Figure 11.8 shows how probes might be applied. Stoddart *et al.* (1997) highlight that if an adult probe is used on the small fingers of infants and children, the pulse oximeter may under-read or over-read due to there being a different path length of tissue for each of the wavelengths. Wong *et al.* (1999) suggest that for infants, the sensor can be taped around the

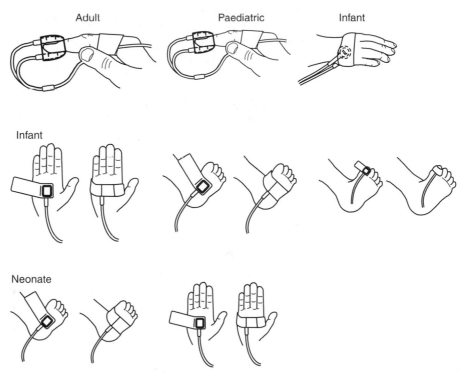

Figure 11.8 Examples of how probes might be applied. (Reproduced with kind permission from Smiths Medical PM, Inc.)

big toe, and the wire taped to the sole of the foot. A sock can then be put over the foot. For children Wong *et al.* (1999) suggest taping the sensor securely to the index finger and taping the wire to the back of the hand. Moyle (1999) warns that though it is tempting to apply extra adhesive tape around the probe, this will both affect accuracy and can cause pressure or thermal damage to the extremity. Also if a finger probe is taped too tightly venous pulsation may occur, leading to measurement error (Le Grand and Peters 1999).

Nails

Accurate pulse oximetry is reliant on the translucence of the body part to which the probe is attached. A study by Peters (1997) found that unpolished acrylic nails do not affect pulse oximetry measurements of oxygen saturation and therefore patients do not need to remove them. However nail varnish can affect SpO_2 readings; the darker the polish the more problematic – blue, black and green are the worst. If it is not possible to remove the nail polish or place the sensor on an unaffected area, the sensor can be placed sideways on the finger rather than across the nailbed, but it may be necessary to tape the sensor in place to prevent movement (Carroll 1997a).

Bright light

Bright lights can also interfere with measurements, and so if phototherapy is being used (e.g. for a jaundiced baby) the probe needs to be covered to protect it from light (Stoddart *et al.* 1997). In bright sunlight or when a bright artificial light is being used, the sensor should also be covered with something opaque (Carroll 1997a).

Movement

Activity

When you next have access to a pulse oximeter, attach the probe to your finger, and then try moving your finger around. What happens to the reading?

Moving or partially dislodging the sensor affects the ability of the light to travel from the light-emitting diodes to the photodetector (Carroll 1997a), and the accuracy of the reading may be affected. When pulse oximeters detect excessive movement they usually alarm as a malfunction, so this is a safe limitation of pulse oximetry as it is obvious. However there is a risk that this desensitises caregivers to true alarms. The technology of newer devices has been designed to prevent movement interfering with readings, but studies to evaluate their effectiveness have had variable results depending on the product used (Bohnhorst *et al.* 2000; Hay *et al.* 2002). Carroll (1997a) notes that rhythmic movements such as **Parkinsonian tremors** or seizures, shivering, exercise and vibrations caused by transport, can all make it difficult for the pulse oximeter to identify which tissue is pulsatile. If possible the sensor should be attached to a part of the body which the patient is most likely to keep still, and if digits are used, they should be kept supported rather than held in the air (Cowan 1997). If a finger-type sensor is used on a continuous basis the cable can be secured to the back of the hand. Carroll (1997a) recommends that using the ear often reduces problems of movement. With small children, the foot or hand may have to be held still for the duration of the reading. A child who is reluctant to co-operate may be encouraged to do so by a parent.

Parkinsonian tremors
A tremor or shaking that occurs in a neurological condition called Parkinson's disease.

Poor peripheral perfusion

For a pulsatile flow to be detected there must be sufficient perfusion in the monitored area (Carroll 1997a). Any condition that reduces pulsatile blood flow to body extremities leads to poor peripheral perfusion. Causes include hypotension (low blood pressure), hypovolaemia (low blood volume), cardiac arrest, or hypothermia. Vasoconstricting drugs, smoking and **peripheral oedema** can also cause poor perfusion, which adversely affects the pulse oximeter signal. If the peripheral pulse is weak or absent pulse oximetry readings will not be precise (Carroll 1997a). Cardiac arrythmias such as **atrial fibrillation**, can interfere with capture of the pulsatile signal, and thus reduce accuracy. If there is a pulse wave displayed on the oximeter, check that it is not dampened as this could indicate a decrease in arterial flow (Carroll 1997a).

Peripheral oedema
Swollen periphery of the body due to excess extracellular fluid.

Atrial fibrillation
An abnormal heart rhythm whereby the atria fibrillate rather than contract, leading to a highly irregular heart rate.

Checking the pulse oximeter's accuracy

To check accuracy you can compare a palpated pulse against the displayed pulse; if they do not correlate then it is likely that the oximeter is not picking up each arteriole pulsation and thus the readings are likely to be inaccurate (Carroll 1997a). The sensor can be moved to an area of higher perfusion, such as the earlobe, or the skin can be warmed. As with any technology, pulse oximeters are not immune to failure. If you think the oximeter may be faulty, you can attach the sensor to your own finger to see if you can obtain a normal reading. Readings can also be checked against arterial blood gas measurement.

Learning outcome 3: Identify when pulse oximetry is used and its advantages

Pulse oximetry has widespread applications, and is recommended whenever there is risk of hypoxaemia (Grap 1998). Assessing hypoxaemia through observation is notoriously inaccurate and unreliable (Le Grand and Peters 1999; Sinex 1999) but it can rapidly lead to tissue damage. The brain is very sensitive to oxygen depletion and visual and cognitive changes can occur when oxygen saturation falls to 80–85 per cent. Other signs of hypoxaemia include restlessness, agitation, hypotension and tachycardia. However, all these signs can be missed or wrongly interpreted.

Cyanosis

A bluish, greyish or purple discoloration of the skin due to presence of abnormal amounts of reduced haemoglobin in the blood.

Cyanosis is the visible sign of hypoxaemia, but is only detected at a saturation of about 75 per cent in normally perfused patients (Hanning and Alexander-Williams 1995). Moyle (1996), when discussing reasons why pulse oximetry has become so commonly used, notes that pulse oximetry can detect hypoxaemia early. Overall, pulse oximetry should be a more accurate and objective measure of hypoxaemia, alerting health professionals at an early stage. It is cheap, non-invasive and can be easily measured during transfer of a patient.

■ **Activity**

Have you seen pulse oximetry used in practice? If so, what care situations was it used in?

You may have thought of the following situations:

Hypoxia

A condition in which inadequate oxygen is available to the tissues to allow normal function.

- **Acute illness**: Pulse oximetry is part of the assessment of anyone who is acutely ill, particularly during initial assessment and management. A study by Summers *et al.* (1998) found that incorporating pulse oximetry into emergency assessment did identify a small, but statistically significant group whose **hypoxia** would otherwise have been missed. It is particularly useful when assessing those with dyspnoea or tachypnoea (Le Grand and Peters 1999), as when Anthony attended A&E with his acute asthma attack. Currently pulse oximeters are not widely available outside acute hospital settings so it is unlikely that Tina's oxygen saturations would be monitored, although if available, it would give the nurses caring for her a useful indication of her oxygenation adequacy.
- **During investigations and surgery**: Pulse oximetry is used during and after procedures and investigations involving general anaesthesia, or sedation, such as during a bronchoscopy.

■ **In-patients with respiratory and circulatory problems**: Patients with respiratory disease, particularly if receiving oxygen therapy, will have SpO_2 monitoring and indeed the amount of oxygen administered may be adjusted according to the SpO_2. Any patients who are at risk of hypoxaemia, such as those with pneumonia, congestive heart failure, COPD exacerbation, acute lung injury and babies like Samir with bronchiolitis, may have continuous SpO_2 monitoring via a pulse oximeter (Rodriguez and Light 1998). Patients whose cardiorespiratory status is unstable, and are undergoing transfer, often have pulse oximetry *in situ*.

■ **In the community**: Pulse oximetry can also be used in the community with people who are at risk of hypoxaemia, for example with chronically ill patients such as those with **cystic fibrosis**. Carroll (1997b) notes the increasing use of pulse oximetry by community nurses and discusses implications. Babies discharged from neonatal units with **chronic lung disease of infancy** may receive oxygen therapy at home, and be monitored by pulse oximetry periodically by the community paediatric team; parents may be asked to monitor SpO_2 overnight to determine oxygen requirements and sleep patterns with and without oxygen (Stoddart *et al.* 1997).

■ **Other advantages**: Pulse oximetry can prevent or reduce the need for arterial blood gas sampling, which is invasive and painful, requiring a skilled practitioner and access to a blood gas analyser. A study involving 152 patients found that use of pulse oximetry led to a significant reduction in unnecessary arterial blood gas analysis (Le Bourdelles *et al.* 1998). Pulse oximetry also provides a continuous measurement rather than intermittent as in arterial blood gas monitoring (Le Grand and Peters 1999), and thus the effectiveness of interventions, such as oxygen therapy and medication, can be evaluated. The impact of mobilisation, physiotherapy and exercise can be assessed (Place 1998) and pulse oximetry may identify whether oxygen therapy is required during these procedures.

Learning outcome 4: Show understanding of the limitations of pulse oximetry

Pulse oximetry complements measurement of other vital signs but it does not replace them (Lowton 1999); oxygen saturations are only a single physiological variable and should not be over-relied upon. Carroll (1997b) advises that the measurement obtained from the pulse oximeter must be interpreted in the light of the whole clinical picture. It has been argued that below 70 per cent the accuracy of pulse oximetry is reduced (Schnapp and Cohen 1990). Moyle (1996) notes that there are safe limitations of pulse oximetry (where the nurse is immediately aware that the device is not functioning properly) and unsafe where the equipment appears to be functioning but the reading is in fact false. It is important to acknowledge the limitations of pulse oximetry. These are summarised in Box 11.3 and discussed below.

Cystic fibrosis
A genetic disease causing oversecretion of a viscous mucus predisposing to respiratory infections.

Chronic lung disease of infancy
A condition seen in some infants who have received intensive respiratory support as neonates.

- Inaccurate at below 70 per cent saturation
- Does not measure adequacy of carbon dioxide elimination
- Does not measure oxygen delivery to the tissues
- Does not measure lung function
- Does not detect hyperoxia
- Cannot distinguish between oxyhaemoglobin, and abnormal haemoglobins
- Does not measure haemoglobin
- Cannot differentiate between venous and arteriole pulsation

Box 11.3 Limitations of pulse oximetry

Stoddart *et al.* (1997) notes that it is the quality of oxygen delivery to the tissues that is of most importance and this depends on cardiac output, tissue perfusion and haemoglobin concentration, not just oxygen saturation of arterial blood. Oxyhaemoglobin saturation could be 99 per cent, but this is of no value if the heart cannot deliver it to the tissues.

Activity — What signs and symptoms might indicate a lack of oxygen to the tissues (hypoxia)?

Signs which you could observe for include the warmth of peripheral areas of the body, colour of skin and tongue, urine output, and mental state (Place 1998).

Cowan (1997) identifies that oxygen therapy may lead to normal readings even though lung function is still impaired. It is also important to remember that pulse oximeters do not measure adequacy of carbon dioxide elimination. The pulse oximeter cannot differentiate between arteriolar and venous pulsation and so in babies with certain cardiac conditions (such as tricuspid valve disease) the pulse oximeter can mistake venous saturation for arterial and give a falsely low reading (Stoddart *et al.* 1997). A further danger with using pulse oximetry in neonates is that hyperoxia, which is dangerous to the retinas of pre-term neonates, and could affect sight, is not detected by pulse oximetry (Stoddart *et al.* 1997). Therefore, in practice, an upper as well as lower SpO_2 limit is established for neonates receiving oxygen, so that the oxygen therapy can be altered appropriately.

Pulse oximeters are unable to differentiate between different forms of saturated haemoglobin (Carroll 1997a). When carbon monoxide is inhaled, carboxyhaemoglobin (COHb) is formed and is absorbed and registered as oxyhaemoglobin, leading to over-estimation of oxygen saturation. Thus for people who have been involved in accidents where there is smoke, or who are affected by carbon monoxide poisoning, pulse oximetry is not recommended. COHb readings are also high in tobacco smokers (Moyle 1996).

Cowan (1997) suggests that people with a low haemoglobin levels may have normal readings even though they may not have enough arterial oxygen to satisfy their needs. This is because the haemoglobin that they do have, even though abnormally low, may be saturated with oxygen, giving a normal but misleading SpO_2. In addition, people with respiratory disease may develop high haemoglobin levels to compensate for their lack of oxygen although the haemoglobin may not be properly saturated with oxygen (Pfister 1995 cited by Cowan 1997). In some types of congenital heart disease there is mixing of oxygenated and deoxygenated blood leading to low SpO_2 readings, although the child is not in fact hypoxic.

Summary

- Pulse oximetry has become increasingly used and has many applications.
- It is non-invasive, easy to apply and provides a continuous measurement.
- It is important to understand the limitations of pulse oximetry and to be aware of its role as complementary to the overall clinical picture.

OBSERVATION OF SPUTUM AND COLLECTION OF SPUTUM SPECIMENS

Adults normally produce about 100 mL of mucus in the respiratory tract daily, but it goes unnoticed as it is usually swallowed (Law 2000). However, in a number of diseases excess mucus is produced, and smoking also stimulates excessive mucus production, which is then expectorated from the lungs and termed sputum (Stocks 1996). Sputum consists of lower respiratory tract secretions, nasopharyngeal and oropharyngeal material (including saliva), microorganisms and cells (Rubin 2002). When sputum is being produced, especially in suspected respiratory disease, a specimen is often required for laboratory examination. You will remember that Tina has been asked to produce a sputum specimen as it is suspected that she has a chest infection.

LEARNING OUTCOMES

By the end of this section you will:

1. Understand how expectoration of sputum can be encouraged, what sputum should be observed for and why.
2. Know how to collect a sputum specimen.

Learning outcome 1: Understand how expectoration of sputum can be encouraged, what sputum should be observed for and why

Clearance of secretions is very important to maintain a clear airway and reduce infection risk (Ruben 2002). However, Law (2000) notes that patients may deny the existence of sputum due to social stigma or lack of awareness. Some, particularly women, feel embarrassed to expectorate, and are more likely to swallow their sputum.

	Activity	How can you encourage patients to expectorate their sputum?

First people need to understand why it is important to clear their secretions. They will be able to cough more easily if in a well-supported, upright position (see Fig. 11.1), and a sputum pot and tissues should be provided. If they are well hydrated, their sputum will be less thick and therefore easier to cough up. A dry mouth makes expectoration difficult, and infected sputum can taste unpleasant, so you need to provide mouthcare. Privacy should be given if there is embarrassment, and nurses should ensure that they do not show any distaste even though they may feel it.

	Activity	How would you describe normal sputum? What do you think might cause sputum to look abnormal?

Normal sputum (or mucus) of healthy individuals is odourless, clear and thin, and is similar in colour and consistency to saliva (Dettenmeier 1992). However, people with chronic respiratory disease, like George, will not have the normal sputum of a healthy individual but have their own baseline which will probably be thicker than usual, and it is likely to be grey, tan or cream rather than clear (Dettenmeier 1992). It is therefore important to be aware of the individual's normal sputum when assessing for abnormalities and George should be alerted to observing his sputum for changes in appearance. Signs of infection are sputum which is green, yellow or rust coloured, and it may also be odorous (Dettenmeier 1992). The presence of purulent green sputum in patients with an acute exacerbation of their COPD is highly associated with infection (Stockley *et al.* 2000). A *Pseudomonas* infection produces thick green sputum with a characteristic odour.

A stringy mucoid specimen often occurs with bronchial asthma (Law 2000). If blood is present the sputum will be rust coloured or red. This is termed **haemoptysis** and may be a sign of infection, but can also be present in cancer, heart failure and pulmonary embolus, and can be distressing to patients. It is important to check that it has actually come from the lungs and has not been vomited (**haemetemesis**) or come from the nose (**epistaxis**). Haemoptysis is worsened by vigorous coughing, chest trauma, chest physiotherapy, anticoagulant therapy and activity.

With young children, you need to ask parents if any sputum has been produced and if so, what it was like in colour and consistency (Woodhams *et al.* 1996). When assessing the amount being produced it is often best to ask in terms of teaspoons, tablespoons or cups. Patients may comment on the taste of the sputum; it may taste unpleasant if infected or taste salty with cystic fibrosis.

Learning outcome 2: Know how to collect a sputum specimen

The goal of sputum collection is to 'obtain fresh, uncontaminated secretions from the tracheo-bronchial tree' (Wilkins *et al.* 2000, p. 112). Although the lower part of the respiratory tract is usually sterile, the upper respiratory tract, nose and mouth, are colonised by large numbers of different bacteria (Wilson 2001).

Activity

Why do you think a sputum specimen might need to be sent to the laboratory?

A sputum specimen may be sent for microbiological examination if infection, including tuberculosis (TB), is suspected, and may also be sent for cytology – examination for abnormal (e.g. cancerous) cells. Box 11.4 outlines the equipment needed and procedure and additional points are discussed below.

It is essential that when a sputum specimen is collected, it has actually come from the lower airways, and has not been cleared from the throat nor is in fact saliva. This needs to be explained carefully to the person, taking into account developmental stage and level of understanding. You can explain that the specimen must come from the 'windpipe'. Sputum is usually more viscous and purulent than saliva; if the specimen appears to be saliva, it should be discarded. A physiotherapist can assist people who are having difficulty expectorating.

Woodhams *et al.* (1996) advise that children of 4–5 years upwards (particularly if they have cystic fibrosis which results in excess secretions being produced) should be able to provide a sputum specimen, if this is explained to them. However obtaining a sputum specimen from younger children will be more difficult and may require help from a physiotherapist. Occasionally suction is needed, possibly using a mucus trap, but this is traumatic for children so would only be used if there is no alternative (Woodhams *et al.* 1996).

When sputum is being sent for testing for TB, the specimen should be at least 10 mL. Three early morning specimens taken on different days are required

---

Equipment needed
- A sterile specimen container with a leak proof lid or cap, and tissues.

Key points
- An early morning specimen is best as bacteria counts are probably highest
- Careful explanation is needed
- The mouth should be rinsed with water and teeth brushed to prevent contamination with oral microbes
- The sputum should be expectorated directly into the labelled container and the lid reapplied immediately

Box 11.4 Key points in collecting a sputum specimen

as *Mycobacterium tuberculosis*, which causes TB, may only be present in small numbers, particularly in the early stages of the disease (Wilson 2001). In small children in whom TB is suspected, early morning gastric washings may be performed in order to collect swallowed sputum.

Testing in the laboratory involves the use of a Gram-stained smear. Most bacteria grow within 24–48 hours, but some bacteria, such as *Mycobacterium tuberculosis*, can take up to 6 weeks to grow (Wilkins *et al.* 2000). Nevertheless, microscopic examination of the sputum can lead to an initial tentative diagnosis. As *Mycobacterium* has very resistant cell walls it is stained using a special dye which cannot be removed by acid or alcohol. This method is termed the 'acid-fast bacilli' or AFB test (Wilson 2001).

Summary

- Nursing measures can encourage expectoration of sputum, which can then be observed for colour, consistency, amount and odour.
- Careful explanations can help to ensure that an uncontaminated specimen of sputum is obtained which can aid with an accurate diagnosis.

OXYGEN THERAPY

Oxygen is a colourless, odourless, tasteless gas which constitutes approximately 21 per cent of atmospheric air at sea level. Oxygen therapy is the administration of supplementary oxygen to enable a higher inspiration of oxygen than is achieved when breathing air. This may be a short-term measure in acute illness (as when Anthony was admitted with acute asthma) or, as with George, long-term therapy for chronic respiratory disease, in which case much support will be required for both the individual concerned and the family.

Note: Correct procedures and local guidelines must be followed for the delivery of oxygen.

LEARNING OUTCOMES

By the end of this section you should be able to:

1. Identify reasons for oxygen therapy and for whom it is needed.
2. Discuss devices for administering oxygen, showing insight into how different concentrations can be achieved.
3. Consider how oxygen therapy can be administered to adults and children who may be frightened or confused.
4. Show insight into important safety aspects of oxygen administration.
5. Explain why humidification of oxygen may be needed and how this can be achieved.

Equipment required will include oxygen delivery systems, comprising masks, nasal cannulae, headboxes and humidification equipment, all of which may be accessible in the skills laboratory.

Learning outcome 1: Identify reasons for oxygen therapy and for whom it is needed

■ **Activity** Reflect on where you have seen oxygen therapy being used within the hospital or community and think of situations where people would benefit from oxygen therapy.

You may have thought of the following situations:

- After a general anaesthetic.
- In emergency situations such as cardiac or respiratory arrest and shock.
- In heart disease where cardiac output is reduced (e.g. **myocardial infarction**).
- In chest injuries following trauma.
- In acute respiratory disease, such as an asthma attack, or bronchiolitis as with Samir.
- In chronic respiratory conditions (such as COPD and cystic fibrosis) where long-term oxygen therapy may be needed, usually for a minimum of 15 hours per day. Dunne (2000) reported improved survival rates in people with COPD who have long-term oxygen therapy. For these patients, like George, oxygen therapy also improves quality of life, as when oxygen demand is increased, such as when carrying out activities like washing and dressing, oxygen therapy helps to reduce breathlessness, and can increase endurance by 30–50 per cent (Rees and Dudley 1998).

Myocardial infarction (MI)
An MI occurs when there is an interruption of blood supply to the myocardium, causing death of tissue and usually resulting in severe chest pain which may radiate to the arms, jaw and/or neck, often accompanied by sweating. 'Heart attack' is the lay term for this condition.

Learning outcome 2: Discuss devices for administering oxygen, showing insight into how different concentrations can be delivered

Key issues are how the oxygen is to be supplied and the devices used to administer it.

Oxygen supplies

In hospital settings, oxygen is obtained either from a cylinder (black with white shoulders) or a wall-mounted piped oxygen supply. Portable cylinders need to be secured in a mobile trolley to avoid damage and to make them easier to move (Sheppard and Davis, 2000a). Replacements need to be ready for use close by. There are a variety of flow meters in use with these, including very low flow meters to be used with infants. If cylinders are in use it is important to regularly check the dial that shows the amount of remaining oxygen, as they can run out quite quickly.

In the home, oxygen must be prescribed and is delivered via an oxygen company. It is usually administered from an oxygen concentrator (McLauchlan 2002), which takes in room air and removes nitrogen through filtration but without depleting the surrounding air. The concentrator runs off electricity (an emergency cylinder is supplied in case of power failure), can deliver up to 4 litres per minute, and is supplied with up to 15 m of tubing, allowing considerable freedom around the home (Baird 2001). George will have this type of arrangement at home.

Delivery devices

The importance of using the correct mask and flow rate when administering oxygen cannot be over-emphasized, but Bell's (1995) study found that this was achieved for only 18 per cent of patients. Different concentrations of oxygen are administered according to clinical need and this affects which oxygen administration device is used. For infants and children like Samir, the method of giving oxygen is selected on the basis of the concentration needed and the child's ability to co-operate with its use (Campbell and Glasper 1995). For adults like Tina who are very breathless and can only mouth breathe, a mask must be used. For all client groups, other than in an emergency situation, concentration of oxygen is prescribed by the doctor according to clinical presentation or through pulse oximetry measurements or blood gas analysis.

Remember that nurses must complete details of oxygen concentration, delivery, commencement and termination of therapy, in patients' notes.

Activity Either in your clinical setting or in the skills laboratory, look at the devices for administering oxygen. How do you think different concentrations are achieved?

Oxygen therapy can be delivered at varying concentrations. These are often measured in percentages, such as 24 per cent, 28 per cent, 35 per cent or 40 per cent, which have been prescribed by the doctor according to the person's requirements. The flow of oxygen is measured in litres per minute using a flow meter. Different devices which you may have found include simple oxygen masks, Venturi masks, nasal cannulae, and non-rebreathing masks (Fig. 11.9). These are all disposable and packaged separately and each individual has their own equipment. For young infants, like Samir, a headbox can be used (Fig. 11.10). Masks need to be cleaned regularly (Sheppard and Davis 2000b), especially if the patient has a productive cough. Equipment should be disposed of according to local policy.

Simple oxygen masks

These are referred to as Hudson, MC (medium concentration) or semi-rigid, and are available in adult and child sizes. The amount of oxygen delivered is adjusted

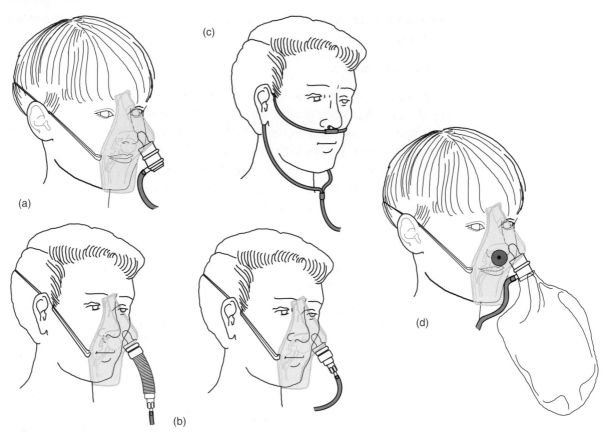

Figure 11.9 Devices for administering oxygen (a) Simple oxygen mask. (b) Venturi masks. (c) Nasal cannulas. (d) Non-rebreathing mask.

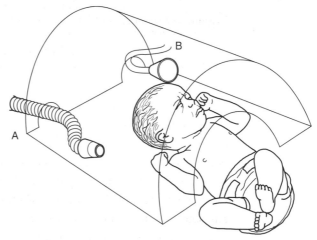

Figure 11.10 Diagram to show positioning of an infant in a headbox for oxygen therapy (original illustration by Faye Riley) (A) Oxygen analyser. (B) Oxygen supply.

only through the use of the flow meter and the exact amount delivered depends on rate and depth of breathing (Porter-Jones 2002). Oxygen can be delivered at 4–15 L per minute, achieving concentrations of 35–70 per cent (Oh 2003). Rates of below 4 L per minute should not be used as, with a low flow rate, rebreathing of carbon dioxide may occur due to exhaled carbon dioxide accumulating within the mask (Oh 2003).

Venturi mask system

In the Venturi oxygen administration system the concentration of oxygen is not significantly affected by the rate and depth of breathing and a set concentration can thus be achieved (Sheppard and Davis 2000a). The mask is supplied with different coloured fittings, each clearly marked with an oxygen percentage and the flow rate that is required. The device ensures that oxygen flow is accurately diluted with entrained air. The nurse can thus administer the exact percentage prescribed by fitting the correct device and setting the correct flow rate.

Nasal cannulae

These are cheap and well tolerated (Vines *et al.* 2000a), and administer oxygen directly into the nostrils rather than into the mouth and nose as masks do. Oxygen flow is only adjusted by use of the oxygen flow meter. Estimated concentration of oxygen achieved ranges from 25 to 40 per cent using a flow rate of 2–6 L per minute (Oh 2003). However, flow rates of more than 4 L per minute are not recommended due to the drying effect on the nasal mucosa (Vines *et al.* 2000a). Nasal cannulae are sometimes used for chronically oxygen-dependent babies, for whom high levels of oxygen may be hazardous, with special low-rate flow meters, which can deliver as little as 250 mL of oxygen per minute.

Activity

For this activity you need access to oxygen administration masks and nasal cannulae in the skills laboratory, and a colleague to use as a patient. Have a go at placing an oxygen mask on a colleague, and then try putting nasal cannulae in place. Look at the diagrams in Fig. 11.9 for guidance as to the optimal positioning. Consider:

1. How can you make the mask and nasal cannulae fit closely?
2. What are the advantages/disadvantages of nasal cannulae?

To make the mask fit comfortably adjust the strap carefully to fit behind the ears. To make the nasal cannulae fit closely move the ends of the tubes through the horizontal piece of tubing across the nose and also the adaptor on the tubing below the chin. Note that if a mask or nasal cannulae are worn for any period of time there is a risk of pressure ulcer development, particularly on the bridge of the nose or behind the ears. Ensuring there is no pressure on the tubing will alleviate this. It is important that masks and cannulae are correctly applied, a good fit and are replaced regularly. Tubing can be supported by gauze to stop sore ears (Jones 1997).

The advantages of nasal cannulae are that people can eat, drink and talk more easily, and procedures such as mouthcare can be carried out without disrupting the oxygen administration. George will find this the most convenient way of receiving his oxygen. With babies, administering oxygen via nasal cannulae allows more freedom to the baby and caregiver, and enables feeding (including breast-feeding) to take place without disruption to oxygen therapy, thus they may be most appropriate for Samir. Also some patients find a mask very claustrophobic. Bambridge's (1993) study found that nasal cannulae were considered comfortable by 90 per cent of patients and were better tolerated than masks.

Administration via nasal cannulae may, however, not be very accurate, as actual intake of oxygen varies according to how much the patient breathes through their mouth, and there are no concentration adjustment devices that can be fitted. With high flow rates there is likely to be discomfort and drying of the nasal mucosa (Oh 2003).

Non-rebreathing masks

These have a large reservoir for oxygen (Vines *et al.* 2000a), with a series of valves to allow the patient to inhale only oxygen and prevent it mixing with expired gases. Concentration of oxygen is determined by the flow meter. They provide a high concentration of oxygen, particularly when required for short periods of time only, for example following surgery.

Headbox (Fig. 11.10)

Some infants best tolerate oxygen therapy when delivered via a headbox, a clear perspex box into which humidified oxygen is delivered when it is placed over the baby's head. Higher percentages of oxygen can be given via a headbox than via cannulae. Care must be taken to ensure that the headbox does not rest on the baby's shoulders or chin. The oxygen concentration in the headbox must be monitored continuously, using an oxygen analyser, to ensure that the prescribed concentration is maintained.

 Activity | What are the advantages and disadvantages of using a headbox to administer oxygen to an infant?

You may have thought of any of these points:

- Most of the baby's care can be performed without interfering with oxygen therapy, although the baby has to be taken out of the headbox for feeding.
- Observation of the baby's colour may be difficult through the headbox due to the humidity.
- The headbox may limit the baby's movement and older infants react vigorously to this.
- The headbox also represents a physical barrier between baby and family and this may be psychologically distressing for all of them. It also limits the extent to which physical comfort in the form of cuddles etc. can be offered to the baby.

All these aspects need to be taken into account when administering oxygen to Samir.

Learning outcome 3: Consider how oxygen therapy can be administered to adults and children who may be frightened or confused

 Activity

Think about how you would approach the following situations:
- A child who is frightened about oxygen therapy and reluctant to co-operate with it.
- A hypoxic adult who is confused and does not want oxygen administered.

Patients who understand how and why they need to use oxygen are far more likely to tolerate such treatment (Baird 2001). Clear explanations are important for all age groups. With children, language appropriate to their level of understanding should be used. Considering level of understanding and learning ability is also particularly important in caring for a person with learning disabilities who needs oxygen therapy, as Anthony would have done when admitted with his acute asthma attack. Demonstration of the mask/cannulae in position on a parent/carer or nurse, and an explanation of the associated sensations and sounds may be reassuring. Encouraging a younger child to position a mask on a doll or teddy may also help to allay fears. Treating oxygen therapy as a game or adventure may promote co-operation, and distraction with toys, stories, etc. can be successful in younger children. Involvement of parents in comforting their child is beneficial to all.

An adult who is confused due to hypoxia may resist oxygen therapy. An important aspect to consider is repositioning to improve ventilation, for example sitting upright in a chair or in bed. Nasal cannulae rather than a mask may be less disturbing. Again, support and explanations from a familiar relative may help.

Learning outcome 4: Show insight into important safety aspects of oxygen administration

The two main hazards associated with oxygen administration are fire, and the delivery of oxygen to people with chronic pulmonary disease, who are carbon dioxide retainers.

Fire hazard

You have probably attended fire lectures where a fire officer has outlined the 'fire triangle' necessary for a fire. Can you remember the three factors? Oxygen, fuel and heat are needed and if one of these is missing the fire cannot start or will quickly go out. Oxygen supports combustion and thus enhances the inflammable properties of other materials such as cigarettes, grease and oil (Sheppard and Davis 2000a). Administration of oxygen could therefore be a fire hazard.

Activity

What precautions will be needed to reduce the risk of fire during oxygen therapy?

You could have thought of:

- No smoking signs.
- No toys or devices that can spark.
- Educating patients and relatives about the risk of smoking during oxygen administration, and of using alcohol-based sprays (e.g. in perfume or aftershave).
- Knowledge of fire procedure and equipment.
- Oxygen cylinders that are used in the home will need to be kept away from gas fires, naked flames and hot radiators (Jones 1997).

Carbon dioxide retainers

A further hazard is that there are certain patients for whom a high percentage of oxygen could be dangerous and actually cause the patient to develop carbon dioxide (CO_2) narcosis leading to coma (Porter-Jones 2002). These are patients who, due to chronic respiratory disease such as experienced by George, continuously retain CO_2. They are termed CO_2 retainers. Children with cystic fibrosis are also potentially at risk from CO_2 narcosis. Normally, rising levels of CO_2 stimulate respiration. However, patients with chronic respiratory disease may continuously have a high level of CO_2 in their blood and therefore their chemoreceptors are no longer stimulated by this. For these patients, the less important hypoxic drive predominates, which means that breathing is only stimulated by lack of oxygen. Patients with chronic respiratory disease are, therefore, normally prescribed only 24–28 per cent oxygen via a venturi mask initially and would only be prescribed a higher amount if indicated by arterial blood gas analysis (Rees and Dudley 1998). When George was first prescribed oxygen it would have been important to establish whether he is a CO_2 retainer.

Learning outcome 5: Explain why humidification of oxygen may be needed and how this can be achieved

Oxygen can be drying to the mucous membranes of the upper airway (Sheppard and Davis 2000b), and this can lead to chest secretions being sticky and difficult to expectorate (Dunn and Chisholm 1998). Dryness to nostrils and mouth can be prevented through good oral hygiene, application of E45 cream and adequate fluid intake. Never use petroleum jelly near oxygen, however, because of its potentially flammable nature (Porter-Jones 2002). If oxygen is to be administered for more than a short period, humidification will be necessary, particularly if the concentration being administered is high for example, over 35 per cent, or at a rate of 4 L per minute or above.

■ Activity

Either in the skills laboratory or in the clinical setting, locate humidification equipment. What sort of water would need to be used do you think and why? What might be hazards associated with using humidification equipment?

As humidification provides a moist environment there is a risk of encouraging bacterial growth. Therefore sterile water needs to be used to minimise bacterial contamination (Porter-Jones 2002), and the water should be changed daily. The bottles themselves should be changed according to the manufacturer's instructions. Cold water systems, where the oxygen is simply bubbled through water at room temperature, are inexpensive and easy to operate as a short-term humidification measure. These systems are noted to be fairly inefficient (Fell and Boehm 1998). In heated-water humidifiers, the oxygen is bubbled across a heated water reservoir. These systems are much more efficient, but there is a risk of mucosal over-heating or burning and excess condensation in the tubing which can reduce oxygen flow (Porter-Jones 2002).

Any humidity supplied to young infants like Samir should be warmed, as cold moist air may cause reflex bronchoconstriction (Carter 1995). However the temperature of the oxygen reaching the baby must be monitored to prevent over-heating. Remember also to explain to patients that humidification may make their face damp, and that the equipment will make a bubbling sound.

Summary

- Oxygen therapy is administered in a wide range of circumstances, to all age groups, and can be a short-term and emergency measure, or a long-term treatment.
- A number of different devices are available for administering oxygen. Nurses must take into account age group, percentage of oxygen prescribed and tolerance when choosing a delivery system.
- The main hazards are combustion and administering a too high percentage to a person with chronic respiratory disease who is a CO_2 retainer. Both these hazards can be avoided by taking necessary care.

ADMINISTERING INHALED MEDICATION

The inhaled route permits medication to go directly to where it is needed in the mucous membranes of the bronchioles, providing an effective method of absorption. As less drug is required, the side effects of the drug used are reduced (Smith 1995). Examples of drugs commonly inhaled are bronchodilators, and steroids for their anti-inflammatory effect.

LEARNING OUTCOMES

By the end of this section you will be able to:

1. Understand why inhalers are used.
2. Accurately explain how to use an inhaler and measure its benefit.
3. Demonstrate knowledge of various types of inhaler, and be able to adapt them in emergency situations.

You may be able to look at different inhalers within the practice setting. Placebo inhalers may be available in the skills laboratory.

Learning outcome 1: Understand why inhalers are used

■ Activity   For what reasons, and by whom, have you seen inhalers used?

You have probably seen inhalers used by both young children and adults. Because asthma is such a common disease – there are 3.5 million people with asthma in the UK alone and 39 million inhalers prescribed in Britain (Weller 2001) – this is probably the commonest reason for seeing inhalers used. Inhalers are also used in COPD and therefore George might be prescribed one too. Inhalers may be used as maintenance therapy as well as in emergency situations where acute dyspnoea and cyanosis occur. (Do you remember what these words mean? They can all be found in the section 'Measuring and recording respirations'.) Inhalers can also be used as prophylactic (preventative) treatment, for example before coming into contact with animal fur, grass, pollen, etc., which may be **allergens** to people with asthma, or before taking strenuous activity where extra oxygen is needed. They need to be taken in a specific order: steroid ones first, then bronchodilators.

Allergen
A foreign substance that initiates an allergic response.

Learning outcome 2: Accurately explain how to use an inhaler and measure its benefit

■ Activity   Instructions for using an inhaler are listed in Box 11.5. Think about how you would actually explain this to an adult and to a child. Try to find someone who uses an inhaler, or if you have access to a skills laboratory, there may be a placebo inhaler so that you can practise the explanation you have developed.

The person should be sitting or preferably standing, to maximise lung expansion, with their head slightly tilted to give them a clear airway. They should clear the respiratory tract by coughing if necessary, and then inhale and exhale deeply before commencing.

1. Check inhaler details (medication and dose) and prescription.
2. Remove the cap and shake the inhaler.
3. Place the mouthpiece into mouth and at the start of a slow deep inspiration, press the canister down, and continue to inhale deeply.
4. Remove the inhaler from mouth and hold breath for 10 seconds, or as long as possible (Vines *et al.* 2000b).
5. Wait several seconds before repeating for a second time if prescribed (note that most people are prescribed two puffs at a time).
6. Record administration on the prescription chart.
7. Wash and dry mouthpiece twice weekly (Vines *et al.* 2000b).

Box 11.5 Instructions for inhaler use

When planning your explanation you need to take developmental stage and learning ability into account. This is especially relevant if your client has a learning disability like Anthony. Demonstration is a useful teaching strategy, particularly with children, but can be used for people of all ages and might be helpful to Anthony. Devices using games (like keeping balls in the air during an inspiration) are available for children to practise technique. The commonest errors have been found to be failure to shake the device, poor co-ordination of actuation and inhalation and absence of breath holding (Dow *et al.* 2001). Duerden and Price (2001) propose that frequent re-assessments and re-education are needed as correct technique usually deteriorates over time. This has implications for all health care practitioners in contact with people using inhalers.

Remember that inhaled medication must always be prescribed and patient details checked as per the drug policy (see Chapter 4). In in-patient settings, the drug should be signed for on the drug administration sheet in the usual way.

Did you know?

■ Fifty per cent of people using inhalers do not do so correctly, and after instruction this only rises to 60 per cent (University of York 2003).
■ An inhaler and spacer, used correctly, are cheaper and more convenient than nebulisers, and can be as effective (Jennings 2002).
■ Accurate inhaler technique is therefore very important!

Measuring the effectiveness of inhalers

What have you read in this chapter that would help you to measure the effectiveness of the inhaled therapy? You may remember that peak flow measurements can be helpful in monitoring effects of inhaled medication (see earlier section). Observation of respiration, including difficulty, rate and sound, are important indicators of whether the medication has been effective. You can also ask the person how they are feeling and observe their colour, mental state and how well they are able to talk.

Learning outcome 3: Demonstrate knowledge of various types of inhaler and be able to adapt them in emergency situations

Activity Think back to inhalers that you have seen and identify different types of devices currently in use.

A detailed overview of the inhaler devices available can be found in Weller (2003). The most commonly used is the metered dose inhaler (MDI) which contains liquid medication under pressure. This is released in the form of a mist when the inhaler is used. MDIs are widely available and comparatively cheap. Other examples which you might have remembered include the diskhaler and

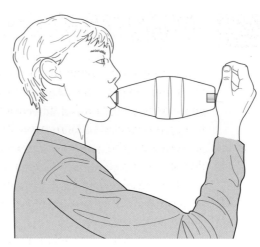

Figure 11.11 The volumatic inhaler.

the rotohaler. With a diskhaler the inhaled particles are contained within a disk and with a rotohaler the particles are enclosed in a capsule. The disk or capsule is then inserted into the inhaler to deliver a metered amount, and activated by inspiration. These are particularly helpful for young children. There appears to be little difference between the effectiveness of different types of inhalers with children; it is as much to do with patient preference (University of York 2003). A recent study revealed a large number of children had inhalers they could not use (Child *et al.* 2002). In adults too, patient preference is crucial, so a good assessment is very important. Another device you have probably seen is a spacer (Fig. 11.11).

Spacers

A spacer, sometimes referred to as a holding device, can be large (e.g. the Volumatic), or small (e.g. the Aerochamber). The spacer holds the medication that has been released, allowing time for the drug to be inhaled through a mouthpiece by activating a one-way valve. The large chamber in the spacer device slows down the speed of the drug leaving the inhaler from 70 to 40 mph and permits the larger particles to stick to the chamber walls (Fink 2000) instead of the mouth where they may cause candida infections (Hunter 1995). The smaller particles in the middle of the chamber then travel on into the trachea and bronchioles for absorption. By filling the chamber with inhaled particles of drug, the person can then breathe these in at their own rate, usually two breaths per inhaled dose, and the particles are less likely to be lost into the atmosphere. Using the spacer is 30 per cent more effective than an ordinary inhaler (Asthma Training Centre 1997). The manufacturers supply detailed instructions for using spacers. It is important that only one puff is squirted into the spacer at a time. Carers of younger children using a spacer and mask while breathing normally (tidal breathing) should allow them to take at least six breaths per puff (Olinsky and Marks 2000).

Why might using a spacer be particularly useful with children?

Spacers are advantageous for children as they remove the necessity to co-ordinate breathing in with activating the canister (Hopkinson 2001). They can therefore be used for giving inhaled medication to very young children. Infants are unable to use the spacer's mouthpiece, but use of an inverted facemask angles the spacer so that the one-way valve falls open, enabling even babies to use a spacer device (Hopkinson 2001). There is a smaller paediatric volumatic available with a soft facemask, which is easier to use. Administration of inhaled medication via a spacer and soft facemask is recommended for children under 5 years (British Thoracic Society 2003).

Large doses of inhaled bronchodilators can be given via an MDI and spacer for emergency treatment of an asthma attack (Olinsky and Marks 2000). It is important that children have easy access to rescue medication in an emergency when at school (Fink 2000). Children may enjoy putting some favourite stickers on the volumatic. Note that spacers can also be used for older people if they are unable to co-ordinate breathing and using the canister. A spacer may also be easier for Anthony to use, for example. Spacers need replacing every 6–12 months, and should be washed in mild detergent, rinsed and allowed to dry naturally on a regular basis. As with any other equipment you should check manufacturer's instructions for advice about usage and maintenance.

Activity If Anthony did not have a spacer and became distressed and dyspnoeic due to his asthma, converting his inhaler into a spacer would help to improve the situation in an emergency. How could you make his ordinary inhaler into a spacer device?

You need a plastic or polystyrene cup and an inhaler. Make a slit in the base of the cup and force the mouthpiece of the inhaler through it. Anthony then needs to hold the open end of the cup over his mouth and face, and you can then press the canister to release the drug into the space made by the cup. Anthony should then breathe in and out slowly at least twice more before the cup is filled with a second metered dose and repeat. This is a useful first aid measure which you can use for any breathless child or adult with asthma if a proper spacer is unavailable.

Summary

- Inhaled medication is frequently prescribed, particularly for people with chronic obstructive pulmonary disease and asthma and a number of different devices are available.
- Inhaled medication is taken both prophylactically and as an emergency measure.

■ Inhalers act directly on the respiratory tract so doses can be lower than when medication is taken systemically.

■ It is very important that inhaler technique is effective so that the correct dose of medication is inhaled.

MANAGING NEBULISED THERAPY

The nebulised route is the passage of medication to the bronchioles directly, as with inhalers, but by vaporising the particles in a stream of air or oxygen. Nebulised particles are much smaller in diameter than inhaled particles (British Thoracic Society 1997). Medication for nebulisers is normally supplied in solution in single-use plastic sealed containers called nebules. As with inhalers, the most common drugs given by nebuliser are bronchodilators and steroids, though they are also now used for antibiotic therapy for patients with cystic fibrosis and HIV.

LEARNING OUTCOMES

By the end of this section you will be able to:

1. Identify indications for nebulised rather than inhaled therapy.
2. Assemble and manage equipment for nebuliser administration and understand the rationale for the care of people receiving nebulised therapy.
3. Decide whether to use oxygen or air to administer a nebuliser.

A nebuliser with mouthpiece and mask attachments should be available in the skills laboratory or you might find them in your practice setting.

Learning outcome 1: Identify indications for nebulised rather than inhaled therapy

Activity

Can you identify the advantages of nebulised therapy over inhaled therapy?

The nebulised route enables bronchodilators to be transported more effectively than inhalers to the bronchioles because the oxygen or air in which it is converted into a vapour reduces the size of the particles, preventing them from sticking to the oral mucosa, and therefore being lost to the respiratory tract. The smaller particles can also travel more easily into the respiratory tract. Link this information to Tina. Can you understand why, in acute asthma, the nebulised route is preferred?

Activity

Think of other people who can benefit from nebulisers.

You could have thought of people who cannot manage to hold and co-ordinate a metered dose inhaler such as young children, some people with learning disabilities who have asthma, and unconscious patients. Nebulised medication can be delivered without a high degree of patient co-operation, for example by a mask, or holding a nebuliser mouthpiece between the lips and breathing normally. Thus nebulisers tend to be given in emergency situations, or where high doses of drug need to be administered in a situation where a person is unable to use other forms of inhaler device (Pearce 1998).

Interesting fact: With good technique, inhalers may be as effective as nebulisers!

Learning outcome 2: Assemble and manage equipment for nebuliser administration and understand the rationale for the care of people receiving nebulised therapy

Activity
Are there any special instructions you would need to give to Tina and Anthony when they are given nebulised therapy?

The following points could all have been considered:

- Optimum position for ventilation. Can you remember this from previous sections? See Fig. 11.1.
- Safety measures if oxygen is being used, which were discussed in the section on oxygen therapy.
- The noise of the nebuliser and the sensation within the mouth need to be explained.

The sensations associated with the nebuliser may be frightening to young children (Jennings 2002). Toddlers in particular may be unwilling to co-operate with a mask. Drug delivery to the lungs is decreased if the child is distressed or crying (British Thoracic Society 2003; Everard 2000; Iles *et al.* 1999). Therefore, in children the routine use of nebulisers should be reserved for those unwilling or unable to cooperate with MDI and spacer (O'Callaghan and Barry, 2000). They are also used during acute episodes to treat those who do not respond to inhalers and for severe exacerbations (British Thoracic Society 2003).

Activity
If you can access nebuliser equipment in the skills laboratory, try fitting the elements together. You need to find a nebuliser unit including a mouthpiece or mask and tubing. Assemble the equipment as in Fig. 11.12 or follow the manufacturer's instructions. Remember that before assembling the equipment for a patient you should wash your hands to reduce the risk of infection.

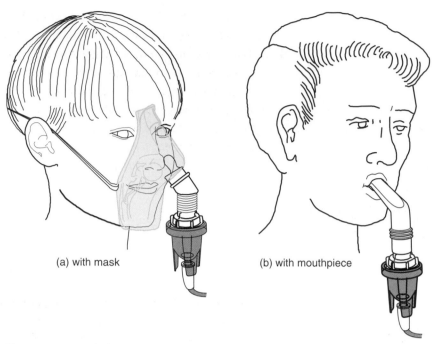

(a) with mask   (b) with mouthpiece

Figure 11.12 Nebuliser equipment.

Nebulised medication must always be prescribed and patient details checked as per the drug policy (see Chapter 4). The drug should be signed for on the drug administration sheet in the usual way. At home Julia and George will not need to do this, but just check the medication before administration.

Activity   Before administering a nebuliser what questions would you need to ask yourself?

You may have considered:

- **Does the peak flow need to be measured first?** This would serve as a baseline for comparison afterwards.
- **Should the person use a mouthpiece or a mask?** Mouthpieces are only used where patients are physically and cognitively able to co-operate with holding it in the mouth. They should then be asked to breathe in and out of the mouth rather than the nose to gain maximum effect. A very breathless patient like Tina may find this too difficult and prefer to use a mask. However, as discussed in the section on oxygen therapy, masks can be distressing to patients. There is no difference in effectiveness when applied correctly.
- **Should I administer the nebuliser via air or oxygen?** See Learning outcome 3 for how you will decide on this.
- **If using a cylinder (either air or oxygen) or piped oxygen what flow rate would be set on the flow meter?** The flow rate must be at least 6 L

per minute (British Thoracic Society 1997), else the particles will not be reduced to the appropriate size for inhalation.

■ **What instructions would I need to give to the person?** The person will need to understand that the mouthpiece or mask must be kept in place and to breathe normally. There is no need to remove to exhale. The nebuliser unit must be kept vertical throughout administration, and continued until all the liquid disappears from the unit, usually 5–10 minutes. It is worth telling the patient to tap the chamber halfway through, to ensure all the solution is nebulised and not left on the chamber wall.

■ **Activity**   After administering a nebuliser, what questions might you ask yourself?

You may have thought of the following:

■ **What should be done with the equipment?** You need to check the manufacturer's instructions as to whether the equipment is 'single use only' or 'single patient use'. If it is 'single use only' it is not suitable for re-using (Gallagher 2002). However if it is 'single patient use', the equipment can all be re-used with the same person, but the nebuliser unit and mouthpiece or mask should be washed in warm tap water at least once daily, dried well and kept covered in a clean place (Jennings 2002). Tubing should not be washed as it cannot be dried properly. George and his wife will need to be instructed about nebuliser cleaning.

■ **How can I evaluate the nebuliser's effectiveness?** You can observe whether the person is still breathless, whether their colour has improved, and whether peak flow readings have increased. You should also consider whether there are any apparent side effects. Nebulised therapy can produce unpleasant side effects.

■ **Activity**   If you know anyone who has used nebulisers ask them to describe any side effects which they encountered.

Adverse side effects can include giddiness, tremor, palpitations, wheeziness and irritable coughing (Dodd 1996). These may be related to the drugs and then dosage may need adjustment. It is also important that the nebules are not too cold as this would cause bronchoconstriction. Mouth infections after prolonged use of certain inhaled drugs may occur too. In addition, if it is a nebulised steroid which is being administered, delivery via a mask may cause irritation to the eyes and skin. Ipratropium bromide, a quite commonly prescribed bronchodilator, can also be irritating to the eyes when given via a mask. Washing the face can prevent irritation, and rinsing the mouth after inhalation of steroids can help to avoid oral candidiasis (Dodd 1996).

Learning outcome 3: Decide whether to use oxygen or air to administer a nebuliser

■ Activity

Think back to the section on oxygen therapy and patients with a hypoxic drive. Do you remember what flow rate is required to administer a nebuliser? If you have seen air used rather than oxygen for administering a nebuliser, can you identify what the rationale could have been?

Remember that if a person is a CO_2 retainer then their breathing is only stimulated by a lack of oxygen. If oxygen is used at 6 litres per minute to administer a nebuliser, what could happen to such a person? Obviously there is a danger, as discussed earlier in this chapter, that CO_2 narcosis may result, and therefore nebulisers for such patients should be administered via air (Porter-Jones 2000), either through an air cylinder (which is grey in colour rather than the black with white shoulders oxygen cylinder) or using an air compressor if available. If a patient requires ongoing nebulisers at home these portable air compressor machines are much more convenient. They extract air from the atmosphere, and are available on prescription. When you are working in a community setting make sure you observe for these.

Summary

- Nebulised therapy is widely used, particularly for people with acute respiratory disease.
- Appropriate decisions must be made as to whether to administer a nebuliser with a mask or a mouthpiece, and via air or oxygen.
- Nurses should be aware of side effects, and how these can be prevented or reduced.

CHAPTER SUMMARY

Respiratory problems can occur within any practice setting, and often arise very suddenly. This chapter aimed to help you to feel confident with measuring respirations, and other frequently used assessment skills – peak flow and pulse oximetry. These skills can appear very straightforward in nature, but it is important to understand what the measurements signify, and how they can be obtained accurately. Encouraging sputum expectoration helps to prevent the development of a chest infection, and nurses should be aware of the significance of the appearance of sputum. Oxygen therapy is administered for a range of people on both a short- and long-term basis. Nurses need to understand the potential hazards, and how it can be delivered safely. Many people with respiratory conditions use inhalers but as they are often used incorrectly, nurses need to understand how they can best be used so that they can educate clients. Nebulised medication is also often prescribed, and nurses need to understand how this can be administered safely.

There are many other specialised respiratory assessment skills and interventions, but the focus of this chapter was to provide a foundation for how you can effectively care for someone with an actual or potential breathing problem. It is particularly important to understand the frightening nature of breathing problems, and to provide psychological support as well as competent technical care.

REFERENCES

Asthma Training Centre 1997. *Asthma Training Centre Learning Package*. Stratford upon Avon.

Baird, A. 2001. Concordance with long-term oxygen therapy. *Practice Nursing* **12**, 457–9.

Bambridge, A.D. 1993. Nasal catheters for oxygen administration. *British Journal of Theatre Nursing Suppl* **2**(10), S11–16.

Bell, C. 1995. Is this what the doctor ordered? Accuracy of oxygen therapy prescribed and delivered in hospital. *Professional Nurse* **10**, 297–300.

Bellamy, D. and Bellamy, G. 1990. Peak flow monitoring. *Practice Nurse* **2**, 406–8.

Bohnhorst, B., Peter, C.S. and Poets, C.F. 2000. Pulse oximeters' reliability in detecting hypoxaemia and bradycardia: comparison between a conventional and two new generation oximeters. *Critical Care Medicine* **28,** 1565–8.

Brewin, A. and Hughes, J. 1995. Effect of patient education on asthma management. *British Journal of Nursing* **4**, 81–2, 99–101.

British Thoracic Society 1997. Guidelines on the management of nebulisers. *Thorax* **52**, supplement 2, S1–24.

British Thoracic Society 2003. British Guidelines on Management of Asthma. *Thorax* **58**, supplement 1.

Campbell, S. and Glasper, E.A. 1995. *Whaley and Wong's Children's Nursing*. London: Mosby.

Carroll, P. 1997a. Pulse oximetry – at your fingertips. *RN* **60**(2), 22–7, 43.

Carroll, P. 1997b. Using pulse oximetry in the home. *Home Healthcare Nurse* **15**, 88–97.

Carter, B. 1995. Nursing support and care: meeting the needs of the child and family with altered respiratory function. In Carter, B. and Dearmun, A. (eds) *Child Health Care Nursing: Concepts, theory and practice*. Oxford: Blackwell Science, 274–305.

Cartridge, M. 1990. *Guidelines for Health Professionals and the Measurement of Peak Flow*. London: National Asthma Campaign.

Child, F., Davies, S., Clayton, S. *et al.* 2002. Inhaler devices for asthma: do we follow the guidelines? *Archives of Diseases in Childhood* **86**, 176–9.

Cote, J., Cartier, A., Malo, J.L. *et al.* 1998. Compliance with peak expiratory flow monitoring in home management of asthma. *Chest (Chicago)* **113**, 968–72.

Cowan, T. 1997. Pulse oximeters. *Professional Nurse* **12**, 744–5, 747–8, 750.

Department of Health 2001. *Valuing People: A new strategy for learning disability for the 21st century*. London: DH.

Dettenmeier, P.A. 1992. *Pulmonary Nursing Care*. St Louis: Mosby.

Dodd, 1996. Nebuliser therapy: what nurses and patients need to know. *Nursing Standard* **10**(31), 39–42.

Donohue, J.F. 1996. Asthma: Indications, benefits, and pitfalls of peak flow monitoring. *Consultant* **36**, 2589–96.

Dow, L., Fowler, L., Lamb, H. and Hall, G.H. 2001. Elderly people's technique in using dry powder inhalers. *British Medical Journal* **323**, 49–50.

Duerden, M. and Price, D. 2001. Training issues in the use of inhalers. *Disease Management Health Outcomes* **9**, 75–87.

Dunn, L. and Chisholm, H. 1998. Oxygen therapy. *Nursing Standard* **13**(7), 57–60.

Dunne, P.J. 2000. The demographics and economics of long-term oxygen therapy. *Respiratory Care* **45**(2), 223–31.

Everard. M, 2000. Trying to deliver aerosols to upset children is a thankless task. *Archives of Diseases in Childhood* **82**, 428.

Fell, H. and Boehm, M. 1998. Easing the discomfort of oxygen therapy. *Nursing Times* **94**(38), 56–8.

Fink, J.B. 2000. Aerosol device selection: evidence to practice. *Respiratory Care* **45**(7), 874–85.

Gallagher, C. 2002. When once is enough. *Nursing Times* **98**(38), 22–5.

Grap, M.J. 1998. Protocols for practice: applying research at the bedside. Pulse oximetry. *Critical Care Nurse* **18**, 94–9.

Hanning, C.D. and Alexander-Williams, J.M. 1995. Pulse oximetry: a practical review. *British Medical Journal* **311**, 367–70.

Hay, W.W., Rodden, D.J., Collins, S.M. *et al.* 2002. Reliability of conventional and new pulse oximetry in neonatal patients. *Journal of Perinatology* **22**(5), 360–6.

Hopkinson, L. 2001. Spacer devices. *Practice Nurse* **21**(6), 22, 24, 26.

Howell, M. 2002. Clinical audit. Pulse oximetry: an audit of nursing and medical staff understanding. *British Journal of Nursing* **11**, 191–7.

Hull, D. and Johnstone, D. 1999. *Essential Paediatrics*, fourth edition. Edinburgh: Churchill Livingstone.

Hunter, S. 1995. The use of steroids in asthma treatment. *Nursing Standard* **9**(38), 25–7.

Iles, R., Lister, P. and Edmunds, A. 1999. Crying significantly reduces absorption of aerolised drug in infants. *Archives of Diseases in Childhood* **81**(2), 163–5.

Jennings, J. 2002. Revisiting nebulisers: cleaning and use. *Practice Nursing* **13**(4), 173.

Jones, S. 1997. Oxygen therapy. *Community Nurse* **3**, 234.

Law, C. 2000. A guide to assessing sputum. *NT Plus* **96**(24), 7–10.

Leach, A. 1994. Making sense of peak flow recordings of lung function. *Nursing Times* **90**(44), 34–5.

Le Bourdelles, G., Estagnasie, P., Lenoir, F. *et al.* 1998. Use of a pulse oximeter in an adult emergency department. *Chest (Chicago)* **113**, 1042–7.

Le Grand, T.S. and Peters, J.I. 1999. Pulse oximetry: advantages and pitfalls. *Journal of Respiratory Diseases* **20**, 195–200, 206.

Lowton, K. 1999. Pulse oximeters for the detection of hypoxaemia. *Professional Nurse* **14**, 343–50.

Matthews, P. 1997. Using a peak flow meter. *Nursing 97* June, 57–9.

McCullen, A.H., Yoos, L. and Kizman, H. 2002. Peak flow meters in childhood asthma: parent report of use and perceived usefulness. *Journal of Pediatric Health Care* **16**(2), 67–72.

McGrath, A.M., Gardner, D.M. and McCormack, J. 2001. Is home peak expiratory flow monitoring effective in controlling asthma symptoms? *Journal of Clinical Pharmacy and Therapeutics* **26**(5), 311–17.

McLauchlan, L. 2002. Supplementary oxygen therapy in the community. *Nursing Times Plus* **98**(40), 50–2.

Moyle, J. 1996. How to guides. Pulse oximetry. *Care of the Critically Ill* **12**(6), insert.

Moyle, J. 1999. Step by step guide. Pulse oximetry. *Journal of Neonatal Nursing* **5**, insert.

O'Callaghan, C. and Barry, P. 2000. How to choose delivery devices for asthma. *Archives of Diseases in Childhood* **82**, 185–7.

Oh, T.E. 2003. Oxygen therapy. In Bersten, A.D. and Soni, N. (eds) *Oh's Intensive Care Manual*, fifth edition. Oxford: Butterworth-Heinemann, 275–82.

Olinsky, A. and Marks, M. 2000. Respiratory conditions. In Smart, J. (ed.) *Paediatric Handbook*. Oxford: Blackwell Science.

Pearce, L. 1998. Know how: asthma inhalers. *Nursing Times* **94**(9) Suppl.

Pedersen, T., Dyrlund Pedersen, B. and Moller, A.M. 2003. Pulse oximetry for perioperative monitoring (Cochrane Review). In *The Cochrane Library*, Issue 4. Chichester: John Wiley and Sons.

Peters, S.M. 1997. The effect of acrylic nails on the measurement of oxygen saturation as determined by pulse oximetry. *Journal of the American Association of Nurse Anesthetists* **5**, 361–3.

Place, B. 1998. Pulse oximetry in adults. *Nursing Times* **94**(50), 48–9.

Porter-Jones, G. 2000. Nebulisers – 2 Administration. *Nursing Times* **96**(37), 51–2.

Porter-Jones, G. 2002. Short-term oxygen therapy. *Nursing Times Plus* **98**(40), 53–6.

Rees, P.J. and Dudley, F. 1998. ABC of oxygen: oxygen therapy in chronic lung diseases. *British Medical Journal* **317**, 871–4.

Rodriguez, R.M. and Light, R.W. 1998. Pulse oximetry in the ICU: uses, benefits, limitations. *The Journal of Critical Illness* **13**, 247–52.

Rubin, B.K. 2002. Physiology of airway mucus clearance. *Respiratory Care* **47**, 761–8.

Scarfone, R.J., Zorc, J.J. and Capraro, G.A. 2001. Patient self-management of acute asthma: adherence to national guidelines a decade later. *Pediatrics* **108**, 2332–8.

Schnapp, L.M. and Cohen, N.H. 1990. Pulse oximetry: uses and abuses. *Chest* **98**, 1244–50.

Seymour, J. 1995. Asthma: peak flow meters. *Nursing Times* **91**(4), 50, 52.

Sinex, J.E. 1999. Pulse oximetry: principles and limitations. *American Journal of Emergency Medicine* **17**, 59–66.

Sheppard, M. and Davis, S. 2000a. Oxygen therapy – 1. *Nursing Times* **96**(29), 43–4.

Sheppard, M. and Davis, S. 2000b. Oxygen therapy – 2. *Nursing Times* **96**(30), 43–4.

Smith, E. 1995. Guidelines for asthma treatment. RCN Nursing Update. *Nursing Standard* **9**(13), 1–8.

Stockley, R.A., O'Brien, C., Pye, A. and Hill, S.L. 2000. Relationship of sputum colour to nature and outpatient management of acute exacerbations of COPD. *Chest* **117**, 1638–45.

Stocks, J. 1996. Respiration. In Hinchliff, S.M., Montague, S.E. and Watson, R. *Physiology for Nursing Practice*, second edition. London: Baillière Tindall, 530–81.

Stoddart, S., Summers, L. and Platt, M.W. 1997. Pulse oximetry: what it is and how to use it. *Journal of Neonatal Nursing* **3**(4), 10, 12–14.

Stoneham, M.D., Saville, G.M. and Wilson, I.H. 1994. Knowledge about pulse oximetry among medical and nursing staff. *The Lancet* **344**, 1339–42.

Summers, R.L., Anders, R.M., Woodward, L.H. *et al.* 1998. Effect of routine pulse oximetry measurements on ED triage classification. *American Journal of Emergency Medicine* **16**(1), 5–7.

University of York 2003. *Inhaler Devices for the Management of Asthma and COPD*. NHS Centre for Reviews and Dissemination **8**(1).

Vines, D.L., Shelledy, D.C. and Peters, J. 2000a. Current respiratory care, part 1: Oxygen therapy, oximetry, bronchial hygiene. *Journal of Critical Illness* **15**, 507–5.

Vines, D.L., Shelledy, D.C. and Peters, J. 2000b. Questions and answers about inhalers. *Journal of Critical Illness* **15**, 563–4.

Weller, T. 2001. Supporting patients through the transition to CFC–free inhalers. *Community Nurse* **7**(2), 39–40.

Weller, T. 2003. Inhaler devices: spoilt for choice. *Nurse 2 Nurse* **3**(3), 17–20.

Wilkins, R.L., Jones Krider, S. and Sheldon, R.L. 2000. *Clinical Assessment in Respiratory Care*, fourth edition. St Louis: Mosby.

Wilson, J. 2001. *Infection Control in Clinical Practice*, second edition. London: Baillière Tindall.

Wong, D.L., Hockenberry-Eaton, M., Winkelstein, M.L. *et al.* 1999. *Nursing Care of Infants and Children*, sixth edition. St Louis: Mosby.

Woodhams, K., Trussler, J. and Wooler, E. 1996. The respiratory system. In McQuaid, L., Huband, S. and Parker, E. (eds) *Children's Nursing*. New York: Churchill Livingstone, 171–87.

Wooler, E. 1994. Asthma in children. *Paediatric Nursing* **6**(10), 29–33.

Woollons, S. 1995. Peak flow meters. *Professional Nurse* **11**, 130–2.

USEFUL WEBSITES

- **Asthma UK** www.asthma.org.uk
- **British Lung Foundation** www.britishlungfoundation.com
- **British Thoracic Society** www.brit-thoracic.org.uk

Managing pain and promoting comfort

Dee Burrows and Lesley Baillie

Clients and patients in all health care settings experience pain and discomfort – whether physical, emotional or spiritual. Recent studies suggest some 72 per cent of hospital in-patients (Brook *et al.* 2002) and a third of those living in the community (Clinical Standards Advisory Group 1999) are in pain at any one time. Managing pain and promoting comfort are therefore essential skills in nursing practice. Many of the skills have already been explored in this book. This chapter, however, aims to bring them together to help you to understand how they may be used deliberately to reduce pain and promote comfort. The first section of the chapter focuses upon pain. Pain and its management are large topics, so the section offers an introduction to provide a foundation for future practice and learning. To develop your understanding and skills further, you need to refer to literature, texts and other sources, some of which are listed at the end of the chapter. The second part of the chapter goes on to look at how nurses promote comfort in a range of settings.

This chapter includes:
- Managing pain in a variety of settings
  - The nature of pain
  - Pain assessment
  - Pain management using medication
  - Other approaches to managing pain
- Promoting comfort using presence, monitoring, touch, talking and physical actions.

Recommended biology reading:
The following questions will help you to focus on the biology underpinning the skills used in pain management. Use your recommended text book to find out:

- What is pain?
- What terminology is used to describe pain?

- Why do we feel pain? Can pain be useful diagnostically?
- What anatomical components are required to 'feel' pain?
- Identify three pain producing substances. Where are they produced?
- What is a nociceptor?
- What effect does myelination have on the transmission of pain messages?
- Where is the substantia gelatinosa? What is its relevance to pain perception?
- What affects pain perception? How does this relate to the gate control theory?
- How does the release of endogenous opiates reduce pain?
- What physical signs may indicate when a person is in pain?

PRACTICE SCENARIOS

The following scenarios illustrate when managing pain and promoting comfort may be needed. They will be referred to throughout this chapter.

Adult

Acute renal failure

This occurs when renal function suddenly ceases leading to oliguria (poor urine output) or anuria (no urine output). It results in high blood urea levels causing loss of appetite, nausea and vomiting.

Pulmonary oedema

This is usually caused by failure of the left ventricle and is a recognised complication of acute renal failure. The resulting increased pulmonary capillary blood pressure leads to fluid entering the alveoli interfering with gas exchange, causing severe breathlessness, orthopnoea and hypoxia.

Sidney Owen, aged 88 years, had always kept very good health and lived independently. However he was admitted as an emergency in **acute renal failure** and 3 days after admission developed **pulmonary oedema**. During the night he was acutely breathless and in his own words 'I thought that I was dying'. But he described how the nurse on duty, Debbie, sat with him: 'She took my hand, which gave me such comfort. It was a great help having her there. She seemed to be there all night!' Sidney made a full recovery but he did not encounter Debbie again – maybe she was doing a temporary shift on the ward. He did not forget her and often talked about that terrible night and the nurse who, by his perception, never left his side and held his hand.

Child

Patience Jackson, aged 9 years, has been admitted to the children's ward with abdominal pain. She was taken to the GP who referred her to the Accident and Emergency (A&E) department. Four doctors have already seen her. She has appendicitis and will need to have an appendicectomy under general anaesthetic. Patience understands what is going to happen and is quite anxious. She has not been in hospital before. Her parents are with her.

Learning disability

Brian O'Connor is a 49-year-old man who has a learning disability. He lives alone in a flat. He works in a local factory tidying and running errands, and he places great value on his work, from which he has never been known to miss a day. Recently he has been acting out of character having been absent from work on several occasions. The factory staff contacted the community nurse for

Peptic ulcer

A necrotic area in the stomach or duodenum extending through the mucosa into the deeper layers. It typically causes burning epigastric pain, and complications include haemorrhage and perforation.

Endoscopy

An investigation using a tube with a light source allowing inspection and biopsy (removal of tissue for examination) of the mucosa of the stomach and duodenum.

Alzheimer's disease

Also referred to as dementia of Alzheimer's type (DAT), this is the most common form of dementia. It is commoner in older people and is thought to result from neurological changes in the brain (Cheston and Bender 1999). Dementia is chronic and progressive in nature, has many causes and commonly presents with memory and language impairment, decline in self-care ability, and behavioural and personality changes (Jacques and Jackson 2000).

Osteoarthritis

A degenerative joint disorder where there is progressive loss of articular cartilage, new bone formation and capsular fibrosis. Main symptoms are pain, stiffness and restricted movement.

learning disabilities, as they were concerned about Brian. On visiting him, the nurse found that he appeared to be unwell and there was evidence of recent vomiting. Although Brian was unable to explain his symptoms the nurse suspected that he might be in pain. The nurse checked his vital signs and contacted the GP. The GP thought Brian might have a **peptic ulcer**, so he was referred for an **endoscopy**. As Brian has no close relatives, the community nurse for learning disabilities is going to accompany him and is preparing him for the procedure using information leaflets.

Mental health

Violet Davies, aged 76 years, has advanced **Alzheimer's disease**. She has been admitted to a nursing home, as her husband is physically and emotionally exhausted and unable to cope. He has refused help in the past as he has been determined to look after his wife, but he has now agreed to her admission. Violet is physically well but she is also known to have **osteoarthritis** in her right hip. She looks permanently worried and agitated and keeps repeating the same phrase over and over again. Mr Davies looks shaky and tearful.

MANAGING PAIN IN A VARIETY OF SETTINGS

LEARNING OUTCOMES

By the end of this section you will be able to:

1. Discuss the nature of pain.
2. Explain the differences between pain threshold, pain tolerance and pain behaviour.
3. Consider the different dimensions of pain that may need to be assessed.
4. Identify appropriate pain assessment tools for different client groups.
5. Demonstrate understanding of the pain ladder and how it can be applied in practice.
6. Explore non-pharmacological approaches to managing pain.

Learning outcome 1: Discuss the nature of pain

Activity

Reflect back on your practice experiences. Write down a few examples of people you have met with pain and the setting that you met them in.

Sadly, pain is all around us. Despite advances in medication management, up to three-quarters of post-operative patients continue to experience moderate to severe pain (MacIntyre and Ready 2002). Figures for pain in the community vary tremendously. It is probable that some 27–40 per cent of people living at home (Census 2001; Clinical Standards Advisory Group 1999) and 70–80 per cent of those in residential care (Closs *et al.* 2003) are experiencing pain at any one time.

It is, therefore, a key element of day-to-day nursing practice in all four branches of care.

Pain is frequently referred to as either acute or chronic. However, the reality is a little more complex. For instance, you may have come across people in acute pain who also have unrelated chronic pain. In addition, in your biology reading you will have learned about A delta and C fibre transmission. If you think about what happens when you twist an ankle, you experience immediate sharp pain as a consequence of A delta fibre stimulation, followed several hours later by deep throbbing pain arising from C fibre stimulation. This is often referred to as fast (A delta fibre) and slow (C fibre) pain. As people's pain is often not clearly defined, viewing pain in this light helps to explain some of the anomalies that can be seen in acute and chronic care settings.

■ Activity

With reference to your biology reading and the scenarios, what factors may affect pain perception? How might these relate to the gate control theory?

You may want to read the following paragraph more than once to ensure that you understand the knowledge underpinning some of the practical skills that will be discussed later in this chapter.

Pain fibres transmit pain impulses as a consequence of stimulation of the nociceptors. These are receptors in the skin, mucous membranes or organs that pick up harmful stimuli. Stimuli may be mechanical, chemical, thermal, electrical, mental, social or spiritual. For example, Sidney is clearly frightened of dying (spiritual stimuli), while Patience's pain is caused by infection (chemical stimuli) and swelling (mechanical stimuli). Both are anxious, which as a mental stimulus may well act through the **limbic system** and descending pathways to open the gate to pain. Brian's ulcer pain also arises from chemical stimulation. Violet's situation is complex, with pain caused by the mechanical stimulation of osteoarthritis and mental, social and possibly spiritual stimulation arising from her Alzheimer's disease. Violet's pain perception may be further enhanced through the **reticular activating system** as a consequence of her agitation. Both ascending and descending influences on the gate are thus reducing the likelihood of the gate closing. Violet's husband, Mr Davies, may also be suffering from social isolation, as well as his mental and physical exhaustion. He may need comforting and active support if he is going to be able to look after his wife at home again in the future.

Some of the examples given above refer to mechanical and chemical stimulation of the nociceptors. This is known as **nociceptive** pain. Pain can also occur as a consequence of peripheral or central nerve damage when it is termed **neuropathic** pain. For example, people with multiple sclerosis may experience neuropathic pain because of demyelination and subsequent scar formation of the nerves. They may also experience nociceptive pain through mechanical stimulation arising from altered muscle balance and muscle spasms (Multiple Sclerosis Trust 2001). Knowledge of these two different types of pain is important if you

Limbic system
A group of brain structures that control the emotional aspects of pain.

Reticular activating system
A network of brain cells concerned with arousal and awareness.

are to understand the different pharmacological and non-pharmacological approaches to pain management discussed later in this chapter.

Defining pain

Activity | Think back to a time when you have experienced pain and write the experience down. Looking at your notes, how would you define pain?

Pain is a complex, personal experience that has been defined in a number of ways. For example, the International Association for the Study of Pain (IASP) defined pain as:

> An unpleasant sensory and emotional experience associated with actual or potential tissue damage, or described in terms of such damage.
>
> *(IASP Subcommittee on Taxonomy 1979, p. 250)*

This definition, which post-dated the publication of the gate control theory, clearly recognises that pain is made up of both physical and psychological components.

A classical definition of pain used in nursing, is that by Margo McCaffery first published in 1968:

> Pain is whatever the experiencing person says it is, existing when the experiencing person says it does.
>
> *(McCaffery 1968, cited in Sofaer 1998, p. 95)*

McCaffery's definition is an operational definition as it aims to guide practice. Nurses who follow this stance believe what the person says about their pain and manage it accordingly. This may appear an obvious statement, as compassion, according to Roach (2002), includes sensitivity to pain (see Chapter 1). However, patients' descriptions are not always believed. Not believing what someone says is, of course, tantamount to calling them a liar. It would be surprising if the population was divided into two groups: honest health care professionals and dishonest clients and patients! As Moskow (1987) points out:

> Pain occurring in unicorns, griffins, and jabberwockies is always imaginary pain, since these are imaginary animals: patients on the other hand, are real, and so they always have real pain.
>
> *(Moskow 1987, p. 68)*

If pain is to be managed effectively so that patients are comfortable, nurses need to be:

- **compassionate** to patients' needs
- willing to listen to their **conscience**
- **confident** in their assessment skills
- **competent** in and **committed** to their chosen pain management strategies
- aware of **comporting** themselves well.

Chapter 1 explains the 6Cs of caring, proposed by Roach (2002) in more detail.

Activity

Return to the notes you made about your experience of pain and the people that you met in practice settings. Was your pain and their's believed? Were you and they treated with compassion? Did the nurses appear to understand the complexity of pain?

To read in detail about the misconceptions surrounding pain it is suggested that you refer to the first half of chapter 3 in McCaffery and Pasero (1999). Before you do so, you might like to examine your own attitudes by completing the scale at the end of this chapter (Appendix 12.1). You can then compare your answers to the views of McCaffery and Pasero (1999). If you are unable to access this text you could try looking up misconceptions, myths, attitudes and barriers in any pain management book that you are able to access.

Learning outcome 2: Explain the difference between pain threshold, pain tolerance and pain behaviour

Activity

1. How often have you or friends commented that someone has 'a high/low pain threshold'? Think for a minute what you meant by this. Jot down your feelings about people with a low threshold and those with a high threshold.
2. Now consider what you understand by the word 'tolerance'.

In pain management, threshold refers to the level at which the population at large perceives a stimulus as painful. In other words, if everything were equal we would all feel pain at pretty much the same level. Pain threshold, therefore, is essentially a physiological measurement.

Pain tolerance refers to the amount of pain an individual can tolerate at any given time. It is linked to our psychological state and is, in essence, an outcome of gate control. To illustrate this, imagine you are sitting in a lecture and are experiencing a really bad headache. What would you do? Perhaps you would take painkillers or go home. You still have your headache but need to get ready for a party. What would you do? It is highly likely that you would go to the party and within a short space of time forget your headache!

Activity

Refer back to the gate control theory to understand more about why and how this happens.

Pain tolerance varies from one individual to the next and within an individual from one minute to the next. Some of the factors that open the gate to pain and thereby increase pain perception are listed in Box 12.1 as 'gate openers'. Those that have the potential to fully or partially close the gate and thereby reduce pain perception are listed as 'gate closers'.

Activity

Look at the scenario of Violet and list the factors that may be influencing her pain perception. Note down an explanation for each factor.

Gate openers	Gate closures
Anxiety	Information
Fear	Relaxation
Worry	Distraction
Tension	Control
Lack of control	Touch
Tiredness	Social interaction
Prolonged pain	Known positive outcome
Recurrent pain	Reassurance
Previous poor experiences	Previous positive experience

Box 12.1 Examples of factors that open and close the gate to pain

You might have come up with:

■ Mr Davies's emotional and physical exhaustion, his desire to support Violet at home and his tearfulness may be transmitted to Violet and increase her worry.
■ The strange and potentially frightening environment may reduce Violet's sense of personal control and enhance her feelings of social isolation.
■ The prolonged nature of Violet's osteoarthritis may have reduced her pain coping strategies.
■ Violet's agitation will prevent her from relaxing and increase her tension.
■ The lack of information about the immediate future may reduce Mr and Mrs Davies's abilities to maintain any sense of cognitive control.
■ Finally, the pathophysiology of Alzheimer's disease may alter Violet's pain experience. This is discussed under learning outcome 3.

Knowing and understanding the factors that reduce pain perception can help guide your approach to pain management. The third concept you need to consider is pain behaviour.

■ **Activity** | Again, thinking about headaches:
1. How do you behave when you have a headache?
2. How does your best friend behave?
3. How do other people you know behave?

Perhaps one of the people you thought of wants attention, while another prefers to be on their own. Maybe one frowns, grimaces and becomes irritable, while someone else tries to relax their facial expression and carry on as normal. As well as non-verbal and social responses, verbal and vocal (e.g. shouting, moaning) responses also vary. These are all different pain behaviours or pain expressions. According to Carr and Mann (2000), pain expression and pain behaviour are learned through our families and culture. In their book *Challenge of Pain*, Melzack and Wall (1996) discuss the influence of culture in relation to the gate control theory. A study by Madjar (1985) highlighted the importance of nurses understanding cultural expression in pain management. She compared post-operative pain behaviours in twenty Anglo-Australian and thirteen Yugoslav-Australian patients and found that although there were no significant differences between vocal and motor behaviours, social and verbal differences were identified. Anglo-Australians were more likely to seek help, including analgesics, but tended to withdraw socially to cope with their pain. Conversely, Yugoslavs preferred company, openly discussed their pain and yet asked for fewer analgesics. Although published some years ago now, these findings have been supported by more recent research.

Activity

1. Think of the different pain behaviours you have seen. List the ones you think Sidney, Patience, Brian and Violet might be adopting?
2. Scenarios often push you into stereotyping (as do handovers). Consider the behaviours you have listed for each scenario and ask yourself why you identified those particular ones.

In summary, an appreciation of the differences between pain threshold, pain tolerance and pain behaviour will help you to understand how people's pain and their reactions to it vary. The next section considers pain responses in greater depth.

Learning outcome 3: Consider the different dimensions of pain that may need to be assessed

Because there are many different factors that influence pain perception and pain behaviour, pain is regarded as a multidimensional phenomenon. A number of different multidimensional frameworks exist to help practitioners assess pain. Deborah McGuire (1992), who is an American nurse, developed one based around six dimensions:

- Physiological
- Sensory
- Affective
- Cognitive
- Behavioural
- Sociocultural.

This framework is outlined below.

Physiological dimension

The physiological dimension of pain deals with the anatomy and physiology of pain perception and the gate control mechanisms. Patience's appendicectomy will cause her to experience acute post-operative pain as a result of the tissue damage arising from the surgical procedure. As well as pain, noxious stimuli will increase sympathetic activity, resulting in raised blood pressure, heart rate, oxygen consumption, muscle tension and sphincter tone in the bladder and bowels

(MacIntyre and Ready 2002). These are frequently cited signs and symptoms of acute pain. However, because of the way the body adapts to stress they normalise long before the pain disappears. (You may wish to refer back to your biology reading on the general adaptation syndrome here.) Physiological signs and symptoms are therefore usually regarded as the least reliable way of measuring pain. However, they may be helpful in situations where verbal assessment is constrained, such as with neonates, unconscious or cognitively impaired patients. As you read in the scenarios, Brian's vital signs were checked by the nurse and would have helped in her general assessment of him. The nurse may have previous recordings of his vital signs which could act as a baseline for comparison.

Sensory dimension

The sensory dimension considers the location, intensity and quality of pain. Acute pain is usually well defined. Patience, for example, would have described her pre-operative pain as being in her lower abdomen either in the centre or on the right. Post-operatively, she is likely to tell you that her pain is localised to the incision site. Brian may be experiencing stomach and back pain, as the pain of peptic ulcers can be referred to the mid or low thoracic spine. Violet's chronic osteoarthritis pain may be more diffuse, radiating into both her back and her knee. Although Sidney's condition is acute, he may have several foci of pain and, as a consequence of toxicity, feel generally uncomfortable.

Both practitioners and the general public tend to think of acute pain as far more intense than chronic pain. However, this is not always the case. Practitioners also have a tendency to rank acute pain so that more credence is given to the pain of a mycodardial infarction (heart attack), for example, than to the pain of a kidney infection. Although there is some minor evidence to suggest that certain pain sensations may be more intense than others, the most important guide is to listen to what the person says about the intensity and quality of their pain. Quality of pain refers to the way pain is described. It is influenced by whether the pain arises from A delta fibre stimulation (sharp pain), C fibre stimulation (deep throbbing or aching pain) or from nerve damage. People with neuropathic pain often describe it as a burning or tingling sensation. Some pain assessment tools help to differentiate the quality of pain in order to inform medication management (see learning outcome 4).

Brian and Violet may be unable to describe their pain because of communication difficulties, confusion or deficits in cognitive processing. In Alzheimer's disease, the disease affects the limbic system, which impacts on the person's ability to explain the quality of their pain. However, the sensory cortex is not involved so patients are still able to perceive pain (Frampton 2003).

| ■ *Activity* | Look at the scenarios again and consider whether you have made any assumptions about the intensity of pain each of the people will be experiencing. On what basis did you make these assumptions? |

You might have listed age, gender, emotional state, cognitive ability, level of understanding, family support, ability to verbalise pain, the acuteness of the pain and so on. Some of these factors, such as emotional state, are known to influence pain perception, while the evidence base for others is less clear. For example, there is considerable debate about whether, as a consequence of A delta fibre demyelination, older people's ability to perceive pain is reduced. If this is the case, it may be one explanation for why older people tend to use C fibre rather than A delta fibre descriptive words to describe their pain (Chakour *et al.* 1996).

Affective dimension

The affective dimension addresses people's emotional responses to pain. In the activity above you may have considered some of the affective factors listed earlier as gate openers or closers. For instance, we know that Patience is 'quite anxious' and that Violet is 'worried and agitated'. We can infer that Sidney was frightened, but the information given on Brian is insufficient to assess his emotional response. One of the affective factors that may be relevant to Brian's experience is helplessness. Studies, such as the classical study by Hayward (1975) on pre-operative information giving and recent work by Arnstein *et al.* (1999) in chronic pain, indicate that the more informed a person, the less helpless they feel, the better able they are to cope with their pain and, in some cases, the less pain they experience. The input from the community nurse for learning disabilities, in explaining to Brian what is happening and preparing him for his endoscopy, should help to decrease feelings of uncertainty and helplessness.

Cognitive dimension

The cognitive dimension explores the way in which pain is influenced by and influences people's thoughts, attitudes, beliefs and preferred cognitive strategies for coping with pain. Sidney's discomfort and pain led him to believe that he was dying, a belief that may well have heightened his pain perception. Patience, on the other hand, understands that she has appendicitis and that the operation will take her pain away. Brian's learning disability and Violet's Alzheimer's disease will affect their cognitive processing of pain and, as such, their understanding (Kovach *et al.* 1999). Strategies for coping with pain are discussed later in the chapter.

Behavioural dimension

The behavioural dimension includes behaviours associated with pain perception and behaviours associated with attempts to control pain. Facial grimacing, moaning, supporting the painful area, rigid posture or restlessness are all recognised signs of acute pain (Cousins and Power 1999). Signs associated with chronic pain include muscle tension, depression, loss of appetite, altered posture, sleeplessness and focus on self. However, just because someone has pain does not mean that they will exhibit pain behaviours. As with physiological signs, acute behavioural signs will normalise as part of general adaptation. Thus if, for example, as Patience recovers from her surgery she appears to be sleeping, or laughing with her parents, it cannot be assumed that she is pain free. Similarly, people with chronic pain do not always display the pain behaviours cited above. The employment of behavioural coping strategies, such as distraction and relaxation, may further emphasise any lack of pain behaviour. As you read in the scenario, Brian's pain and discomfort was exhibited through his changed behaviour.

It is precisely because the physiological and behavioural signs are unreliable that pain experts emphasise the importance of verbal pain assessment. However, these signs are helpful if verbal assessment is limited or impossible. Kovach *et al.* (1999) developed a categorical index of the behaviours associated with discomfort and pain in people with Alzheimer's disease. The most frequently occurring signs were tense body language, sad facial expression, fidgeting, repetitive verbalisations and verbal outbursts. Agitation, which is one of Violet's symptoms, was also listed.

Sociocultural dimension

The sixth and final of McGuire's (1992) dimensions is the sociocultural dimension. This deals with family, cultural, societal and environmental influences on pain. Children learn about pain, pain behaviours and coping strategies from their families and peer groups. In addition, the meaning of pain and the expression of pain differ between ethnic groups and cultures (Moulin 1998, Smith-Stoner 2003). Many years ago, one of the writers was about to give an opiate injection to a non-English speaking man who was screaming. His son arrived and informed the staff that this behaviour was a way of letting out the devils that were causing the problems – a practice that was apparently common in the man's cultural group. Within 10 minutes he was quite relaxed and peaceful. This anecdote demonstrates the importance of capturing the patient or client's perspective.

In summary, McGuire's (1992) framework offers a guide and knowledge base for the different aspects of pain that can be helpful when assessing and managing pain.

Learning outcome 4: Identify appropriate pain assessment tools for different client groups

Pain is assessed in a variety of ways in different clinical settings. It is a key aspect of pain management and research has consistently demonstrated that accurate pain assessment leads to effective pain management. All patients and clients should, therefore, have their pain assessed and recorded at the beginning of each episode of care and at suitable intervals thereafter.

Pain intensity

In busy acute settings there are times when it may be appropriate to simply ask a patient:

- 'Do you have any pain?'
- 'Where is the pain?'
- 'How bad is the pain?'

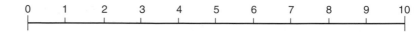

Figure 12.1 A numerical analogue scale.

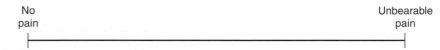

Figure 12.2 Visual analogue scale.

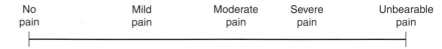

Figure 12.3 Verbal analogue scale.

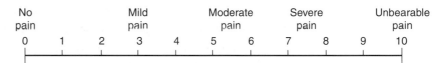

Figure 12.4 Combined verbal and numerical scale.

To help patients respond to this last question, some nurses and doctors ask, 'On a 0–10 scale, with 0 being no pain and 10 being the worse pain you can imagine, what is your pain?' Imagining a 0–10 scale when you are anxious, experiencing intense pain and possibly feeling very ill can be difficult. It is more effective to show the patient a scale and to ask them to point to the level that their pain is at. Figure 12.1 is an example of this type of **numerical analogue scale**.

Other types of scales are the **visual analogue scale** (Fig. 12.2), the **verbal analogue scale** (Fig. 12.3) and combined **verbal and numerical scale** (Fig. 12.4). The latter tends to be the easiest to use, with some 96 per cent of cognitively sound adults able to visualise pain intensity in this way. Pain intensity in chronic pain can also be measured using these scales. However, other dimensions of pain must also be assessed.

Categorical scales are also popular measurement tools. An example is shown in Fig. 12.5. These scales can be used either as verbal rating scales by recording the words or as numerical rating scales by assigning a number to each level as shown in Fig. 12.5. Categorical scales are simple to explain and complete. However, they lack the degree of sensitivity that can be obtained with the analogue scales.

Other types of relatively simple scales include the colour analogue scale that shades from, for example, white for no pain, through to dark red for worst possible pain. While this type of measurement tool may be useful in situations where there are language barriers, it should be noted that the meaning of colour varies from one culture to another. It may, therefore, be necessary to adapt the colour for use with different ethnic groups.

Pain intensity

None	0
Mild	1
Moderate	2
Severe	3

Figure 12.5 Categorical pain assessment scale.

Several researchers and practitioners have developed and adopted faces scales to use with children in pain. These tools have a smiling or neutral face at one end of the scale and a frowning or crying face at the other end. For further discussion of paediatric pain assessment, Boyd (2003) offers a review of tools available for neonates, while Clarke (2003) focuses upon children.

Stuppy (1998) used the Faces Pain Scale (Bieri *et al.* 1990), which uses oval, frowning faces rather than the more common round, crying faces with adults. She found that subjects were able to differentiate easily between the varying levels of pain and found the scale more acceptable than the childlike round faces. However, a recent study by Closs *et al.* (2003) suggested that fewer than 50 per cent of adults with moderate to severe cognitive impairment are able to understand the Faces Pain Scale. This study compared five assessment tools (categorical, visual, numerical, colour and Faces Pain Scale) with care home residents. All residents with mild cognitive impairment and 68 per cent with moderate to severe impairment were able to complete the categorical scale. For the numerical scale the figures were 96 per cent and 58 per cent respectively. The visual and colour analogue scales scored similarly to the Faces Pain Scale.

Activity	Make some notes on how you would approach Violet to assess her pain, taking into account ways of communicating with people who have Alzheimer's disease and how you could explain the categorical scale to her and her husband.

The tools mentioned above are all restricted to measuring pain intensity. Similar scales can also be used to measure pain distress, pain relief and anxiety.

Body charts can help to identify the location of pain and, when used with a categorical or numerical scale, can provide insight into the areas that are the most painful. It is important to be aware that just because someone is complaining of pain in one area of their body does not mean to say that they do not have pain elsewhere. In post-operative settings, it is not unusual for nurses to give morphine in response to a patient's complaint of pain, when the problem is a post-intubation sore throat or long-standing back pain, rather than incisional pain. Many people with chronic pain also have multiple pain foci.

Multidimensional pain assessment

Multidimensional pain assessment tools are useful for people with complex care needs and those experiencing chronic pain. One of the best known tools is the McGill Pain Questionnaire (MPQ) (Melzack and Katz 1999), which is available in both a long and short form. Through the use of descriptor words, the MPQ enables practitioners to identify the nature and quality of pain (see learning outcome 3, sensory dimension) and thereby best approaches to pain management (see learning outcomes 5 and 6). Pain diaries can also be a useful way of gaining insight into the activities and factors that enhance and reduce people's pain.

Psychological and coping strategies assessment

There are many tools available to assess the psychological components of pain and the ways in which people cope with their pain. These measurements are generally administered by pain experts and tend to be used in out-patient and chronic care settings.

Figure 12.6 shows the Pain Strategies Questionnaire (PSQ). The tool was developed from the strategies recorded by 200 adults attending surgical out-patients' clinics for the first time. The tool was then used in a randomised control trial to test whether identifying and supporting patients' own strategies in the hospital setting would reduce patients' post-operative anxiety, pain and distress, as well as a number of other outcomes (Burrows 2000). The study findings are discussed under learning outcome 6.

■ **Activity**   Complete column A of the Pain Strategies Questionnaire (Fig. 12.6).

Depending upon your past experience of pain, you may or may not have been aware of some of the strategies that you use when you are in pain. We will consider how you might support patients' own strategies later in the chapter.

Non-verbal pain assessment

The emphasis on pain being a subjective experience has led society to assume that those who cannot verbally and fluently describe their pain do not have pain (Anand and Craig 1996). The community nurse for learning disabilities who visited Brian used her expertise to identify that he was probably in pain. She did this without using a formal assessment tool.

■ **Activity**   Reflecting upon what you have learned so far in this chapter, how do you think the nurse concluded Brian was in pain?

Although the verbal description is the gold standard of pain assessment, health care practitioners have to be open to considering behavioural responses as indicators of pain in those who cannot communicate their pain. Brian's behaviour had altered. He might also have been groaning, grimacing, curled over or holding his stomach, and he might have been sweating with a raised blood pressure

Pain strategies questionnaire

Many people use strategies at home to help relieve pain. We have found that if you continue to use them in hospital it can help to reduce the amount of pain you experience. Please help us to find out what you use by filling in the table below and handing this sheet to your nurse:

Please place a ✓ in column A, against all of the strategies that you use when in pain.

In column B, please place a ✓ against any of the strategies you would like to use in hospital.

Strategy	Column A	Column B
None/not sure		
Painkillers (state which if known)		
Distraction e.g. TV, reading etc.		
Relaxation		
Breathing exercises		
Imagery (using your senses to imagine a place or experience)		
Music		
Massage		
Warmth		
Cold		
Resting alone: e.g. lying down, trying to sleep, peace & quiet PLEASE STATE WHICH		
Grin & bear, mind over matter, positive thinking		
Mobilising: e.g. walking, moving about, exercise PLEASE STATE WHICH		
Positioning: e.g. changing position, support painful area PLEASE STATE WHICH		
Treatment: e.g. seeking medical attention to treat the cause or pain, advice or information PLEASE STATE WHICH		
Reassurance: e.g. talking about the pain, physical contact with someone else, confidence in someone else PLEASE STATE WHICH		
General help with activities		
Other: PLEASE STATE WHAT		

Thank you for completing this questionnaire

Figure 12.6 Pain strategies questionnaire (Burrows 2000). (Reproduced with kind permission of Dee Burrows).

and pulse. In addition, the nurse would have known how Brian usually communicates and how he communicates pain either verbally or non-verbally.

In summary, there are a variety of approaches to pain assessment. Each has its place with different client groups and different dimensions of pain. Whatever the approach, the response should be recorded so that it can be compared with the pain experienced following an intervention. In acute pain settings recordings should be made at rest and upon movement: Patience, for example, may well stay quite rigid if she experiences pain following her surgery. As deep breathing, leg movements and mobilisation are important to post-operative recovery and the prevention of complications, it is imperative that pain does not prevent movement and rehabilitation. The same goals are equally important for Sidney, Brian and Violet.

Activity Investigate what pain assessment tools are used in your locality for different client groups.

Learning outcome 5: Demonstrate understanding of the pain ladder and how it can be applied in practice

Analgesics
Drugs for relieving pain: painkillers.

Analgesia
Pain relief.

Knowledge of pharmacology and **analgesic** management may help to enhance **analgesia**, decrease anxiety and promote comfort.

The World Health Organization (1996) suggests that analgesic administration should be based on the pain ladder, where simple analgesics are used for mild pain, weak opioids for moderate pain and strong opioids for severe pain. Drugs from different levels of the ladder can be co-prescribed and administered as patients move from one level to another. Other key principles in analgesic management include:

- Assessing pain at the beginning of each episode of care and at appropriate intervals thereafter
- Giving analgesics before or as soon as the pain begins
- Giving sufficient and regular analgesics to ensure patient comfort
- Assessing pain relief
- Never letting pain get out of control.

Activity Why should you never let pain get out of control?

You may have come up with a number of ideas, such as the fact that it is inhumane, places hospitalised patients at risk of physical complications, places community patients at risk of depression and so on.

Pharmacological management of pain is a team effort, involving the patient/client, their family, the doctor, pharmacist, nurse and others. Nurses should:

- Listen to patients and their relatives
- Record patients' pain assessments

Table 12.1 Commonly used analgesics and their position on the ladder

Drug	Location on ladder	Administration	Side effects
Paracetamol	Simple analgesic: Helpful for mild pain. Effect often underestimated	Adult: 1–2 500-mg tablets every 4 hours. Maximum 8 per day, unless otherwise directed	Rare. Potentially fatal liver damage following overdose
Codeine	Weak opioid: Helpful for moderate pain	Adult: 30–60 mg	Constipation. Initial drowsiness/dizziness not unusual
Morphine	Strong opioid: helpful for severe pain	Adult: varies. Note 10 mg IM/IV is equivalent to 30 mg oral	Most commonly nausea and vomiting. May also experience light-headedness, confusion, pruritus, constipation. Respiratory depression

■ Manage and evaluate pain
■ Work with relevant members of the multidisciplinary team towards effective pain control
■ Ensure that their knowledge is sufficient to achieve patient comfort
■ Work to educate patients/clients.

Patients should be encouraged to request analgesics, take sufficient analgesics to enable them to carry out appropriate activities and ask for more analgesics if their pain continues.

Table 12.1 gives an example of an analgesic from each level of the ladder.

 Activity — Make a list of the analgesics used in your locality. Think about their location on the ladder, dosages and side effects.

You may find that you come across drugs such as co-codamol, co-dydramol and co-proxamol. These drugs combine paracetamol with a weak opioid. Although popular in the community, research by McQuay and Moore (1998) suggests that there is little, if any, advantage to combination drugs. Indeed co-proxamol was shown to be no more effective than 1 g of paracetamol. You might like to talk to a pharmacist about their views on these drugs.

Studies suggest that around 20 per cent of doctors and nurses fear that patients will become addicted to painkillers (Carr and Mann 2000). In fact, hospital-prompted addiction occurs in less than 0.5 per cent of admissions (Ferrell *et al.* 1992). Addiction is caused by cravings, and this is another reason why we should ensure that patients receive sufficient analgesics to be comfortable. It is interesting to note that in Patience Jackson's scenario there is no mention of analgesics being administered either in A&E or on the ward. Not only is fear of prompting addiction a problem in health care generally, but it appears particularly prevalent in relation to children and older people.

Routes of analgesic administration

> **■ Activity**   List the different routes for administering analgesics that you have come across.

You may have included patient controlled analgesic (PCA) systems on your list. Patient controlled analgesia is an approach to pain management in which the patient controls the dose and frequency of analgesic up to a predetermined limit. When practitioners refer to PCA, they generally mean the intravenous system that delivers opioids when the patient presses a demand button. These systems are most commonly used in surgical settings and their management is covered by local protocols.

> **■ Activity**   Look up your local protocol for PCA. List the recordings that must be made by nurses and why.

The concept of PCA is an important one. It acknowledges the patient as the expert on their pain and as a partner in pain management. People living at home manage their pain on a day-to-day basis, purchasing over the counter painkillers or visiting their GP for prescriptions. On admission to hospital, the power and control for medication management is frequently transferred to doctors and nurses.

Entonox is a 50:50 mixture of nitrous oxide and oxygen delivered through a hand-held mask or mouthpiece. If the patient becomes drowsy (as a consequence of the drug), their hand and therefore the delivery set will fall away. As such, entonox is another form of patient controlled analgesia. It is effective for mild to moderate short-lasting pain and is used by paramedics, in A&E and for procedural pain (BOC Medical 2001; MacIntyre and Ready 2001).

Epidural space
The space between the spinal canal and dura mater.

Epidurals are another route for administration, involving the infusion of a local anaesthetic, with or without an opioid, through a fine catheter into the **epidural space** (MacIntyre and Ready 2001).

> **■ Activity**   Look up your local protocols for entonox and epidurals. List the recordings that must be made by nurses and why.

Non-steroidal anti-inflammatory drugs

Non-steroidal anti-inflammatory drugs (NSAIDs) reduce inflammation and are effective for mild to moderate pain. They are commonly used post-operatively in combination with analgesics and are also the drug of choice in conditions such

Drugs	Examples
Antidepressants	Amitriptyline, imipramine, dothiepin
Anticonvulsants	Carbamazepine, sodium valproate, gabapentin

Box 12.2 Examples of antidepressants and anticonvulsants used in neuropathic pain management

as arthritis. Ibuprofen 400 mg and diclofenac 50 mg have been shown to be as effective as 10 mg intramuscular morphine in the treatment of acute pain (McQuay and Moore 1998). Side effects include gastric irritation, bleeding and renal failure.

Analgesics and NSAIDs are useful drugs in the management of nociceptive pain. However, other drugs are needed for the treatment of neuropathic pain.

Drugs for neuropathic pain

True analgesics have a limited effect on neuropathic pain. However, the analgesic properties of antidepressants and anticonvulsants have been found to be useful. Unfortunately, because many health care practitioners are unaware that these drugs may be used to treat pain, it is not uncommon for patients with neuropathic pain to hear themselves labelled as 'depressed epileptics' because of the medication they are taking. It is worth finding out, therefore, why someone is taking their medication, rather than assuming the obvious. Chapter 2 discusses how such labelling of patients affects interactions between nurses and patients.

Box 12.2 shows some of the common antidepressants and anticonvulsants used in pain management.

Resources

There are many resources to help nurses develop their pharmacological knowledge. These include standard pharmacological and pain management texts, specialist texts such as that by MacIntyre and Ready (2001), websites such as the British National Formulary (BNF) site (www.bnf.com), pharmaceutical literature, journal articles and nursing, medical and pharmacist colleagues. Understanding the way a drug works can be a rewarding addition to a nurse's knowledge base and practice.

Learning outcome 6: Explore non-pharmacological approaches to managing pain

Non-pharmacological approaches to pain management include a variety of technical, taught, self-generated, comfort care and complimentary strategies. The latter include acupuncture, which is available through the NHS, reflexology, massage and aromatherapy, but it is beyond the remit of this chapter to discuss these approaches.

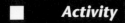 **Activity**   Look at the strategies that you ticked in Fig. 12.6. As a nurse, how might you support someone who wanted to use these strategies in a hospital setting?

The study by Burrows (2000) found that identifying and supporting patients' self-generated strategies reduced post-operative anxiety, opiate consumption, pain and distress. Much of the literature (e.g. Seers and Carroll 1998; Sindhu 1996) on non-pharmacological strategies suggests that nurses should teach imagery, relaxation, distraction and exercises and administer massage, heat and cold. In fact, the evidence for the efficacy of taught strategies remains relatively weak, although further studies are currently underway. In chronic pain management there is a fairly long history of working with patients to develop their own strategies. Studies suggest that this may be more effective than using taught strategies (Rokke and al'Absi 1992).

In the activity above, you might have come up with some of the ideas offered in Table 12.2.

Table 12.2 Examples of supporting patients in using their own pain-relieving strategies

Identify the strategies the person uses	*Understand how the strategy works*	*Work with the person to enable them to use their strategy in the clinical setting*
Distraction	Focusing on something other than pain. Useful for brief periods. Can increase self-control and reduce pain intensity	May include watching TV, reading, listening to music, visits from family and friends. Example: if a patient says they watch television help them to the day room
Relaxation	Directs attention away from pain. Useful for mild to moderate pain. Can reduce muscle tension, distress, anxiety and fatigue	Find out the person's technique. Support them with it if asked. Ensure periods of relative peace and quiet to enable them to use the strategy
Imagery	Using imagination to create mental pictures. Directs attention away from pain by imaging sights, sounds, odours, taste and feel, e.g. a garden on a warm summer's day. Can alter pain experience e.g. when visualising cool water trickling over a hot painful area	Find out the person's preferred image. Talk them through it if asked. Ensure periods of relative peace and quiet to enable them to use the strategy
Warmth	Promotes relaxation and comfort, reduces muscle tension	Hot water bottles cannot be used in hospital settings for safety reasons. Heat pads and warm water are alternatives
Cold	May help reduce inflammatory pain. Should not be used over wounds, as cold will decrease healing rates	Provide cold flannels, water, ice or cold packs. Even better show the patient/family where to access them in the clinical area
Positioning	Eases stiffness and enhances comfort	Help person to adopt most comfortable position, using own special pillows or cushions

The nurse's caring role in the context of people using self-generated strategies is to support the person to use their strategies effectively when the experience of illness and a strange environment may disrupt their expertise. This may mean being compassionate to the person's needs by simply giving them permission to use the technique, being confident in offering ideas on how to adapt the strategy to a clinical setting, being committed to reminding the person to use their strategy, and/or being competent to work with them to rehearse and use their techniques.

■ **Activity** — List the constraints that you are aware of in your locality in terms of allowing patients and clients to use their own strategies in clinical settings. Give some thought as to whether the rationale for any barriers is sound.

Hospital policies can sometimes present barriers, but in a break with ward protocol, one of the authors was recently allowed access to a ward microwave to heat up a wheat pack for relieving back pain following unrelated surgery. The above focus upon self-generated strategies is not to deny the utility of nurses taking the lead in introducing techniques to patients. However, not all strategies are appropriate for all people, in all situations. For example, touch and massage can be painful for people with neuropathic pain as their A beta touch fibres may also be damaged. Conversely gentle stroking or a hand massage may calm someone who is agitated in A&E or during procedural pain.

■ **Activity** — Consider which non-pharmacological strategies you might use with each of the people in the scenarios and why. How do these link to the different dimensions of pain and promotion of comfort care?

There are many other non-pharmacological approaches to pain management, some of which you are likely to come across during your pre-registration studies. For most patients, the most effective approach is to listen to what the person says about their pain and its effect on their activities, to work with the multidisciplinary team to combine pharmacological and non-pharmacological strategies and to monitor the effectiveness of pain relief. The next section of this chapter moves on to look in more detail at ways of promoting comfort.

Summary

- Pain is a subjective, multidimensional experience, unique to each individual.
- Nurses need to differentiate between the terms pain threshold, tolerance and behaviour.
- Effective pain assessment is the key to successful pain management and pain assessment tools can facilitate communication about pain.
- Pain management comprises both pharmacological and non-pharmacological approaches. As people generally have their own pain-coping strategies, these should be incorporated into pain management.

PROMOTING COMFORT

Actions that promote comfort are 'familiar, provide warmth, and help us to feel safe, snug, sheltered, protected, and to feel less vulnerable and exposed' (Morse *et al.* 1994, p. 194). People are usually able to promote their own comfort, but when they are unwell, physically or mentally, their usual ways of seeking comfort may not be possible. Promoting comfort, therefore, is a fundamental skill all nurses need to develop.

LEARNING OUTCOMES

By the end of this section you will be able to:

1. Discuss the nature of comfort and promoting comfort.
2. Demonstrate the use of presence to provide comfort.
3. Identify how monitoring can promote comfort.
4. Consider how touch can be used in comfort care.
5. Explore how talking can be used to promote comfort.
6. Select physical actions that can be used to promote comfort.
7. Integrate a number of strategies for promoting comfort in different circumstances.

Learning outcome 1: Discuss the nature of comfort and promoting comfort

Activity

Think back to the scenarios at the start of this chapter. Do you think the four people are experiencing comfort or discomfort, and if so, in what way?

All the people in the scenarios appear to have some discomfort. Sidney has physical discomfort, especially as he is struggling to breathe, and his fear of dying is a psychological discomfort. Patience is experiencing physical discomfort due to her pain, but also psychological discomfort as she is anxious. Brian has physical discomfort due to his pain, and his nausea and vomiting, but he might also have psychological discomfort as he will not understand why he is feeling unwell, and will be missing his work and colleagues. Up until the nurse visited, Brian had been unable to seek help, and this could have added to his psychological discomfort. Violet certainly appears to be suffering discomfort and it might be assumed that this is mainly psychological due to her change of environment and her mental condition. However it might also be physical – she could be in pain due to her osteoarthritis or need to pass urine but be unable to express this verbally. There could be other reasons too – she could be too hot or too cold, or hungry or thirsty. It is important not to make assumptions about the reasons for people's apparent discomfort.

For each of these people there are a variety of reasons why they are experiencing discomfort and nurses therefore need to use a range of strategies to promote their comfort. Promoting comfort should not assume a passive role for patients but may include self-care strategies (Morse 1992). Many nursing actions essential for patient comfort (e.g. an injection, repositioning) can actually cause discomfort in the short term. Several writers have acknowledged that for an acutely ill person total comfort may not be possible. For example Morse *et al.* (1994) argue that 'Total comfort is an elusive gold standard for the sick, for the very nature of illness disrupts the body – to be sick is to be without comfort' (p. 194). They therefore suggest that nurses should aim to maintain patients within their own comfort range. In Sidney's scenario, he expressed that he felt comforted by Debbie, and her care helped him to endure his discomfort. However he clearly did not achieve total comfort.

Comfort care is the action taken to promote comfort; this may be successful to a greater or lesser degree. Kolkaba (1995) states that when comfort care is successful patients feel well cared for and comforted because the care was efficient, individualised, targeted to the whole person and creative.

Bottorff *et al.* (1995) observed that comforting strategies are embedded in practice and are often devalued. Yet they are a significant part of nurses' work.

Activity

Sidney's scenario mentions only that the nurse held his hand and this was comforting. Can you think of anything else that the nurse, Debbie, might have been doing which could have added to his feeling of being comforted?

The fact that Debbie was holding Sidney's hand implies that she was actually there with him. 'Being there' or 'Presence' is well recognised as a comfort strategy. It is also safe to assume that Debbie was not only with Sidney and holding his hand but was also actually checking and monitoring his condition. This would also have been comforting as it would have helped Sidney to feel safe. It is also likely that she used some physical actions, such as repositioning Sidney in a better position for breathing. Debbie would also have talked to Sidney, perhaps using comforting phrases like 'You're doing well', or giving him explanations about what was happening to him. Thus in promoting comfort for Sidney, Debbie used:

- Her presence
- Monitoring
- Touch
- Talking
- Physical actions.

In the next sections each of these comfort care strategies are looked at in more detail.

Learning outcome 2: Demonstrate the use of presence to provide comfort

Presence is about 'being there' – with someone who is in distress and needs comfort. Zerwekh's (1997) description of presence suggests planned, professional nursing action; presencing is referred to as a 'fundamental nursing intervention' (p. 260), involving 'deliberate focused attention, receptivity to the other person, and persistent awareness of the other's shared humanity' (p. 261). Davidson (1992) argues that it is a 'mark of one's humanity to be able to just be with someone, no matter what state they are in, without needing to act on them in some way'(p. 203). Studies have confirmed that the presence of nurses is a source of comfort (Clukey 1997; Gilje 1993). When Brian goes for his endoscopy, the community nurse for learning disability will provide a comforting presence.

Activity	Think about when you have sat with someone who is distressed, either in nursing or in everyday life. Were you comfortable doing this or was it difficult in anyway?

It is not always easy to be with someone who is in distress. This is particularly so if you are not able to relieve their discomfort, and in some circumstances this is not possible. If someone has received bad news, for example about a diagnosis or death of a loved one, nothing you can say or do can take that away. Nurses often feel more comfortable when they can 'put things right': relieve mental distress, pain, vomiting or breathlessness. If they are unable to do this, simply being with a person who, despite medication and other measures, continues to be suicidal, in pain, vomiting or acutely breathless, can engender feelings of helplessness in nurses.

Often the presence of a relative or friend (rather than a nurse) is the best source of comfort. Morse *et al.* (1994) give the example of a man with depression and how he gained comfort from support given by family and friends. In the past hospitals have been less than welcoming to relatives being present during procedures but nowadays their presence, if desired by the patient and themselves, is generally unquestioned, although they may not be actively supported. When relatives/friends are providing comfort by being present, the role of nurses is then to support this person to be with their loved one, remembering that they may find it difficult to be there.

It is well accepted that for children the presence of parents is the most important element in promoting comfort (Broome 2000; Pederson 1994; Woodgate and Kristjansen 1996). Parents have a trusting relationship with their child, know their vocabulary and coping strategies, and their style of comforting is familiar. However they may find being with their distressed child an uncomfortable experience and need support and comfort from nurses in turn. Nurses must enable them to be present as a source of comfort without becoming exhausted and overburdened.

Activity	For Patience's parents to stay with her and comfort her, what support do you think they might need from nurses?

Patience's parents will be anxious about their daughter's condition and her operation. It will help them if nurses give explanations about what to expect, guide them in ways of supporting Patience, and go to the bedside regularly to check that they are all managing rather than leaving them alone, therefore 'being there' for the whole family. In particular when Patience goes to theatre, having her parents present in the anaesthetic room will comfort her, but they must be informed as to what will happen, at what point it will be best for them to leave and what will happen next. For example they might be told that she is likely to be in theatre and recovery for about an hour so this might be a good point for them to pop home or have a meal in the hospital canteen. Nurses would then be addressing their comfort needs too.

Broome (2000) argues that health care professionals have a responsibility to teach parents to support their children during painful procedures, and indeed a leaflet and video serving this purpose is described by Pederson (1994). Yet Woodgate and Kristjanson (1998) found that some nurses considered it the parents' 'duty' to comfort their child experiencing post-operative pain and spoke negatively of them if they were unable to do so, rather than considering that the parents might need support to fulfil their comforting role. While parents are practised in comforting their children in everyday situations, they may need additional help in situations when their child is acutely unwell.

Learning outcome 3: Identify how monitoring can promote comfort

Monitoring, referred to as 'vigilance' by Hawley (2000) and as 'surveillance' by Walker (1996), is about observing and checking a distressed person's mental and/or physical condition. It is easy to see how monitoring might be combined with 'being there': presence. A number of research studies have identified that monitoring is perceived as a comforting action, for example:

- Women recovering from hip surgery felt comforted by being closely monitored and checked on regularly (Kralik *et al.*'s 1997).
- Mental health patients felt comforted by nurses checking on them and following through with them (Weissman and Appleton 1995).
- Frightened people with a sudden illness or injury and a need to 'feel safe' found surveillance by nurses comforting (Walker 1996).

This comfort measure might involve taking physiological measurements but also includes observing the person's appearance, asking about symptoms, and carrying out pain assessment as described earlier in this chapter. Hawley (2000) found that patients felt comforted knowing that a nurse was watching over them, ready to respond to any change in their condition.

Nurses who are monitoring people need specific knowledge and skills – to be able to select, carry out and interpret physiological measurements and observations, and act on these as appropriate. In relation to Roach's 6Cs of caring (Roach 2002) (explained in Chapter 1), this comfort measure particularly relates to competence, commitment and confidence. Competent and confident nurses, who show commitment to monitoring their patients, inspire confidence in the frightened and distressed people they are caring for.

Activity

Drawing on other chapters of this book and your experience in nursing to date, think about what things you might do when monitoring someone after an operation (like Patience).

With Patience, monitoring would include checking her respiration, oxygen saturation, her other vital signs, and her fluid balance. Checking her pain level would also be very important (as explained in the section on pain assessment earlier in this chapter). You would also ask her about how she feels generally, for example she might experience nausea or have a dry mouth. Did you remember that she has a wound? You would therefore check the wound dressing for any bleeding. Some patients with surgical wounds have drains and so you would then check for wound drainage too. Remember that as Patience's parents are present, monitoring also involves checking on how they are managing with the situation.

Learning outcome 4: Consider how touch can be used in comfort care

In the scenario of Sidney it was Debbie's use of touch that he recalled about her comforting actions. There are two main types of touch used in nursing care: instrumental touch and comforting touch. **Instrumental touch** is the type used while carrying out other nursing actions, for example when repositioning someone or taking their pulse. As care increasingly uses technology this type of touch is diminishing, for example there is minimal touch involved in using electronic equipment to measure pulse or blood pressure, and using hoists to move patients. **Comforting touch** is touch that is used with the intention to comfort. Moore and Gilbert (1995) suggest that nurses should be encouraged to use comforting touch consciously and intentionally. It is easy to see how using comforting touch could be combined with other comfort measures: presence, and also monitoring. For example Debbie could have been observing Sidney's breathing while holding his hand. In Chapter 1 Box 1.3 gives an example of how both instrumental touch (used to assist with washing and dressing) and expressive touch (touching the shoulder) were used to bring comfort to one of the authors of this chapter post-operatively.

The use of touch to comfort is well supported by research (Bush 2001; Chang 2001; Hawley 2000; Morse and Proctor 1998; Walters 1994). In a vividly described example Smith-Regojo (1995) recalls stroking the forehead of a man dying from a severe burn; she later found out that the man did not speak any English, thus highlighting the importance of touch to communicate comfort, rather than words.

Activity

Think back to a recent experience where you were comforting someone. Did you use touch? If so, how did you use it? How comfortable do you feel about using touch to comfort? Now ask three close family members or friends about how they would feel about nurses using touch to comfort them.

People vary in how comfortable they feel about using and receiving touch; some people are much more 'touchy' than others. Some nurses use touch a great deal and feel very comfortable to use touch in a variety of ways, while others shy away from using touch. Many people respond well to touch as a means to comfort them but nurses should be sensitive to any non-verbal cues that suggest touch is unwanted by patients. Touch has cultural significance and also has different meanings and rules according to the gender of those involved (Giger and Davidhizar 1999). Giger and Davidhizar (1999) go on to suggest that the 'message conveyed through touch depends on the attitude of the person involved and on the meaning of touch both to the person touching and to the person being touched' (p. 31). As with any other care, you should evaluate the effect, so look for how touch is responded to. For example does it make the person calmer or more agitated? Does the person whose hand you are holding grasp it tightly or snatch their hand away? In some situations it is appropriate to ask: 'Would you like to hold my hand during this [procedure]?' Also be aware that in some care situations use of touch could be misconstrued, and some people might view touch as an invasion of privacy and personal space.

| ■ *Activity* | In the scenarios, Debbie used touch to comfort Sidney by holding his hand. Now think about Brian, Patience and Violet and identify ways that touch might have been used to comfort them. |

When the community nurse for learning disabilities first visited Brian to find out what was wrong, she might have used touch by placing a hand on his arm, for example, or she might have held his hand when sitting down with him trying to find out what was wrong. Depending on the closeness of the relationship she has established with him (which might have been over some years) she may even have given him a hug. This form of close touch is not uncommon in a variety of nursing settings but is obviously not appropriate in every situation and its use would be based on the nurse's professional judgement. For Patience, her family can use touch in whatever way she responds to, which might well be holding her with their arms around her, or stroking her face. When she first starts to wake up from the anaesthetic, before her parents are present, recovery room nurses might gently stroke her hand or forehead. For Violet, holding her hand might be the most appropriate way to use touch but putting an arm around her shoulders might also be comforting. Her husband might use either of these strategies to comfort her. The scenario suggests that he also needs comforting, and so nurses could use similar types of touch for him too.

In relation to infants, different forms of touch have been identified: holding hands, stroking, rubbing, holding, patting, rocking and squeezing (Morse *et al.* 1993). But many of these are applicable to other age groups too. Bottorff *et al.* (1995) suggest that touch can be used purely for comforting by holding a hand or stroking to reassure, soothe or calm people in acute distress. But they also identify 'connecting touch', which might be a light touch prior to a nurse leaving the bedside to reinforce interest in the patient or reassure them.

Learning outcome 5: Explore how talking can be used to promote comfort

Studies in a range of settings have supported the role of talk in comforting, for example:

■ Walters' (1994) study identified talking and listening to critically ill patients as important in comfort care, even with unconscious patients.

■ Weissman and Appleton (1995) found that for mental health patients, being kept informed helped to enhance comfort.

Hawley (2000) identified four types of comforting talk which emergency room patients described nurses using:

■ Reassuring talk, for example phrases like 'Don't worry, we'll take care of you'.

■ Coaching talk, helping patients to stay in control and cope with pain and anxiety, for example.

■ Explanatory talk, such as giving information and answering questions.

■ Empathetic talk, which conveyed understanding and caring.

A pattern of talk – 'comfort talk' – has been identified (Morse 1992; Morse and Proctor 1998), which nurses use to help patients get through difficult situations or painful procedures. This appears to be what Hawley (2000) refers to as 'coaching'. Penrod *et al.* (1999) describe comfort talk being used during nasogastric tube insertion in order to gain patient co-operation. Comfort talk is slow and rhythmic, with short simple sentences and uses phrases such as 'We're almost there' 'You're fine' along with other emotionally supportive statements (Proctor *et al.* 1996). Morse and Proctor (1998) suggest that comfort talk aims to help patients to endure the situation, allow an information exchange and communicate a sense of caring. They emphasise that nurses' comfort talk is accompanied by being face-to-face with the patient, holding the patient's hand and focusing on their eyes. Thus appropriate non-verbal communication (looked at in Chapter 2) is also important. Morse and Proctor (1998) suggest that comfort talk could actually reduce mortality and morbidity, as comfort is often about encouraging patients to accept procedures, and thereby patients will be less distressed and shocked, and in less pain.

 Activity

Think about Brian undergoing his endoscopy. This involves asking him to swallow a tube. He will be administered an anaesthetic spray to his throat (which tastes unpleasant) and might also be given a muscle relaxant. Think about phrases that might be used by a nurse who is supporting him during this procedure, using each of Hawley's four categories: reassuring, coaching, explanatory and empathetic.

Examples in each category include:

■ **Reassuring**: The nurse might say: 'Don't worry, it'll soon be over', 'You'll be fine'.

- **Coaching**: The nurse could say 'Okay Brian, swallow the tube, well done, keep swallowing, keep swallowing, you're doing really well'. They should be aware that someone with a learning disability may take longer to process these instructions. This also applies to anyone who has had sedation.

- **Explanatory**: When the spray is administered the nurse could say 'Brian, open wide now. We're going to spray the back of your throat to make it numb for you. It tastes a bit horrible, but then your throat will go numb'. When the tube is about to be passed, the nurse could say 'Brian, we need to put this tube down through your mouth into your stomach so we can look down it and see what's making you sick. In a moment we're going to ask you to swallow the tube'.

- **Empathetic**: The nurse might say 'Brian, I'm sorry, I know this is uncomfortable for you'.

The tone used to say phrases like those above is just as important as the words chosen.

Patients and families can also find comfort from a friendly and informal social exchange on an equal footing about everyday topics. Such chat can provide distraction and lighten the atmosphere (Bottorff *et al.* 1995) and for the patient – or relative – who is feeling wretched, being 'chatted to' – as one human being to another – can be comforting. Taylor (1992) refers to the comforting nature of 'ordinariness' and how this represents a shared humanity between nurses and patients. Bottorff *et al.* (1995) identified the gentle use of humour as an often used strategy for comforting.

■ *Activity*	Think about topics for 'ordinary' conversation with Sidney, the next morning after his bad night, when he is able to talk but still feeling frightened.

Developing the confidence to chat to a variety of people in different circumstances and different settings develops with practice, so do take every opportunity, both at work and outside work. Items in the news can provide good material, so try to listen to the news regularly, or read the newspaper. However be careful about bringing up highly political issues or expressing strong opinions. The best items to discuss are ones that are slightly amusing or eccentric perhaps. Of course the weather is always a very acceptable topic of conversation!

You can often draw cues for 'ordinary' conversation from simply being observant. For example, Sidney might have a photograph on his locker, perhaps of children or animals. You could ask him, 'Who are the children in the photo? They look lovely children'. He might respond by saying they're his grandchildren, and you can then follow it up with, 'So do they live far away?', and so on. It can be appropriate to offer information about yourself. For example, if Sidney had a dog, you might tell him that you have a dog yourself, and discuss the nice things about having a dog. Be alert of course for if he doesn't seem to want to talk – perhaps he is too tired, but many people do appreciate having an interest shown in them, even when they don't feel well. Children often have a favourite cuddly toy, and this is always a good starting point for conversation, so if Patience is cuddling a soft toy you might admire it and ask if it has a name.

Talking can also be used in techniques to promote relaxation such as guided imagery and distraction. You considered these strategies in relation to pain relief earlier in this chapter. The literature identifies these comfort measures mainly in relation to children (Pederson 1994) and pain management, but they can successfully be used with adults, and in other circumstances where comfort is needed. Kolkaba and Fox (1996) present a study where guided imagery, in the form of a tape with background music and talking was used successfully with women undergoing radiotherapy for breast cancer. The use of music in itself was found to be comforting in a study by McCaffrey and Good (2000). The use of play, reading stories, blowing bubbles and games are all frequently described in relation to children as distraction measures. Stephens *et al.* (1999) state that parents instinctively use techniques such as singing to comfort their children. Nurses can support parents in using any comforting techniques that they would normally use.

Learning outcome 6: Select physical actions that can be used to promote comfort

Activity

What physical actions have you used in practice, or seen used, to promote comfort?

There are a wide range of physical actions nurses take in order to promote comfort. You might have included:

- **Administering medicines**: Obvious examples of medicines that promote comfort include analgesics (which you looked at earlier in this chapter), antiemetics (to prevent nausea and vomiting), antipyretics (to reduce high temperature), bronchodilators (via nebulisers or inhalers) and oxygen to reduce dyspnoea, and sedatives. However many prescribed medicines also reduce discomfort from unpleasant symptoms. Examples include drugs to regulate the heart rate and rhythm, thus stopping palpitations, aperients to treat constipation, and antibiotics which relieve fever-related symptoms like headache, aching and malaise.
- **Repositioning**: Assisting a breathless person into a sitting position well supported by pillows (see Fig. 11.1 in Chapter 11) or in a chair, turning people to provide relief from pressure (see Chapter 5), and positioning limbs to prevent contractures, are all examples of using repositioning to promote comfort.
- **Providing a comfortable bed**: For a person who is in bed for all or part of the day a comfortable bed and appropriate bedding are fundamental. A comfortable, pressure-relieving mattress (see Chapter 5) should be

provided. Clean, unwrinkled bedlinen, covers that are not too hot, too heavy or too cold, and sufficient supportive pillows are all essential.

- **Assisting with hygiene**: Chapter 7 covers all aspects of this in detail, and attention should be paid to mouth care, hair care and shaving, as well as the skin. For people who are able, a warm bath can be comforting. Hygiene is an important comfort measure for people who are vomiting, like Brian. Teeth cleaning, mouthwashes, hand and face washes, and changing of clothes might make him feel more comfortable.

- **Assisting with elimination**: Incontinence causes both physical and psychological discomfort. Chapter 8 looked in detail at assisting people with elimination, and promoting continence and managing incontinence in ways that promote comfort.

- **Providing food and drink**: Hunger and thirst cause discomfort, as you will almost certainly have experienced yourself at some point. Chapter 9 looks in detail at how people can be assisted with eating and drinking. For people who are nil by mouth, like Patience was pre-operatively and Brian was when preparing for his endoscopy, it is important to explain why they cannot eat and drink and to offer mouthwashes to reduce the discomfort of a dry mouth.

- **Modifying the environment**: You need to be observant about whether the environment is too hot or too cold for the people you are caring for. Patients who are just sitting can quickly become cold. Windows can be opened or closed and fans used to modify environmental temperature. Also pay attention to reducing excessive or unpleasant noise. Music, if to people's choice, can be comforting, as can a pleasant décor, plants, and pictures. The psychological environment is also important in promoting comfort. A calm, confident and relaxed atmosphere where there is good teamwork can all engender comfort too.

In many instances people may not request the physical actions listed above due to communication difficulties or because they feel unable to ask, so nurses need to be proactive in assessing people's needs for these comfort measures. The way in which physical actions are carried out is also significant. In Kralik *et al.*'s (1997) study patients described being given physical care which, although it left them free of pain, physically comfortable and clean, did not leave them feeling cared for because of the depersonalised manner in which it was carried out. It is easy to see how physical actions could be combined with other aspects of comfort care: talking, monitoring, presence and touch.

Learning outcome 7: Integrate a number of strategies in promoting comfort in different circumstances

In the previous sections a number of different strategies to promote comfort were discussed but it has already been highlighted that combining strategies is necessary in comfort care. Competent physical actions and monitoring of patients' conditions are expected as fundamental aspects of the nurse's role but in order to provide comfort these need to be integrated with presence, touch and talking. These latter measures are ones that nurses often feel they do not have time for but the art of comfort care is about smoothly integrating a number of measures.

Activity

Identify how the use of presence, monitoring, talking, touch and physical actions could be integrated to promote comfort if Brian, when recovering from his endoscopy, appears agitated and uncomfortable.

The community nurse for learning disability should sit with him and hold his hand (**presence** and **touch**), explain where he is and that his test is all over, reassuring him that he is fine (**talking**). Brian's vital signs will be checked by the endoscopy staff for any abnormality (**monitoring**). **Physical actions** include trying to find out if his throat is sore and offering analgesics. It will be important to communicate with Brian effectively to do this and the community nurse who knows Brian will be able to use her knowledge of how he communicates to find out his needs. He might want to get dressed into his own clothes, wash his hands and face, clean his teeth, and sit up in a chair. He might feel ready for a drink and a biscuit, or maybe he wants to go to the toilet.

Summary

- Promoting comfort is a key role of nurses in many different settings, and is fundamental to caring.
- Promoting comfort requires a holistic approach and the integration of presence, monitoring, touch, talking and physical actions, encompassing a range of skills and knowledge, as applicable for each individual.

CHAPTER SUMMARY

Throughout this book practical nursing skills have been contextualised within a philosophy of caring. Chapter 1 introduced Roach's 6Cs of caring and these were returned to in this final chapter which has looked at some fundamental aspects of nursing: managing pain and promoting comfort. Nurses have an important role in promoting comfort, a role recognised by Florence Nightingale who wrote in 1854: 'The benefits which this Institution [hospital] ought to afford to the sick are perhaps best seen when we are enabled to give comfort in the time of danger and to lessen the agony of death' (Verney 1970, p. 24). Pain management is a huge topic with a developing theoretical base and this chapter's material aimed to provide a firm basis from which to build your nursing practice. Both pain management and promoting comfort require nurses to integrate a range of skills, with an appropriate attitude and a sound underpinning knowledge base.

REFERENCES

Anand, K.J.S. and Craig, K.D. 1996. Editorial: new perspectives on the definition of pain. *Pain* **67**(1), 3–6.

Arnstein, P., Caudill, M., Mandle, C.L. *et al.* 1999. Self efficacy as a mediator of the relationship between pain intensity, disability and depression in chronic pain patients. *Pain* **80**, 483–91.

Bieri, D., Reeve, R.A., Champion, G.D. *et al.* 1990. The faces pain scale for the self-assessment of the severity of pain experienced by children. *Pain* **41**, 139–50.

BOC Medical 2001. *Entonox: Controlled Pain Relief. Reference Guide.* Manchester: the BOC Group.

Bottorff, J.L., Gogag, M. and Engelberg-Lotzkar, M. 1995. Comforting: exploring the work of cancer nurses. *Journal of Advanced Nursing* **22**, 1077–84.

Boyd, S. 2003. Assessing infant pain: a review of the pain assessment tools available. *Journal of Neonatal Nursing* **9**(4), 122–6.

Brook, P., Collins, P.D., Briggs, J. and Nichols, B.J. 2002. Point prevalence study of pain in a district general hospital. *Annual Scientific Meeting 2002 Poster Abstracts.* London: The Pain Society.

Broome, M.E. 2000. Helping parents support their child in pain. *Pediatric Nursing* **26**, 315–17.

Burrows, D. 1997. Action on pain. In Thomson, S. (ed.) *Nurse Teachers as Researchers: A reflective approach.* London: Arnold, 86–117.

Burrows, D. 2000. Engaging patients in their own pain management: an action research study. Unpublished PhD thesis, Brunel University.

Bush, E. 2001. The use of human touch to improve the well-being of older adults: a holistic nursing intervention. *Journal of Holistic Nursing* **19**, 256–70.

Carr, E. and Mann, E. 2000. *Pain: Creative approaches to effective management.* Basingstoke: Macmillan Press.

Census 2001. *Health, Disability and Provision of Care.* National Statistics Online: www.statistics.gov.uk/census2001/profiles/commentaries/health.asp. Accessed 1 November 2003.

Chakour, M.C., Gibson, S.J., Bradbeer, M. and Helme, R.D. 1996. The effect of age on A delta- and C-fibre thermal pain stimuli. *Pain* **64**, 143–52.

Chang, S.O. 2001. The conceptual structure of physical touch in caring. *Journal of Advanced Nursing* **33**, 820–7.

Cheston, R. and Bender, M. 1999. *Understanding Dementia: The man with the worried eyes.* London: Jessica Kinsley.

Clarke, S. 2003. Orthopaedic practice: an impression of pain assessment. *Journal of Orthopaedic Nursing* **7**, 132–6.

Clinical Standards Advisory Group 1999. *Services for Patients with Pain.* London: Stationery Office Books.

Closs, S.J., Barr, B., Briggs, M. *et al.* 2003. Evaluating pain in care home residents with dementia. *Nursing and Residential Care* **5**(1), 32–3.

Clukey, L. 1997. *'Just Be There': The experience of anticipatory grief.* Rush University, College of Nursing DNSC.

Cousins, M. and Power, I. 1999. Acute and postoperative pain. In Wall, P.D. and Melzack, R. (eds) *Textbook of Pain*, fourth edition. Edinburgh: Churchill Livingstone, 447–92.

Davidson, B. 1992. What can be the relevance of the psychiatric nurse to the life of a person who is mentally ill? *Journal of Clinical Nursing* **1**, 199–205.

Ferrell, B.R., McCaffery, M. and Rhiner, M. 1992. Pain and addiction: an urgent need for change in nursing education. *Journal of Pain and Symptom Management* **7**, 117–24.

Frampton, M. 2003. Experience assessment and management of pain in people with dementia. *Age and Ageing* **32**(3), 248–51.

Giger, J.N. and Davdhizar, R.E. 1999. *Transcultural Nursing: Assessment and intervention*, third edition. St Louis: Mosby.

Gilje, F.L. 1993. A phenomenological study of patients' experiences of the nurse's presence. PhD thesis, University of Colorado Health Sciences Center.

Hawley, M.P. 2000. Nurse comforting strategies: perceptions of emergency department patients. *Clinical Nursing Research* **9**, 441–59.

Hayward, J. 1975. *Information: A prescription against pain*. London: Royal College of Nursing.

IASP (International Association for the Study of Pain) Subcommittee on Taxonomy 1979. Pain terms: a list with definitions and notes on usage. *Pain* **6**, 249–52.

Jacques, A. and Jackson, G.A. 2000. *Understanding Dementia*, third edition. Edinburgh: Churchill Livingstone.

Kolkaba, K.Y. 1995. Comfort as process and product, merged in holistic art. *Journal of Holistic Nursing* **13**, 117–31.

Kolkaba, K. and Fox, C. 1996. The effects of guided imagery on comfort of women with early stage breast cancer undergoing radiation therapy. *Oncology Nursing Forum* **26**, 67–72.

Kovach, C.R., Griffie, J. and Muchka, S. 1999. Assessment and treatment of discomfort for people with late-stage dementia. *Journal of Pain and Symptom Management* **18**, 412–19.

Kralik, D., Koch, T. and Wotton, K. 1997. Engagement and detachment: understanding patients' experiences with nursing. *Journal of Advanced Nursing* **26**, 399–407.

MacIntyre, P.E. and Ready, L.B. 2002. *Acute Pain Management*, second edition. Edinburgh: W.B. Saunders.

Madjar, I. 1985. Pain and the surgical patient: a cross-cultural perspective. *Australian Journal of Advanced Nursing* **2**(2), 29–33.

McCaffery, M. and Pesaro, C. 1999. *Pain Clinical Manual*, second edition. St Louis: Mosby.

McCaffrey, R.G. and Good, M. 2000. The lived experience of listening to music while recovering from surgery. *Journal of Holistic Nursing* **18**, 378–90.

McGuire, D. 1992. Comprehensive and multidimensional assessment and measurement of pain. *Journal of Pain and Symptom Management* **7**, 312–19.

McQuay, H. and Moore, A. 1998. *An Evidence-based Resource for Pain Relief*. Oxford: Oxford University Press.

Melzack, R. and Katz, J. 1999. Pain measurements in persons in pain. In Wall, P.D. and Melzack, R. (eds) *Textbook of Pain*, fourth edition. Edinburgh: Churchill Livingstone, 409–26.

Melzack, R. and Wall, P. 1996. *Challenge of Pain*. Harmondsworth: Penguin.

Moore, J.R. and Gilbert, D.A. 1995. Elderly residents: perceptions of nurses' comforting touch. *Journal of Gerontological Nursing* **21**, 6–13.

Morse, J.M. 1992. Comfort: the refocusing of nursing care. *Clinical Nursing Research* **1**, 91–106.

Morse, J.M. and Proctor, A. 1998. Maintaining patient endurance: the comfort work of trauma nurses. *Clinical Nursing Research* **7**, 250–74.

Morse, J.M., Solberg, S.M. and Edwards, J. 1993. Caregiver–infant interaction. Comforting post-operative neonates. *Scandanavian Journal of Caring Sciences* **72**, 105–11.

Morse, J.M.; Bottorff, J.L. and Hutchinson, S. 1994. The phenomenology of comfort *Journal of Advanced Nursing* **20**, 189–95.

Moskow, S.B. 1987. *Human Hand and other Ailments*. Boston: Little, Brown & Co.

Moulin, P. 1998. Social representations of pain. *European Journal of Palliative Care* **5**(3), 93–6.

Multiple Sclerosis Trust 2001. *Multiple Sclerosis. Information for health and social care professionals*. Letchworth: Multiple Sclerosis Trust.

Pederson, C. 1994. Ways to feel comfortable: teaching aids to promote children's comfort. *Issues in Comprehensive Pediatric Nursing* **17**, 37–46.

Penrod, J., Morse, J.M. and Wilson, S. 1999. A blend of comforting strategies and a form of team comforting were used during nasogastric tube insertion. *Journal of Clinical Nursing* **8**, 31–8.

Proctor, A., Morse, J.M. and Khonsari, S. 1996. Sounds of comfort in the trauma center: how nurses talk to patients in pain. *Social Science Medicine* **42**, 1669–80.

Roach, S.M. 2002. *Caring, the Human Mode of Being: A blueprint for the health professions*, second revised edition. Ottawa: Canadian Hospital Association Press.

Rokke, P.D. and al'Absi, M. 1992. Matching pain coping strategies to the individual: a prospective validation of the cognitive coping strategy inventory. *Journal of Behavioral Medicine* 15, 611–25.

Seers, K. and Carroll, D. 1998. Relaxation techniques for acute pain management: a systematic review. *Journal of Advanced Nursing* **27**, 466–75.

Sindhu, F. 1996. Are non-pharmacological nursing interventions for the management of pain effective? – A meta-analysis. *Journal of Advanced Nursing* **24**, 1152–9.

Smith-Regojo, P. 1995. 'Being with' a patient who is dying. *Holistic Nursing Practice* **9**, 1–3.

Smith-Stoner, M. 2003. How Buddhism influences pain control choices. *Nursing* **33**(4), 17.

Sofaer, B. 1998. *Pain: Principles, Practice and Patients*, third edition. Cheltenham: Stanley Thornes.

Stephens, B.K., Barkey, M.E. and Hall, H.R. 1999. Techniques to comfort children during stressful procedures. *Accident and Emergency Nursing* **7**, 226–36.

Stuppy, D.J. 1998. The Faces Pain Scale. *Applied Nursing Research* **11**(2), 84–9.

Taylor, B.J. 1992. Relieving pain through ordinariness in nursing: A phenomenologic account of a comforting nurse-patient encounter. *Advances in Nursing Science* **15**(1), 33–43.

Verney, H. 1970. *Florence Nightingale at Harley Street: her reports to the governors of her Nursing Home 1853–4*. London: J.M. Dent & Sons Ltd.

Walker, A.C. 1996. The 'expert' nurse comforter: perceptions of medical/surgical patients. *International Journal of Nursing Practice* **2**, 40–4.

Walters, A.J. 1994. The comforting role in critical care nursing practice: a phenomenological interpretation. *International Journal of Nursing Studies* **31**, 607–16.

Weissman, J. and Appleton, C. 1995. The therapeutic aspects of acceptance. *Perspectives in Psychiatric Care* **31**, 19–23.

Woodgate, R. and Kistjanson, L.J. 1996. A young child's pain: how parents and nurses 'take care'. *International Journal of Nursing Studies* **33**, 271–84.

World Health Organization 1996. *Cancer Pain Relief*, second edition. Geneva: World Health Organization.

Zerwekh, J.V. 1997. The practice of presencing. *Seminars in Oncology Nursing* **13**(4), 260–2.

USEFUL WEBSITES

- **Abbott Laboratories** www.abbott.com
- **American Academy of Pain Management** www.aapainmanage.org
- **American Pain Society** www.ampainsoc.org
- **AstraZeneca** www.Astra.com
- **Baxter** www.Baxter.com
- **The British Pain Society** www.britishpainsociety.org
- **Dee Burrows** http://www.deeburrows.co.uk/
- **International Association for the Study of Pain** http://www.iasp-pain.org/
- **Medscape** www.medscape.com
- *Nursing World* www.nursingworld.org
- **Pain.com** www.pain.com

APPENDIX 12.1 – ATTITUDE TO PAIN QUESTIONNAIRE (BURROWS 1997)

	Strongly agree	Agree	Unsure	Disagree	Strongly disagree
1. Nurses can determine accurately the amount of pain a person will suffer from knowledge of the surgery					
2. Talking to patients preoperatively about pain helps reduce pain post-operatively					
3. Analgesics are always the best way of reducing pain					
4. Using pain assessment charts provides a more accurate picture of the patient's pain					
5. All real pain has an identifiable physical cause					
6. Education on pain management helps nurses recognise when patients are in pain					
7. It is best that patients should not know what is happening to them as this may cause anxiety					
8. Patients who have had surgery (of any type) in the past, know what to expect with regard to post-operative pain					
9. Patients should expect to suffer some pain					
10. A person's age affects their tolerance to pain					
11. Anxiety increases the perception of pain					
12. Patients complaining of pain 2–3 hours after an injection should be encouraged to wait a little longer for their next injection					
13. Nurses most often underestimate the severity and existence of a person's pain					
14. Patients who refuse analgesics when they are in pain are not acting in their own best interests					
15. Some ethnic groups can tolerate more pain than others					

	Strongly agree	Agree	Unsure	Disagree	Strongly disagree
16. It is possible to control pain post-operatively					
17. Talking and listening to patients can reduce their pain					
18. Patients should receive post-operative analgesics on a PRN basis only					
19. Nurses always make accurate inferences about the severity and existence of a person's pain					
20. Relaxation and distraction techniques are effective measures in relieving pain					
21. The person who uses his/her pain to obtain benefits or preferential treatment does not hurt as much as he/she says he/she does and may not hurt at all					
22. Patients should receive post-operative analgesics on both a regular and PRN basis					
23. What the person says about his/her pain is always true					
24. Patients who refuse analgesics show a great sense of character					
25. Nurses are better qualified and more experienced to determine the existence and nature of a person's pain than the person him/herself					
26. Patients should receive analgesics on a regular basis only					
27. All persons can and should be encouraged to have a high tolerance to pain					
28. Nurses learn enough about pain during their training to manage patient's post-operative pain effectively					
29. Care should be taken when giving controlled drugs post-operatively as patients easily become addicted					
30. A person's pain can always be detected by their behaviour and physiological signs					

Odd numbered questions and question 30 taken from Davis, P. 1988. Changing nursing practice for more effective control of post-operative pain through a staff initiated educational programme. *Nurse Education Today* **8**(6), 325–31.

Index

Notes: page numbers in **bold** refer to figures, page numbers in *italics* refer to tables, page numbers in ***bold italics*** refer to margin tones